T2-FHQ-649

THE MEDICAL CLINICS OF NORTH AMERICA

VOLUME 65 / NUMBER 1
JANUARY 1981

SYMPOSIUM ON
ACUTE MEDICAL ILLNESS

Lawrence Sherman, M.D., and
Howard Kolodny, M.D., *Guest Editors*

W. B. SAUNDERS COMPANY — Philadelphia · London · Toronto

W. B. Saunders Company: West Washington Square
Philadelphia, PA. 19105

1 St. Anne's Road
Eastbourne, East Sussex BN21 3UN, England

1 Goldthorne Avenue
Toronto, Ontario M8Z 5T9, Canada

Library of Congress Cataloging in Publication Data
Main entry under title:

Symposium on acute medical illness.

(The Medical clinics of North America; v. 65, no. 1)
1. Medical emergencies.   I. Sherman, Lawrence.   II. Kolodny, Howard.
III. Series: Medical clinics of North America; v. 65, no. 1.   IV. Title:
Acute medical illness. [DNLM: 1. Acute disease.   2. Emergency medicine.
3. Critical care. W1 ME252R v. 65 no. 1 / WB105 S989]
RC60.M4 vol. 65, no. 1   [RC86.7]   616s   [616'.025]
                                                     80–21952

The Medical Clinics are also published in other languages,
by the following:

Spanish   Nueva Editorial Interamericana, S. A. de C. V., Cedro 512,
                 Apartado 26370, Mexico 4, D.F., Mexico

Italian   Piccin Editore, Via Porciglia, 10,
                 35100 Padua, Italy

Greek   Anglo-Hellenic Agency, 5 Koumpari Street,
                 Athens 138, Greece

Portuguese   Editora Interamericana do Brazil Ltds.,
                 Av. Venezuela 131 2. Andar, Rio de Janeiro

Turkish   Guven Bookstore, Mudafaa Cad. 16-B, P.O. Box 145,
                 Kizilay, Ankara

THE MEDICAL CLINICS OF NORTH AMERICA   ISSN 0025-7125
January 1981   **Volume 65 – Number 1**

© 1981 by W. B. Saunders Company.   Copyright under the Uniform Copyright Convention.
Simultaneously published in Canada.   All rights reserved.   This publication is protected by
copyright.   No part of it may be reproduced, stored in a retrieval system, or transmitted in
any form or by any means, electronic, mechanical, photocopying, recording, or otherwise,
without written permission from the publisher.   Made in the United States of America.

The Medical Clinics of North America (USPS 337-340) is published every other month by W. B. Saunders
Company, West Washington Square, Philadelphia, Pennsylvania 19105, at Hampton Road, Cherry Hill, New
Jersey 08002. Subscription price is $29.50 per year. Second class postage paid at Cherry Hill, New Jersey
08002. POSTMASTER: Send address changes to W. B. Saunders Company, West Washington Square, Phila-
delphia, Pennsylvania 19105.
   This issue is Volume 65, Number 1.
   The editor of this publication is Doris J. Holmes, W. B. Saunders Company, West Washington Square,
Philadelphia, Pennsylvania 19105.

Library of Congress catalog card number 80-21952.

Contributors

LEONARD A. ARBEIT, M.D., Instructor in Medicine, State University of New York at Stony Brook, Stony Brook, New York

SELIM BARUH, M.D., Physician-in Charge, Diabetes, Queens Hospital Center Affiliation of the Long Island Jewish-Hillside Medical Center; Assistant Professor of Medicine, School of Medicine, State University of New York at Stony Brook, Stony Brook, New York

EDWARD H. BERGOFSKY, M.D., Professor of Medicine, State University of New York at Stony Brook, School of Medicine, Stony Brook, New York

GERALD F. FLETCHER, M.D., Director of Internal Medicine, Georgia Baptist Medical Center; Professor in Medicine (Cardiology), Emory University School of Medicine, Atlanta, Georgia

SANDOR A. FRIEDMAN, M.D., Chief, Department of Medicine, Coney Island Hospital; Professor of Medicine, State University of New York, Downstate Medical Center, Brooklyn, New York

ROBERT A. GREENWALD, M.D., Chief, Division of Rheumatology, Long Island Jewish-Hillside Medical Center, New Hyde Park; Associate Professor of Medicine, State University of New York at Stony Brook, Stony Brook, New York

DAVID GROB, M.D., Director, Department of Medicine, Maimonides Medical Center; Professor of Medicine, State University of New York, Downstate Medical Center, Brooklyn, New York

HANS W. GRÜNWALD, M.D., Chief, Division of Hematology, Queens Hospital Center Affiliation of the Long Island Jewish-Hillside Medical Center, Jamaica; Associate Professor of Medicine, Health Sciences Center, State University of New York at Stony Brook, Stony Brook, New York

ADAM HUREWITZ, M.D., Assistant Professor of Medicine, State University of New York, Stony Brook School of Medicine, Stony Brook, New York

KANDHASAMY JAGATHAMBAL, M.D., Assistant Attending, Division of Hematology, Department of Medicine, and Physician in Charge of Coagulation, Queens Hospital Center Affiliation of the Long Island Jewish-Hillside Medical Center, Jamaica, New York

HOWARD D. KOLODNY, M.D., Professor of Clinical Medicine, School of Medicine, State University of New York at Stony Brook; Attending Physician, Long Island Jewish-Hillside Medical Center, Jamaica, New York

CHERYL L. KUNIS, M.D., Instructor in Medicine, New York University Medical Center, New York, New York

JEROME LOWENSTEIN, M.D., Professor of Medicine, New York University School of Medicine, New York, New York

CATHERINE T. MARINO, M.D., Physician-in-charge, Division of Rheumatology, Queens Hospital Center Affiliation of the Long Island Jewish-Hillside Medical Center, Jamaica; Assistant Professor of Medicine, State University of New York at Stony Brook, Stony Brook, New York

SHELDON MARKOWITZ, M.D., Fellow in Endocrinology, Queens Hospital Center Affiliation, Long Island Jewish-Hillside Medical Center, Jamaica, New York

PREM MISRA, M.D., Physician-in-Charge, Division of Gastroenterology, Department of Medicine, Queens Hospital Center Affiliation of the Long Island Jewish-Hillside Medical Center; Assistant Professor of Medicine, State University of New York at Stony Brook, Stony Brook, New York

PATRICK MURPHY, M.D., Fellow in Medicine (Cardiology), Emory University School of Medicine, Atlanta, Georgia

SAMUEL PERRY, M.D., Assistant Professor of Psychiatry, Cornell University Medical College; Consultation-Liaison Division, New York Hospital, New York, New York

FRED ROSNER, M.D., Director of Medicine, Queens Hospital Center Affiliation of the Long Island Jewish-Hillside Medical Center; Professor of Medicine, Health Science Center, State University of New York at Stony Brook, Stony Brook, New York

THOMAS D. SABIN, M.D., Director, Neurological Unit, Boston City Hospital; Associate Professor of Neurology and Psychiatry, Boston University School of Medicine; Lecturer in Neurology, Harvard University School of Medicine, Tufts University School of Medicine

RICHARD R. SCHNEIDER, M.D., Instructor of Medicine, Mount Sinai School of Medicine, City University of New York; Director, Cardiac Invasive Laboratory, Mount Sinai Hospital Services–City Hospital Center, Elmhurst, New York

STANLEY G. SECKLER, M.D., Professor of Clinical Medicine, Mount Sinai School of Medicine, City University of New York; Chief, Department of Medicine, Mount Sinai Hospital Services–City Hospital Center, Elmhurst, New York

LAWRENCE SHERMAN, M.D., Associate Director of Medicine, Queens Hospital Center Affiliation, Long Island Jewish-Hillside Medical Center, Jamaica; Professor of Medicine, School of Medicine, State University of New York at Stony Brook, Stony Brook, New York

HOWARD M. SIMONS, M.D., Instructor in Dermatology, Hospital of the University of Pennsylvania, Philadelphia; Physician in Chief, Dermatology, Abington Memorial Hospital, Abington, Pennsylvania

MILTON VIEDERMAN, M.D., Professor of Clinical Psychiatry, Cornell University Medical College; Director, Consultation-Liaison Division, New York Hospital, New York, New York

STEPHEN W. WEINSTEIN, M.D., Associate Professor of Medicine, State University of New York at Stony Brook, Stony Brook, New York

Contents

>   Patients who respond irrationally to acute medical
>   illness and to proper treatment can be very frustrating.
>   Examples include the patient who refuses treatment,
>   becomes confused and pulls out catheters or intra-
>   venous lines, or experiences overwhelming panic
>   after a myocardial infarction. A conceptual model for
>   categorizing such behavior is presented, and some
>   practical suggestions for the management of typical
>   maladaptive responses are offered.

>   The terms coma, semicoma, stupor, and somnolence
>   all refer to pathological depression of normal alertness
>   or consciousness, while the acute confusional state
>   refers to a disturbance in the content of consciousness.
>   These two common problems are grouped together
>   because of the overlap in diagnostic considerations
>   and initial therapeutic approach. Special techniques
>   are also required in the bedside examination used for
>   evaluating the confused or obtunded patient.

>   Two therapeutic directions are available for the
>   management of the adult respiratory distress syn-
>   drome. The first is the alleviation of the effects of

acute respiratory failure through assisted oxygenation and mechanical ventilation. The second is the suppression of the amplification response which remains the source of continuing lung injury.

Richard R. Schneider and Stanley G. Seckler

Acute chest pain probably compels more people to see a physician than any other pain. Unfortunately, its evaluation is a difficult matter even for the most astute physician. The more common etiologies are discussed in detail.

Gerald F. Fletcher and Patrick Murphy

Acute care situations today involve many areas of patient care in addition to intensive care units: the emergency room, the emergency setting in the field, operating and recovery rooms, and so forth. Patients in these areas may have problems that justify the use of procedures such as electrical cardioversion, insertion of a Swan-Ganz catheter, intravenous insertion of a pacemaker, pericardiocentesis, and intra-aortic counterpulsation. These procedures must be used judiciously and only after proper subjective and objective assessment.

Sandor A. Friedman

An established aneurysm is subject to a vicious cycle. As blood flows through the ectatic segment, turbulence develops and forward velocity decreases. Thrombus formation and increased wall pressure result and, in turn, cause the aneurysm to dilate further. Clinical manifestations depend on location and size. Current concepts in diagnosis and management of the most common true aneurysms as well as dissecting aneurysms of the aorta are discussed.

Sheldon Markowitz, Lawrence Sherman,
Howard D. Kolodny, and Selim Baruh

Pituitary apoplexy refers to a neuroendocrine emergency produced by hemorrhage or infarction of the pituitary gland—usually an adenomatous gland. This is a well-defined syndrome that occurs in 5 to 10 percent of patients with pituitary tumors. Common clinical features include sudden headache, visual disturbances, changes in sensorium, nausea and vomiting, nuchal rigidity, and fever. Once considered rare and uniformly fatal, the syndrome is now recognized more frequently and is considered treatable.

Selim Baruh, Lawrence Sherman, and
Sheldon Markowitz

Diabetic ketoacidosis can present with a wide range of altered sensorium, from quasi-normal consciousness to deep coma. A pH less than 7.1, extreme hyperglycemia and hyperosmolality, extreme total body water and electrolyte depletion, and cardiovascular collapse all imply poor prognosis.

Kandhasamy Jagathambal, Hans W. Grünwald, and
Fred Rosner

Successful management of patients with defective hemostasis and bleeding depends on accurate diagnosis, which in turn depends on an understanding of the normal mechanisms required to keep the hemostatic systems in balance. Normal hemostasis, the clinical manifestations of various bleeding disorders, and the diagnostic approach to and management of these disorders are reviewed.

Leonard A. Arbeit and Stephen W. Weinstein

The focus of this review is the subcategory acute tubular necrosis, and the goal is to integrate current knowledge of the pathophysiology based upon what is known about human and experimental acute tubular necrosis with the clinical manifestations of the disease. A rationale for prevention and treatment of these groups of diseases is offered.

Cheryl L. Kunis and Jerome Lowenstein

Although extracellular potassium represents only 2 percent of total body stores, changes in the extracellular concentration are associated with significant changes in the transcellular potassium gradient which result in alterations in cellular function. An understanding of the factors which determine the distribution of potassium between cells and the extracellular space and of the mechanisms responsible for homeostasis, provides a framework for the rational treatment of life-threatening hyperkalemia.

Catherine T. Marino and Robert A. Greenwald

Acute or subacute onset of monoarticular or pauciarticular arthritis may result from crystal deposition within the joint, infection, or trauma. Arthrocentesis with examination of synovial fluid often provides a rapid diagnosis when crystals are found with the polarizing microscope or bacteria are identified by gram stain.

David Grob

A variety of disorders may affect one part or another of the neuromuscular or motor system. Weakness occurs in almost all disorders and is usually the presenting complaint. In some disorders there is also atrophy and, in a few, stiffness, spasm, pain, tenderness, or abnormal movements.

Prem Misra

Hepatic encephalopathy, defined as a neuropsychiatric syndrome characterized by intellectual deterioration, altered state of consciousness, and neurologic abnormalities in a patient with advanced liver disease or portasystemic shunting, is a complication of both acute and chronic disease such as viral hepatitis, drug or toxin-induced liver disease, acute fatty liver of pregnancy, or cirrhosis of the liver.

Howard M. Simons

Anaphylaxis, toxic epidermal necrolysis, and erythema multiforme frequently result from exposure to adverse or hostile environmental factors. Accurate diagnosis and subsequent treatment of these life-threatening conditions require thorough understanding of occasionally subtle cutaneous changes. This discussion puts heavy emphasis on diagnostic clues that can be gleaned from history, signs, and symptoms.

RECENT SYMPOSIA

March 1980
   NONINVASIVE CARDIAC DIAGNOSIS II

May 1980
   INFECTIOUS LUNG DISEASES

July 1980
   HEMATOLOGIC DISORDERS

September 1980
   CUTANEOUS SIGNS OF SYSTEMIC DISEASE

November 1980
   INFLAMMATORY BOWEL DISEASE

FORTHCOMING SYMPOSIA

March 1981
   BODY FLUID AND ELECTROLYTE DISORDERS
   LAURENCE H. BECK, M.D., *Guest Editor*

May 1981
   OBSTRUCTIVE LUNG DISEASES
   RICHARD A. MATTHAY, M.D., *Guest Editor*

July 1981
   CLINICAL ALLERGY
   MICHAEL F. MULLARKEY, M.D., *Guest Editor*

September 1981
   ANTIMICROBIAL THERAPY
   BURKE A. CUNHA, M.D., *Guest Editor*

November 1981
   GASTROINTESTINAL MOTILITY DISORDERS
   MARVIN M. SCHUSTER, M.D., *Guest Editor*

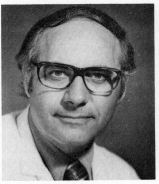
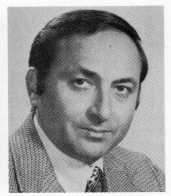

Foreword

LAWRENCE SHERMAN, M.D.
Guest Editor

HOWARD D. KOLODNY, M.D.
Guest Editor

Management of the acutely ill patient presents a continuing challenge to the clinician. The introduction of sophisticated monitoring equipment and life support systems, the development of new treatment methods, and the greater understanding of pathophysiological mechanisms require physicians to expand their information base. Obviously a a single issue of *The Medical Clinics* could not possibly encompass the entire field of emergency medicine; it would be difficult enough adequately to review recent advances in emergency care. The editors sought to select topics of current interest that review new treatments or procedures, or—in some instances—provide a new and better understanding of patients and disease processes.

There is much to learn and to use in this issue. The opening article on management of emotional reactions to acute medical illness reminds us of the great emotional demands that an acute physical illness places on each patient. The closing article on acute life-threatening dermatologic disorders emphasizes the continuing challenges to health presented by adverse or hostile environmental factors. The articles in between stress the essentials of care needed for recognizing and treating major acute illnesses involving the cardiovascular, pulmonary, endocrine, hematopoietic and gastrointestinal systems.

The purpose of this symposium on Acute Medical Illness, as in the earlier symposium we edited some years ago, is to help the doctor on the spot proceed knowledgeably and with all deliberate speed. We thank the contributors for sharing their knowledge and experience. Because of their labors each reader will find these articles to be useful sources of patient care information, and will be able to turn confidently to the symposium as a welcome reference when he or she becomes that doctor on the spot.

1

    We are happy to acknowledge the assistance provided by Berenice
Florman and Barbara Poskrop in helping us coordinate the many elements of this issue.

LAWRENCE SHERMAN, M.D.
HOWARD D. KOLODNY, M.D.
Guest Editors

Long Island Jewish-Hillside Medical Center
New Hyde Park, New York

Management of Emotional Reactions to Acute Medical Illness

Samuel Perry, M.D., *
and Milton Viederman, M.D.†

During an acute medical illness, psychological issues are not the physician's primary concern. Providing potentially life-saving treatment must take precedence. Most patients respect this priority and until the crisis passes are willing to accept the doctor's procedures, explanations and reassurance. Problems in medical management arise when psychological issues cannot be deferred, such as when a patient refuses treatment, or becomes confused and pulls out his catheter, or experiences an overwhelming panic after a myocardial infarction.

To help the physician deal with such problems, we will present a model conceptualized as three successive but partially overlapping tasks which confront the patient during an acute illness.[15] Although we recognize that this categorization is oversimplified and does not do justice to the complexities of human behavior, we find this scheme useful as a framework for practical suggestions about the management of patients who respond to illness maladaptively (Table 1).

As physicians we tend to forget the demands an acute physical illness places on the patient who must suddenly alter his sense of himself, his relationships with others, and his view of the future. Most patients successfullly weather the stages we will describe, but each causes a disturbance in homeostasis.

The first psychological task individuals must accomplish is to acknowledge to themselves and to others that they are ill. Second, they must permit themselves to depend on others for care. Third, as their condition improves, they must resume normal functioning. Individuals may have difficulty at any of these three stages. We shall discuss the demands placed upon patients at each stage and the associated maladaptive responses, and then suggest appropriate approaches to management of the problems that may arise.

*Assistant Professor of Psychiatry, Cornell University Medical College; Consultation-Liaison Division, New York Hospital, New York, New York
†Professor of Clinical Psychiatry, Cornell University Medical College; Director, Consultation-Liaison Division, New York Hospital, New York, New York

Supported in part by National Institute of Mental Health Grant 2 TO 1 MH14747-04.

Table 1. *Psychological Tasks and Common Maladaptive Responses
during Acute Medical Illness*

PSYCHOLOGICAL TASKS DURING ACUTE MEDICAL ILLNESS	COMMON MALADAPTIVE RESPONSES
Stage 1: Acknowledgment of illness	Denial Panic Psychosis
Stage 2: Regressive dependency	Noncompliance Signing out against advice Overdemandingness Confusion and agitation
Stage 3: Return to normal functioning	Premature return to functioning Reluctance to return to functioning

ACKNOWLEDGMENT OF ILLNESS

Stage 1. The individual must acknowledge to himself and others that he is ill, but not be overwhelmed. This task appears simpler than it is. To function effectively, everyone must to a certain extent push his vulnerabilities out of awareness. Those who are constantly preoccupied with their inevitable mortality or who monitor their every ache and pain are involuted and ineffectual. However, when serious illness strikes, every individual must confront what he tends daily to disavow: his susceptibility, his limitations, and his eventual death. Along with modifying this perception of himself, the acutely ill individual must also suddenly modify the way he relates to others. Not only must he reveal his limitations, but he must expose to caretakers aspects of himself which are potentially embarrassing and usually kept private: the body's nakedness, excretions, smells, noises, and so on.

Patients who have difficulty with the psychological task of this stage may use global denial, become flooded with panic, or become psychotic when they sense they may be seriously ill.

Denial

As an individual acknowledges that he is sick, he must find some way to handle the accompanying fear. Most people can diminish their fears by using adaptive mechanisms which should not be confused with denial. For example, in experiencing the onset of crushing chest pains,[14, 18] some patients say to themselves that the heart attack is only mild (minimization); some accurately describe the symptoms and their presumptive diagnosis but keep the emotional impact out of awareness (isolation of affect); some believe the hospitalization will provide a much needed rest (rationalization); some attribute the problem to gastric distress, take an antacid, and then call a doctor (displacement); and some are well aware of what has happened but consciously keep this awareness out of view unless so reminded (suppression).

These devices are usually temporary and acceptable ways of coping. Though the staff may fear that the patient suddenly will be overwhelmed when he realizes the full seriousness of his illness, no data support such concern.[9] In fact, some studies suggest that patients have a better prognosis if they are able to decrease their anxiety in these ways.[6, 7, 10, 13] As a general rule, the patient's defenses against anxiety need not be challenged unless they in some way interfere with his medical management.

Problems arise when patients handle their fears by global denial, i.e., by not acknowledging that they are ill and by refusing treatment. This denial unconsciously defends against the threat of illness by repudiating a piece of reality. Attempts to convince the denying patient about the seriousness of his illness often backfire because such confrontations only increase the underlying fear and the need for denial. The following vignette illustrates a different approach.

A 42 year old man was brought to the Emergency Room by his wife because of chest pain. The electrocardiogram indicated a widespread infarction, but the man insisted the pain was caused by spiced chili and that he was going home. The wife and the intern tried to convince him about the dangers of this action until, out of frustration, they threatened: "If you walk out of here, you're liable to drop dead in the street." In reaction, the man's fears and need for denial increased and a psychiatric consultation became necessary.

The psychiatrist took a different tack. In a calm manner he diminished the underlying fear: "You've made it through the most dangerous first few hours and now convalescence can begin;" "The heart muscle is now soft like setting cement but will harden as it heals;" "It's a good thing you've come to the hospital where you can be observed and helped at once if any unsuspected complication should occur;" and so on. As the man felt reassured, the need for denial diminished. The psychiatrist could then address the surfacing panic in a manner similar to what we will suggest below. Even after agreeing to be admitted, the patient was medicated to diminish the likelihood that the fear and subsequent denial might reoccur over the next few days.

Panic

Some anxiety always accompanies an awareness of being ill. Problems in management occur if this anxiety becomes excessive and does not respond to simple reassurance and explanation. When panic interferes with history-taking, diagnostic procedures, and monitoring and threatens to induce autonomic lability, arrhythmias, or respiratory complications, psychological intervention becomes necessary.

The management of a panic reaction has two components: emotional support and pharmacotherapy. Emotional support begins with an understanding that panic emerges because the patient fears that he will not be able to cope with some event in the immediate or distant future. The physician should elicit *specifically* what the patient fears might happen. Vague answers should not be accepted, but rather pursued. For example, if the patient simply responds that he is afraid he will die, the doctor should try to determine the meaning of this fear for this particular patient at this particular time: "Yes, in some way all patients are afraid of dying, but for various reasons. What about the thought of dying is especially frightening to you?" When pressed to elaborate, patients may describe concerns about being abandoned, suffering intractable pain, becoming crippled, losing their minds, leaving their families, and so forth. The patient will benefit not only by being understood and attaching his overwhelming fear to an idea, but also by providing the physician an opportunity to offer reassurance directed at the specific fear rather than global comments as "I'm sure everything will be all right." Blanket statements of this kind are often perceived as impersonal and cause the physician to lose his credibility, because no one can be certain that all will be well.

With the patient's particular fear in mind, the physician can be more authentic and specific when offering hope and reassurance. For example, if a patient with chest pain is afraid he will die because his father died of a heart attack, the doctor can point out that identification with a dead parent is common and does not in itself imply a poor prognosis; or if a patient is afraid that cancer means unremitting pain, the doctor can indicate that most cancers are treatable, some are curable, and many powerful medicines for pain are currently available. This kind of discussion will help allay the panic if a tone of equanimity is combined with an indication that the patient's fears have a personal meaning and rationale.

Some patients become so flooded with anxiety that medication is necessary before such an exchange can take place. Unless a patient is in such a panic that he is no longer rational, benzodiazepines are the drugs of choice. They may be given by mouth or with caution intravenously; their intramuscular absorption is erratic. After two or three days — because tissue saturation will have occurred and because the half-life is quite long — only a bedtime dosage is required with a repeat dose available during the day at the nurse's discretion.[8]

The physician should not rely solely on medication for relief of anxiety. The patient will feel more helpless if he believes the drug is doing all the work and that he would lose control without it. Instead, the physician should ask how the patient has coped with stress in the past — by trying to think positively, by using prayer, by leaning on his wife, by understanding the intricacies of the problem, whatever. The physician can then state that the medication will relieve the anxiety sufficiently for the patient to use similar coping mechanisms again, mechanisms which the physician will then encourage and support.

Psychosis

When a patient's panic is so extreme that he becomes irrational, combative, or delusional, antipsychotic medication is necessary. Benzodiazepines can make these patients worse. Many of them use a heightened vigilance to protect themselves against imagined threats; when sedated, they feel even more frightened and become more suspicious, confused and hostile. Among the antipsychotics, haloperidol is preferred over the phenothiazines because of its decreased sedative, anticholinergic and hypotensive effects. The recommended initial dose is 1 to 10 mg parenterally and then adjustment at half-hour intervals until adequate tranquilization has been achieved. The patient can be maintained on a single oral or a parenteral nightly dose of one half the total daily dose given during this rapid tranquilization.[2]

REGRESSIVE DEPENDENCY

Stage 2. The individual must depend on others for care. More is involved in allowing oneself to become a "patient" than is apparent. The functioning adult realizes that he cannot rely on others to meet his every need, that healthy skepticism as opposed to blind trust protects against disappointment and exploitation, and that to a large extent everyone must take control of and be responsible for his own life. However, when acutely ill, this same individual is expected to regress and temporarily to modify his mature way of operating: as a patient he is expected to depend more on others, to trust those he may not know, to accept what he cannot fully understand, and to relinquish some control and even responsibility for what happens to him.

Some patients cannot appropriately place themselves in the care of others. Specifically, they will not comply with procedures, they become unduly suspicious, may sign out against advice or, at the other extreme, may become overdependent and demanding. Other patients cannot cooperate because of confusion secondary to an organic mental syndrome.

Noncompliance

Patients are reluctant to relinquish control and to place themselves trustfully in the care of others for many different reasons. No single approach is sufficient. The psychological management must be tailored to fit the psychodynamics of the individual patient. To illustrate the need for flexibility, four cases will be presented; in each, the plan of management was based on the underlying reason for the noncompliance.

Noncompliance to Defend against Humiliation. A 54 year old influential bank president was admitted to the ICU after his first myocardial infarction. On the third day he started removing the leads of his cardiac monitor and carrying his intravenous bottle to the staff's bathroom rather than using the bedside commode, which he found "disgraceful." The nursing staff wanted a stop to his arrogant behavior, but the internist realized that this man — who spent his life maintaining a proper image — could not suddenly change character and comfortably place himself in a humiliating position. Choosing the "executive" bathroom was this patient's way of maintaining his pride and autonomy. This need to be in control was a long-standing character trait which had its roots in his early struggles with an overprotective and controlling mother.

The internist wisely chose to compromise rather than engage in a disruptive power struggle. He told the patient that his behavior might cause the staff to lose respect for him. He then suggested that the patient not waste his energy locking horns over the matter, but instead spend his convalescent time catching up on more important affairs. His dictating machine could be brought from the office to the ICU and his secretary could check in daily with the mail and go over the office activities. Although the patient used the dictating machine only once and for the most part ignored the events at the office until his recovery, his self-esteem was restored and the noncompliance stopped.

Noncompliance to Defend against Helplessness. A 43 year old woman was admitted for an exacerbation of lupus erythematosus. In two days she had infuriated the staff by smoking in her room. When the rheumatologist asked about this behavior, she confided that smoking was the one thing she could do all by herself — even after she had become a complete cripple. Following this lead, this physician who had treated the patient for years realized the noncompliance was based on a fear of becoming completely helpless and dependent on others. He told the patient she could smoke only if she wheeled herself into the solarium. He also gave the patient responsibility for documenting on paper the fluctuations in her symptoms, the response to different medications, and her daily intake and output. This maneuver, along with his general tone, indicated that he expected the patient to take more responsibility for her treatment. When the patient felt she was no longer totally dependent on the staff and had "a mind of her own," the need for noncompliance stopped.

NONCOMPLIANCE TO DEFEND AGAINST FEARS OF EMASCULATION. A 27 year old professional ball player was hospitalized for acute hepatitis requiring rest and observation. After the first week his usual "macho" style had escalated. He was exercising in the hall, pinching the nurses, and exposing himself while resting in bed. One evening his beer-drinking friends became rowdy during visiting hours. The staff became even more incensed and on the following day wanted the patient transferred or discharged. A psychiatric consultation was requested.

The psychiatric interview indicated that this man viewed his illness as an emasculating experience: he felt rundown, his muscles were not as taut, and he wondered aloud how he would perform "on the field and in bed" after he left the hospital. The psychiatrist acknowledged that being ill often made a patient feel more like a boy than a man and added, "I'm sure it's not easy for a guy like you to feel strapped down"; and "Taking it easy for now is going to be one of the hardest games you'll ever have to play." The psychiatrist also recommended that the nurses act more admiringly toward the patient by joking that he should not do push-ups off the ceiling and by asking about his athletic accomplishments. He further suggested that they not ignore the patient's exposed genitals but rather expect him to cover up because "sick or well, he's still a man."

The nurses were at first understandably hesitant to accept these suggestions but realized that some give and take would be necessary. As long as the patient was generally cooperative, some leeway could be granted on smaller issues to insure that necessary treatment could proceed. After the patient's sense of manliness was reinforced, the provocative behavior decreased and was not a problem by the time of discharge.

NONCOMPLIANCE BASED ON A MISTRUST OF OTHERS. A 41 year old truck driver was admitted for gastrointestinal bleeding. On the fourth day his condition was no longer critical, although the cause of the bleeding had not yet been determined. That evening he walked into the nurses' station and demanded his clothes to go home. The staff was not completely surprised because from the onset the patient had been furtive and suspicious.

When the attending psychiatrist arrived, he did not challenge the patient's judgment or rights. He stated that the option to leave was always available and should not preclude the patient's telling his side of the story. This approach was based on an understanding that the patient had always been a loner who harbored bitterness and resentment. To expect this man to change character suddenly and become accepting and trusting was unreasonable. Instead, the doctor kept a respectful distance, was firm and completely honest, and implied that he did not require that the patient trust him blindly — trust would take time to build.

The patient felt more comfortable with this matter of fact approach and revealed his reasons for wanting to leave: the male nurse who gave baths was "creepy," the nurses were "all sweetsie pies," and the aides barged into rooms without so much as knocking. A debate over these issues would have been futile, particularly since the patient's perceptions were not totally inaccurate. Furthermore, the doctor realized that the situation could be changed more easily than this man's longstanding mistrust of others. The need for further medical care warranted some compromise. He told the patient — and later the nurses — that an effort would be made to have the staff knock before entering, that the male nurse would be assigned to other patients, and that everyone would be less intrusive. The patient was reminded that the option to leave was still available if these modifications did not improve his situation. Although the patient never warmed up to the staff, he felt less trapped and invaded, and stayed to receive further treatment.

Signing Out against Advice

The threat to sign out is rarely a sudden act. The decision has usually been reached in desperation after a series of misunderstandings.[1, 17] The first step toward resolution is to allow the patient to air his grievances. The angry and frightened patient must feel he has an ally. To form this alliance, the physician conveys his respect for the patient's position even if he does not fully agree with the patient's perception of what has occurred. After the resentment has been expressed, the physician can deal with the underlying anxiety by determining *specifically* what the patient fears.

Patients threatening to leave the hospital rarely respond to rapid tranquilization or statements that they must sign a sheet of paper and will not receive further care if they leave against advice. These threats make the patients more mistrustful and they become more intent on leaving. Instead, the patient should be given more — not less — autonomy; for example, he may be offered the opportunity to decide within reasonable medical limits when he should take his medicine, or he may even be offered an overnight pass to decompress an otherwise impossible situation.

Managing the patient is only half the problem. Usually the staff is also angry and must be given an opportunity to voice their complaints before they will accept some compromise. The staff may feel less incensed if they appreciate that the patient's behavior is his automatic and characteristic way of acting outside the hospital and should not be taken as a personal attack.

If these maneuvers fail, physicians should understand the legal rights of patients who refuse treatment. Although laws vary from state to state and each case is decided on an individual basis, certain general principles can be helpful. Medical patients have the legal right to leave the hospital at any time if they are competent, that is, if they understand what they are doing and the possible consequences to their health. They are required by law to sign nothing. If they are restrained, the physician may be charged with "false imprisonment" or with "battery" (the unpermitted, unprivileged touching of another person).

The situation is different in an emergency or if the patient is incompetent. When a physician acts in good faith during a life-threatening emergency and no relative opposes him, legal judgment usually will not be made against the physician. Negligence could be charged if the physician does not act under the circumstances. If the situation is not an emergency, the patient must be declared incompetent in order for the physician to proceed against the patient's will. Competency is a legal and not a medical term. Physicians cannot declare a person incompetent, and all patients are considered competent unless deemed otherwise by the court. If a patient refuses treatment because he is confused — in delirium tremens, agitated postoperatively, assaultively demented, or psychotic — the doctor may protect the patient's bodily integrity by customary methods, including restraint. A detailed mental status report in the chart should have quotes from the patient revealing that he does not understand the nature of his illness, the treatment, or the potential danger of the absence of treatment. A consent from the next of kin should be obtained if possible. When the physician suspects that legal problems may occur after the medical crisis has passed, a petition should be filed to have the court declare the patient incompetent and to appoint a guardian. In the absence of family, the hospital administrator may act as the petitioner to the court.

The Overdemanding Patient

In contrast to those who refuse care, some patients become too dependent and demanding. They expect a nurse to come the moment the buzzer is pushed, for the doctor to spend hours at the bedside answering questions, for the food to be comparable to that found in a gourmet restaurant, and for every twinge of discomfort to be relieved upon request.

The first step in management is for the caretakers to acknowledge that these patients can be infuriating. Failure to recognize the resentment will eventually lead to an explosion, which will have a more destructive effect on the treatment than if the anger had been recognized earlier. The second step is to determine the basis for the behavior. Some patients fear they will die if left alone, others feel entitled to superb care because they are ill, others are afraid they will be neglected as they have been in the past, and so on. After the basis for the demandingness has been explored and the patient has the sense that he has been understood, the third step is to confront the patient tactfully and explain that his behavior has had an effect opposite to what he would like. If the pattern continues, his level of expectation will inevitably result in alienation and the resentment in the staff will lead to his receiving less attention than might otherwise be the case. The fourth step is to work out an agreement with the patient and set reasonable limits, such as what self-care the patient is expected to perform and how often the nurses will visit at regular intervals rather than on demand. These limits should be made explicit; some testing will no doubt follow. If necessary, these guidelines can be written down as a "private contract" which conveys special concern and appeals to the patient's sense of entitlement.[19]

Confusion and Agitation: The Organic Mental Syndrome

The inability of patients to depend appropriately on others is not always based on characterologic issues. Particularly with the acutely ill, uncooperativeness may derive from an organic mental syndrome. An organic basis for aberrant behavior should be highly suspected in patients who: (1) are not alert; (2) cannot give the date or name the hospital; (3) cannot register three items and recall them a few moments later; (4) cannot follow a three-stage command; and (5) cannot draw the face of a clock.[4, 11, 16] The diagnosis may be evident when the patient's impaired sensorium combined with anxiety and a strange environment leads to confusion and agitation: he begins screaming, pulling out pacemakers or sutures, and then tries to climb over the bed rails.

When prompt tranquilization is required, haloperidol, 1 to 10 mg parenterally, is the drug of choice with repeat doses every half-hour as described above. Medication alone is not sufficient. The physician must then search for a treatable cause of the organic problem: drug reaction, metabolic deficiency, impaired cerebral perfusion, subdural hematoma, and so forth.[5]

During this investigation, the staff — preoccupied with medical problems and frustrated with the delirious patient who does not respond to reason — may rely on heavy sedation and restraints. This approach is unsatisfactory. Oversedation can cause increased confusion, hypotension, cardiac toxicity and insufficient ventilation with a predisposition to atelectasis and pneumonitis. Restraints can cause increased belligerence, suspiciousness, uncooperativeness, and excessive exertion, increased arterial and venous pressure, and restricted mobility.

Recognizing the limitations of restraints and sedation, the treating staff can use psychological maneuvers to influence the delirious patient. Because confusion and not necessarily inherent hostility causes the organic patient to become defiant and uncooperative, the goal is to diminish this confusion by organizing his world and by correcting misperceptions; for example: "Mr. John Smith, I am your nurse. You are in the hospital to get treatment for your heart condition. The medicine causes you to feel light-headed and confused. You are not losing your mind and the confusion will disappear. At times your imagination plays tricks on you so that you see and hear things which are not there. This machine counts the heartbeats. No, it cannot read your mind. This tube puts medicine into your arm; it is not a snake. I know how frightened you become when you do not understand what is happening. I will not let you hurt yourself." These organizing comments cannot be made all at once. The impaired attention span and defect in recent memory cause the patient to forget what has been told him. In an abbreviated form, similar remarks must be repeated over and over again at the bedside if they are going to prevent the outbursts from recurring when the confusion returns.

Because the required psychological maneuvers are time-consuming, the staff should consider having one or two close relatives share this responsibility. The selected relatives can be instructed to treat the confused patient as if he were a young child awakening from a frightening nightmare and needing to be touched, comforted, reassured, and to have his misperceptions corrected. This activity has the additional merit of relieving the helplessness family members often experience when they have nothing productive to do for the patient. If relatives are not available or suitable to participate at the bedside, a nightly phone call around 10:00 P.M. may orient the patient sufficiently to prevent severe agitation during the night ("sundowning"). The family also can be told to bring a clock, a calendar, and a few familiar items (such as photos from the bedroom dresser) to help maintain the patient's orientation. Soft music and light may be used during the night when sufficient stimulation might not otherwise be present. Patients with an organic mental syndrome require a carefully titrated quantity of stimulation and become agitated with too much or too little. This range may be quite narrow and the proper dosage must be determined empirically for each individual patient.

RETURN TO NORMAL FUNCTIONING

Stage 3. The individual must resume functioning as his medical illness improves. As the patient improves, his preoccupation with bodily sensations and withdrawal from worldly responsibility is expected gradually to decrease along with his inclination to depend on others. This stage, like the previous two, will be influenced by the patient's personality and by sociocultural factors. The physician naturally considers the residual physical limitations and does not expect all patients to return to normal in the same way or at the same rate.

We will discuss below patients who fall outside this acceptable range, specifically, those who return to normal activities prematurely and those who remain in a dependent state longer than their medical conditions indicate.

Premature Return to Normal Functioning

Physicians are accustomed to having convalescent patients ask repeatedly when they may go home. These inquiries do not pose a problem unless the patient presses for premature resumption of activity. Such pressure often stems from fears of becoming chronically dependent and from a need to be reassured that one is improving and will be able to resume a normal life. Because of these concerns, such patients may respond adversely to statements such as, "You still need to let us take care of you because you are not yet over a very serious illness." Instead, the physician can emphasize how maturely the patient has handled his illness and the positive features of his recovery: "You've done a responsible job getting well up to this point. Your tests show continuing improvement. To make sure you are even stronger for what lies ahead, I want your recovery to be more complete. I realize that waiting is difficult for someone so impatient to be well."

A note of caution about these eager patients: because they are uncomplaining, stoical, and grateful about their care, they often elicit admiration from the staff, who then unwittingly may participate in their suppression of fears, sadness, and doubts about the future. The physician must be alert to the presence of these feelings and recognize that palpitations, anxiety attacks, irritability or nightmares around the time of discharge may indicate that the patient needs an opportunity to discuss such concealed feelings about his illness. The physician can facilitate this discussion by mentioning that it is perfectly normal to have some anxieties about a physical illness and by inquiring *which* anxieties have been generated in the patient. Concerns about sexual performance are rarely volunteered, so the physician may have to introduce this topic.

Reluctance to Return to Normal Functions

Relinquishing the dependent role is very difficult for patients who have secretly longed for such gratification. They may develop new symptoms at the time of discharge, or challenge the doctor's reassurance that the physical crisis has passed. For those patients afraid to face the future, the best treatment is prevention. The physician should not assume that all patients are looking forward to leaving the Coronary Care Unit, to being weaned from the respirator,[3] or to being discharged from the hospital. Most patients have some concerns about whether they are completely well, whether the symptoms will suddenly return, or whether they will die because they are no longer being closely monitored. Studies have shown an increase in anxiety and catecholamine excretion in cardiac patients shortly after transfer from the CCU and a decrease in cardiovascular complications when patients are adequately prepared.[12] Finally, some patients may be more willing to give up the sick role if they believe they are not required to give up simultaneously their dependency upon the physicians to whom they have grown attached. Such patients are reassured when the doctor outlines his plan to follow the patient after discharge and offers an appointment in the near future. These patients may be less clinging when they are convinced they will not be abandoned by their physicians.

CONCLUSION

Patients who respond irrationally to acute medical illness and to proper treatment can be very frustrating. We have presented a conceptual model to categorize such behavior and have offered suggestions about the management of typical maladaptive responses. Practicing physicians are well aware of the complexity of the behavior of patients and will realize that we have oversimplified in the service of exposition. Nevertheless, we hope this article will offer a framework for thinking about such problems and will change an inherently frustrating situation to one that evokes curiosity and reflection.

REFERENCES

1. Albert, H. D., and Kornfeld, D. S.: The threat to sign out against medical advice. Ann. Intern. Med., 79:888–891, 1973.
2. Anderson, W. H., Kuehnle, J. C., and Catanzano, D. N.: Rapid treatment of acute psychosis. Amer. J. Psychiat., 133:1076–1078, 1976.
3. Feeley, T. W.: Problems in weaning patients from ventilators. Resident Staff Physician, 22:51–55, 1976.
4. Folstein, M. F., Folstein, S. E., and McHugh, P. R.: Mini-mental states: A practical method for grading the cognitive state of patients for the clinician. J. Psychiat. Res., 12:189–198, 1975.
5. Fox, J. H., Topel, J. L., and Huckman, M. S.: Dementia in the Elderly — A search for treatable illnesses. J. Gerontol., 33:557–564, 1975.
6. Froese, A., Hackett, T. P., and Cassem, N. H.: Trajectories of anxiety and depression in denying and non-denying acute MI patients during hospitalizations. J. Psychosom. Res., 18:413–420, 1974.
7. Gentry, W., Doyle, Foster, R. N., et al.: Denial as determinant of anxiety and perceived health status in the CCU. Psychosom. Med., 34:39–44, 1972.
8. Greenblatt, D. J., and Shader, R. I.: Benzodiazepines in Clinical Practice. New York, Raven Press, 1974.
9. Hackett, T. P., Cassem, N. H., and Wishnie, H. A.: The Coronary Care Unit. An appraisal of its psychological hazards. New Eng. J. Med., 279:1365–1370, 1968.
10. Hackett, T. P., and Weisman, A. D.: Denial as a factor in patients with heart disease and cancer. Ann. NY Acad. Sci., 164:802–817, 1969.

11. Jacobs, I. W., Bernhard, N. R., Delgado, A., et al.: Screening for organic mental syndrome in the medically ill. Ann. Intern. Med., 86:40–46, 1977.
12. Klein, R. F., Kuber, V. A., Zipes, D. P., et al.: Transfer from a Coronary Care Unit. Arch. Intern. Med., 122:104–108, 1960.
13. Miller, W., and Rosenfeld, R.: A psychophysiological study of denial following acute myocardial infarction. J. Psychosom. Res., 19:43–54, 1975.
14. Moss, A. J., et al.: Delay in hospitalization during the acute coronary period. Amer. J. Cardiol., 24:259, 1969.
15. Parsons, T.: The Social System. Glencoe, Illinois, Free Press, 1951.
16. Robbins, E., and Stern, M.: Assessment of psychiatric emergencies. In Glick, R. A., Meyerson, A. T., Robbins, E., et al., eds.: Psychiatric Emergencies. New York, Grune and Stratton, 1976.
17. Schlauch, R. W., Reich, P., and Kelley, M. J.: Leaving the hospital against medical advice. New Engl. J. Med., 300:22–24, 1979.
18. Simon, A. B., et al.: Components of delay in the pre-hospital setting of acute myocardial infarction. Amer. J. Cardiol., 30:475–482, 1972.
19. Simons, R. D., Morris, J. I., Frank, H. A., et al.: Pain medication contracts for problem patients. Psychosomatics, 20:118, 1979.

Consultation-Liaison Division
The New York Hospital
525 East 68th Street
New York, New York 10021

Coma and the Acute Confusional State in the Emergency Room

*Thomas D. Sabin, M.D.**

These two common problems are grouped together because of the overlap in diagnostic considerations and initial therapeutic approach for the two disorders. There are also special techniques required in the bedside examination used for the evaluation of the confused or obtunded patient. The terms coma, semicoma, stupor, and somnolence all refer to pathological depression of normal alertness or consciousness, while the acute confusional state refers to a disturbance in the content of consciousness.

COMA

PATHOGENESIS

Alertness requires normal function of the ascending reticular activating system.[8] This is a highly complex polysynaptic region in the very core of the upper pons and the midbrain which divides into both thalamic regions and ultimately becomes widespread within the hemispheres. A great variety of specific afferent systems contribute some portion of their neuronal activity into this system as they pass through these brain stem structures. Pathologic decrease in consciousness is so common because of the vulnerability of this ascending reticular activating system. This vulnerability is both anatomic and biochemical.

The structural problem becomes manifest in unilateral supratentorial space-occupying lesions when the medial or uncal portion of the temporal lobe is forced through the tentorial notch beside the midbrain. This distorts the reticular activating substance in the core of the midbrain and thereby causes a decrease in alertness. This distortion is the basis for the depressed state of consciousness which occurs early in the process of herniation from supratentorial mass lesions.

Director, Neurological Unit, Boston City Hospital, Associate Professor of Neurology and Psychiatry, Boston University School of Medicine; Lecturer in Neurology, Harvard Medical School and Tufts University School of Medicine, Boston, Massachusetts

Two additional accompaniments of uncal herniation are of diagnostic importance. The herniated uncus also causes compression of the oculomotor nerve. The parasympathetic pupillomotor fibers which course along the periphery of the oculomotor nerve are first compressed and this results in a dilated pupil which is unresponsive to light.

When the herniated uncus forces the midbrain against the narrow rigid contralateral tentorial margin, then motor fibers within the midbrain may be affected and signs of upper motor neuron deficits appear on the *same* side as the supratentorial mass lesion causing the herniation. In fatal cases an actual groove in the midbrain is seen (Kernohan's notch). The most striking example of a supratentorial mass lesion which may be associated only with ipsilateral upper motor neuron signs is a subdural hematoma. Here the mass lesion is dispersed over the hemisphere and as it enlarges it may produce little in the way of focal effects on the subadjacent cortex. When herniation occurs, obtundation and ipsilateral motor findings related to Kernohan's notch are commonly found. This phenomenon is the basis for the clinical maxim that the side of pupillary dilatation is a more accurate predictor of the side of a supratentorial mass lesion than the side of the hemiparesis. When there is bilateral herniation of supratentorial structures, the midbrain is still affected, as it is forced caudally and elongated in the anteroposterior direction by bilateral uncal compression.

If the brain stem is sectioned below the level of the upper pons a disturbance in alertness does not occur. Once the ascending reticular system has become bilaterally distributed at the level of the thalamus, a unilateral destructive lesion will fail to cause obtundation. While distortion of the ascending reticular activating system in the midbrain is the major anatomic basis for pathologic states of obtundation, critically located small focal lesions from the upper pons rostral to the mesencephalic-diencephalic junction may also cause obtundation. Thus, small infarcts which destroy the reticular core of the brain stem[15] cause states of prolonged coma.

The pharmacologic or biochemical vulnerability of the reticular activating system is reflected in the appearance of obtundation in nearly every variety of severe metabolic disturbance as well as being the major action of numerous pharmacologic agents. Administration of intravenous barbiturates rapidly produces obtundation without causing focal neurologic signs such as aphasia, cortical blindness, or sensory loss. Yet regional arterial perfusion of barbiturates as in the Wada test indicate that these other areas of the nervous system are vulnerable to barbiturates. The most common causes of obtundation are exogenous or endogenous toxins. The numerous synapses in the ascending reticular activating system may be the basis for the striking selective production of obtundation by so many classes of drugs and toxins. The distinction between an intracranial structural process versus an extracranial metabolic or toxic encephalopathy is the primary diagnostic step in evaluating a patient with coma.

Early Management of the Comatose Patient

Sometimes treatment must be undertaken before even these basic diagnostic distinctions are made. The overriding concern becomes the immediate treatment of any remediable causes of permanent brain damage. A simple way of keeping these entities in mind is to recall the essential requirements for brain metabolism. These include adequate oxygen, circulation to get the oxygen to the brain, glucose for substrate, as well as a cofactor based on thiamine to metabolize the glucose. Thus, the patient must be guaranteed an adequate airway, respiratory exchange, and general circulation. If there is any possibility that the patient has been nutritionally deprived, 100 mg of intravenous thiamine should be given. Thiamine must be administered prior to glucose, since a glucose load in a thiamine-deficient patient may result in acute Wernicke's encephalopathy and the possibility of sudden death with circulatory collapse.[1] After blood is obtained for the various diagnostic studies (including glucose levels) the patient may be given 25 gm of intravenous glucose as a 50 per cent solution. If there is a suspicion of drug ingestion, naloxone (Narcan) may be administered as part of these early diagnostic and therapeutic maneuvers. The patient is positioned so as to prevent aspiration. If there is any possibility that the coma is due to head injury the patient ought to be handled as though there were also a cervical fracture in order to prevent injury to the spinal cord. Someone should always be with the comatose patient. As soon as these initial urgent needs are satisfied, a rapid general medical and neurologic examination is performed.

Examination of the Comatose Patient

The importance of looking for subtle signs of head injury on the emergency service must be emphasized. Certain weapons of the street such as a stocking filled with sand can create devastating brain lesions but leave only a slight bogginess or an area of petechiae on the scalp which can be identified only if the patient's hair and scalp are carefully searched.[14] The neurologic examination of the comatose patient is quite different from the routine neurologic examination. In the most common conditions associated with coma there tends to be a rostral-caudal deterioration in nervous system function as the process worsens. This is the case with both structural intracranial processes and toxic-metabolic encephalopathies. Rostral-caudal deterioration refers to the sequential loss of certain functions beginning with the cerebral cortex, then the upper brain stem, midbrain, pons, and finally the medulla. A rapid assessment of the anatomic level in a given patient can be made by examination of the state of consciousness, pupils, eye movements, respirations, and remaining motor functions.[10, 13] Small disparities in the level of functioning remaining in these areas are common, but large disparities may be of great diagnostic importance.

The level of consciousness is evaluated by repeated efforts to wake the patient and gain his attention. An imprecise array of terms, such as stupor, semicoma, etc., have been used to describe the spectrum of normal alertness to unconsciousness. These terms are best avoided. The records should describe the patient's behavior. In the diencephalic stages of obtundation, varying degrees of consciousness will be noted but the patient is comatose in the midbrain, pontine, and medullary stages of rostral-caudal deterioration.

Examination of the pupils is usually a fairly straightforward matter, and the size, symmetry, and response to light should be recorded. If there is an expanding supratentorial mass or widespread edema causing midline herniation then both pupils tend to be small in the diencephalic stage. A magnifying glass may be necessary to see if the pupillary response to light has been preserved. If the supratentorial mass is laterally placed and the incus herniates through the tentorial notch, then the compression of the pupil or motor fibers on the periphery of the third cranial nerve will cause early pupillary dilatation and the pupil will become unresponsive to light. The pupillary signs of third nerve dysfunction appear before the paralysis of extraocular muscles. The diencephalic stage is then characterized by either unilateral pupillary dilatation with unilateral herniation syndromes or with symmetric small pupils which respond to light in midline herniation or most toxic-metabolic encephalopathies. Once the deterioration involves the midbrain, the pupils are no longer reactive to light in herniation syndromes and tend to be in the midposition, and may not change in the pontine and medullary phases of deterioration. The agonal dilatation of unresponsive pupils has been attributed to a widespread release of norepinephrine throughout the anoxic body tissues.

The state of extraocular movements is another valuable way of establishing the level of remaining nervous system function. With pathologic drowsiness in the diencephalic stage the so-called doll's eyes maneuvers become overly facile. When a normal conscious individual has his head passively turned to the right, the eyes will move to the right. In an obtunded individual they will move to the left. This release of vestibular reflexes has been labeled the doll's eye phenomenon. Drowsiness may also cause phorias which have been latent to become tropias. Divergent squints often appear most exaggerated, with upward deviation of the eyes. In the mesencephalic stage of deterioration, the eyes no longer move easily with the doll's head maneuver and a stronger stimulus may become necessary. Conjugate deviation of the eyes to the stimulated side can be induced by instilling icewater in the external ear canal. A maximal stimulus consists of 40 ml of icewater instilled over a 30 second period. One should be careful that no perforation in the drum or other process in the external ear is present that might be adversely affected by this irrigation. In the mesencephalic stage of dysfunction the eyes can still be conjugately drawn to the side of stimulation, although if third nerve structures are sufficiently damaged there may be a deficit in adduction.

Once the pons and medulla have been destroyed there is no response in the eye movements to doll's head or ice water caloric stimulation.

When the patient's head is at 35° to the horizontal and both ears are simultaneously stimulated with warm water at 44° C there is conjugate upward deviation of the eyes if the midbrain centers for vertical gaze are intact. The comatose patient may present with tonic conjugate deviation of the eyes. In an acute hemisphere lesion destruction of the fibers from the frontal center for contralateral conjugate gaze results in a relative overactivity of the contralateral intact center causing deviation of the eyes toward the injured hemisphere. If there is an associated hemiplegia then the eyes will be deviating away from the side of the hemiplegia and toward the side of the lesion. These fibers cross in the midbrain and with lesions in the brain stem conjugately deviate away from the side of the lesion and therefore toward the hemiplegia.

The respiratory pattern is another useful marker for the level of remaining nervous system function. The respirations at the diencephalic stage of rostral-caudal deterioration may be normal or show periodic respiration including Cheyne-Stokes respirations. Central neurogenic hyperventilation with continued respiratory rates of about 40 and appropriate changes in blood gases may occur with midbrain dysfunction. When pontine damage is superimposed on the midbrain syndrome then central neurogenic hyperventilation disappears and may be replaced by breathing that is apparently more normal. A pause at inspiration (apneustic breathing) is characteristic of pontine level lesions. As the pons is destroyed then breathing becomes ataxic, irregular and unpredictable. At this point respiratory arrest is imminent.

Motor system function must be tested quite differently from the usual neurologic examination. Usually spontaneous movements or the movements in relationship to painful stimuli can be observed. A hemiplegia is easy to recognize in the diencephalic stage. Bilateral decorticate posture may rarely be seen in the diencephalic stage. This consists of a posture of adduction at the shoulder with flexion at the elbow, wrists and fingers with extensor posturing of the lower extremities. There is a stage short of decorticate posturing where there is fairly facile movement away from the painful stimuli but the range of passive movement in these limbs is limited by counterholding (gegenhalten).

In the midbrain stage of deterioration, decerebrate postures appear. Decerebration rarely appears in a florid full-blown form but more often only fragments of the posture appear and then only in response to noxious stimulation. The examiner should place the semiflexed upper extremities across the patient's abdomen and then provide a painful stimulus to the sternum. If the patient consistently reaches after the painful stimulus with only one limb then one can determine that the opposite side is hemiplegic. If the patient's arms extend away from the painful stimulus even by a few centimeters one should suspect decerebration and, thus, dysfunction at the mesencephalic level. This is especially suspicious when the extension is accompanied by even slight internal rotation of the forearm. When the patient moves the limb toward the painful stimulus at the sternum a second stimulus at the iliac crest will ascertain that the patient is not simply demonstrating decorticate posturing but is actually reaching for the noxious stimulus.

As the midbrain is destroyed and pontine dysfunction appears, decerebration will disappear and the limbs will become flaccid. No movement will appear with noxious stimulation. Disappearance of decerebration is often mistaken for improvement. The limbs remain flaccid in the medullary phase of deterioration. With these parameters of examination in mind, one can quickly establish what level of nervous system function remains and begin consideration of the major diagnostic categories.

DIFFERENTIAL DIAGNOSIS OF COMA

One of the initial diagnostic decisions is whether the alteration in consciousness is due to a process which is primarily intracranial or extracranial. Extracranial processes are those systemic toxic and metabolic states which cause suppression of the ascending reticular activating system. The intracranial processes are subdivided into those in which focal signs are likely versus those in which no focal signs may be anticipated.

The major categories of intracranial processes with focal brain dysfunction include trauma, intracranial intraparenchymal hemorrhages, tumors, certain forms of infection, and brain infarction.

Trauma

Concussion refers to a transient loss of consciousness. The patient with concussion alone is usually already recovering consciousness by the time the accident floor is reached. If there is associated contusion of the brain, unconsciousness may be more lasting, and blood may be found in the spinal fluid, in addition to focal signs such as hemiplegia, aphasia, or other signs of cortical injury. When rotational forces during trauma cause the frontal lobes to come down upon the cribriform plate, contusion of the olfactory bulbs occurs and anosmia is found. One of the major problems in head trauma is the detection and treatment of hematomas in the brain parenchyma or subdural or epidural space. The CT scan has greatly simplified this problem in acute situations, but the CT scan may not reveal a chronic subdural hematoma.

From 2 to 6 weeks after the trauma the clot may resolve into a fluid which is isodense with brain on CT scans. Thus, one may see only a shift without any lesion, or if the subdural hematomas are bilateral there may not even be a shift but the ventricular size may be unusually small (the "hypernormal" CT scan). An apparently negative CT scan in an appropriate clinical setting should not dissuade the physician from the diagnosis of subdural hematoma. An isotope scan may reveal a lesion when the CT scan has failed to do so. An arteriogram may occasionally be necessary to pursue this diagnosis fully.

Since the mass lesion is a widely dispersed force over the convexity of one side of the brain there may be no focal cortical signs, but the distortion of the ascending reticular activating system secondary to the mass effect causes drowsiness and this may be the only feature present in the patient with chronic subdural hematoma.

Hemorrhage

Spontaneous hemorrhages into brain parenchyma are growing less common as the assiduous treatment of hypertension is becoming more widely practiced. While brain hemorrhages may occur in a variety of bleeding diatheses such as anticoagulation, end stage leukemias, hepatic disease, and so forth, the major association is still with hypertension.

Hypertensive hemorrhages tend to occur in four sites. The lateral ganglionic area of the hemisphere is most common and results in conjugate deviation of the eyes away from the hemiplegia, severe headache, hemiplegia, and signs of progressive uncal herniation with rostral-caudal deterioration. These hemorrhages are usually too deeply situated to be helped by surgical treatment.

The thalamus is a second common site of hypertensive hemorrhage and also causes headache and hemiplegia. The hemorrhage frequently dissects into upper midbrain structures and this may explain why the eyes are often conjugately deviated toward the hemiplegia. A rarer, but highly characteristic tonic downward convergence of the eyes has also been reported with thalamic hemorrhage.[3]

Pontine hemorrhage is usually fatal within 48 hours. Since the initial lesion is in the pons, the clinical picture is different from that seen with rostral-caudal deterioration. There is bilateral flaccid paralysis of the limbs, and the doll's eye maneuver or the ice water caloric test will fail to cause lateral conjugate eye deviation but some vertical gaze may remain, owing to intact midbrain centers. Peculiar vertical conjugate eye movements "ocular bobbing" may be witnessed. The eyes drift downward and then more rapidly elevate upward, slightly above the resting level before descending once again to the resting level. The movements often occur in brief bursts. Pontine hemorrhage is usually also associated with pinpoint pupils, resulting from destruction of the descending sympathetic fibers at a time when midbrain parasympathetic fibers are still functioning. The pinpoint pupils respond to light so minimally that a magnifying glass may be necessary to see the constriction.

The prompt diagnosis of hypertensive cerebellar hemorrhage is most important because of the possibility of surgical intervention. An acute cerebellar mass can compress medullary respiratory centers and cause sudden death. Surgical evacuation of cerebellar hemorrhages can be lifesaving.[12] Cerebellar hemorrhage presents with acute ataxia, nausea, vomiting, and severe headache. On examination both truncal ataxia and hemiataxia may be present. Nystagmus is usually present and there may be forced deviation of gaze opposite the side of the hematoma. A CT scan will reveal high density blood in the cerebellar hemisphere. On occasion the onset of these hemorrhagic syndromes can be ingravescent and the whole syndrome may take several days to appear.

Tumors

Most intracranial tumors are diagnosed early enough nowadays so that patients do not present with coma in the emergency room. Certain special situations, however, should be kept in mind by the emergency room physician.

Tumors in the midline of the neuraxis either within or outside the ventricular system may cause very little in the way of neurologic symptoms or signs until spinal fluid flow is obstructed, and then obtundation with acute hydrocephalus and rapid deterioration in clinical status occurs. Posterior fossa herniation is a totally different problem from the supratentorial herniation with its orderly rostral-caudal deterioration of function. Mass lesions in the posterior fossa may present with respiratory arrest as the first manifestation of foramen magnum herniation. The tempo of investigation for patients suspected of harboring posterior fossa mass lesions should reflect this possibility. Papilledema will usually be present in these patients. Since papilledema takes about 24 hours to develop fully, it will not be seen in massive acute hemorrhages, but if the patient has had a slowly growing tumor, he is more apt to have papilledema when seen with an acute deterioration in level of consciousness. Midline posterior fossa or intraventricular tumor-associated hydrocephalus should be treated with emergency ventricular drainage or ventriculostomy.

Pituitary adenomas can present with acute coma when spontaneous hemorrhagic necrosis of the tumor occurs. Patients with pituitary apoplexy have headaches, visual loss and stiff neck, obtundation, extraocular palsies, and acute hypotension. The recognition and treatment of the acute hypoadrenal state caused by the failure of ACTH production is an essential lifesaving maneuver which the emergency room physician must be aware of. An enlarged sella seen on the plain skull films will serve as an important clue to the diagnosis of pituitary apoplexy. If massive doses of steroids stabilize the patient's vital signs then surgical decompression of the optic chiasm may be considered. The CT scan has proven to be extremely useful in diagnosing most intracranial tumors.

Cerebral abscess usually presents as a mass lesion. The appearance is often characteristic on CT scan. A small bulb of air in the low density center of a lesion with a ring-like enhancement is diagnostic of abscess. Brain abscesses by themselves do not give rise to fever and the spinal fluid may be normal.

Hemispheric infarcts may acutely produce lethargy or confusion, but unilateral lesions seldom cause complete coma. An exception occurs when a massive acute hemisphere infarction resulting from a carotid embolus results in severe brain edema. In this circumstance herniation and fatal rostral-caudal deterioration of brain function can occur in 1 to 2 hours. Small infarcts of the brain stem can interrupt the reticular activating system and produce lasting coma.[15] In the "locked-in" syndrome, extensive paralysis occurs because of bilateral destruction of the motor pathways in the basis pontis.[6] The patient is conscious but the medical staff may not realize it unless they develop a code using eyeblinks to communicate with the patient.

In certain other intracranial processes causing coma, such as meningitis, encephalitis, and subarachnoid hemorrhage, no focal signs may be present. The physician is vitally dependent upon careful examination of the spinal fluid for the correct diagnosis. Focal signs may be present but are then a bonus for the diagnostician. Aneurysms of the posterior communicating artery often cause an acute third nerve palsy. Bacterial meningitis may cause cerebral thrombophlebitis with hemiplegias and focal seizures. Similarly, the predilection of the herpes simplex virus for the temporal lobe will often assist in the diagnosis of that variety of viral encephalitis.

This category of intracranial processes without obvious focal signs should serve as a forceful reminder that every comatose patient must have a spinal fluid examination performed unless there is a contraindication for lumbar puncture. If the patient is deemed too ill for a lumbar puncture, then some other diagnostic procedure must be substituted on an emergency basis. A CT scan prior to lumbar puncture is often a reasonable arrangement, if the CT scanner is available on an emergency basis.

The extracranial processes which cause coma can also be divided into two broad categories: Those encephalopathies arising as a result of endogenous metabolic derangements and those that are due to exogenous toxins. The differential diagnosis of the endogenous metabolic derangements consists of a listing which includes the failures in all the body's vital organ systems. All major dysfunctions in these systems ultimately lead to coma. This proves to be a simple device to retain a logical scheme for an approach to the endogenous metabolic encephalopathies and is reflected in section IIIB of Table 1.

The toxic encephalopathies are most commonly due to purposeful ingestions of drugs, but prescribed drugs must not be forgotten especially in the increasingly large elderly population who are unusually sensitive to the sedative effects of many drugs in the modern therapeutic armamentarium. Some sedative drugs have special effects on the eyes which may help with the diagnosis. Doraden may cause large pupils which are unresponsive to light. Morphine causes pupilloconstriction. Atropine-like effects will cause dilated fixed pupils. Severely obtunded patients with drug overdose may be capable of brushing away painful stimuli and even muttering a few sounds but may have absent eye movements even with ice water caloric stimulation. This disparity in rostral-caudal levels is highly suggestive of sedative drug overdose. A toxic screen and an emergency electroencephalogram which shows characteristic effects of sedative medication will be useful in confirming the diagnosis.

Endogenous metabolic encephalopathies usually will have no focal signs, but exceptions occur when clinically inapparent earlier lesions once again become manifest as metabolic derangement occurs. A patient who has had an old cerebral infarct with complete recovery may have his hemiplegia reappear when he begins to develop carbon dioxide narcosis because of chronic pulmonary disease. Focal seizures apparently arising from the supplementary motor area with fencing postures and groping movements of the extended arm have proven to be highly suggestive of nonketotic hyperosmolar coma.

One of the most important practical distinctions between the toxic-metabolic encephalopathies and the intracranial processes relates to the pupillary light response. In all of the toxic-metabolic encephalopathies except anoxic encephalopathy and those caused by drugs which have

Table 1. *Some Causes of the Acute Confusional State**

I. Central nervous system disorders
   A. Conditions mimicking confusion
      1. Korsakoff syndrome
      2. Fluent aphasia
      3. Denial syndromes
   B. Conditions causing acute confusion
      1. Mass lesions (tumors, hematomas, granulomas)
      2. Infections (viral, bacterial, parasitic spirochetal, meningitis, encephalitis, or abscess)
      3. Deficiency states (niacin, thiamine, vitamin B_{12})
      4. Epilepsy (postictal states, psychomotor seizures)
      5. Trauma (concussion, contusion; epidural, subdural, or intracerebral hematomas)
      6. Cerebrovascular disease (subarachnoid hemorrhage, infarction of lingual gyrus, nondominant parietal lobe or mesial temporal lobe)
      7. Heat stroke
      8. Dementing disorders (especially liable to confusion with even trivial general medical illness, head injury, or simply a change in environment)
II. Psychiatric disorders
   A. Acute schizophrenia
   B. Acute manic and paranoid states
   C. Homosexual panic
   D. Ganser's syndrome
III. Extracranial disorders
   A. Exogenous intoxications
      1. Alcohol, barbiturates
      2. Tranquilizers
      3. Belladonna derivatives
      4. Psychotomimetics
      5. Others: ergot, salicylates, caffeine, heavy metals
      6. Withdrawal syndromes
   B. General medical diseases
      1. Disturbances of hydration, electrolytes, and osmolarity
      2. Cardiovascular disturbances (hypotension, congestive heart failure, hypertensive encephalopathy)
      3. Pulmonary failure (carbon dioxide narcosis anoxia)
      4. Hepatic encephalopathy
      5. Uremia and the postdialysis syndrome
      6. Endocrine disorders: hypoglycemia, thyroid adrenal, and pituitary syndromes
      7. Porphyria
      8. Vasculitides
      9. Acute infections outside the central nervous system
     10. Toxemia of pregnancy

---

*Modified after Safran, A. P., and Sabin, T. D.: Confusion. *In* Schwartz, G. R., et al., eds.: Principles and Practice of Emergency Medicine. Philadelphia, W. B. Saunders Co., 1978, pp. 511–517.

specific effects on the pupil, pupillary response to light will be spared regardless of the stage of rostral-caudal deterioration.

Decerebration does occur in the toxic-metabolic encephalopathies and should not be considered diagnostic of structural brain disease. Metabolic encephalopathy is often accompanied by widespread involuntary small amplitude myoclonic jerks in the musculature. The patient should be examined with an oblique light for several minutes, as the muscle twitches are often not otherwise apparent.

Clearly the full discussion of all the causes of coma is beyond the scope of this article which may serve only as a model for an approach to the comatose patient. Diligent support of all such patients by the emergency room physician is mandatory so that reversible causes of coma can be found. Even those patients who appear to be in extremis may make useful recoveries.

ACUTE CONFUSION

CLINICAL FEATURES

Confusion is the result of a defect in the moment to moment attentional mechanisms. These are mechanisms that determine the sequence of integration of stimuli into the conscious life of the individual. The acute confusional syndrome is also known in the psychiatric literature as an acute organic brain syndrome or acute toxic psychosis.[5, 7] Disorientation is not the sine qua non of the acute confusional state. The major feature is a failure to maintain normal sequential thought, and this is a reflection of the inability to rank the priority of stimuli. The consequent failure in the designation of behavioral priorities causes an immediate and drastic disintegration of adaptational interaction with the environment. Thus, the confused patient does not appear on the emergency floor on his own volition but is usually brought there by a concerned family member or by the police.

The patient's general behavior and speech reflect the inappropriate sequencing of ideas. He may present a wide range of abnormal behaviors including assaultiveness, motor hyperactivity, hallucinations, somnolence, extreme states of panic or fear. There is a great danger that a patient in an acute confusional state may be labelled as having a psychiatric problem and the underlying organic disorder may be missed. The state of alertness of the confused patient may be normal, depressed or hyperalert. Hyperalert confusional states are most commonly associated with withdrawal states. The hypoalert confusional states overlap with obtundation or coma, as discussed above. Despite the obvious aberrant thinking of the confused patient, the examiner will occasionally be surprised to get valid diagnostic information regarding drug ingestion or past illnesses which may be relevant to the present problem. Memory for the patient's past life may be intact during the period of confusion. The patient has no insight into his confused state and is unaware of his disordered thinking. When the patient recovers from the confusional state, there is ordinarily no memory of the period of acute confusion.

Detailed neurologic examination of the patient with acute confusion is extremely difficult. One feature that such patients have that may be mistaken for a focal finding is nominal aphasia.[2] Confused patients often have a word-finding difficulty and circumlocutory phrases will appear in their spontaneous speech. Speech comprehension and repetition is otherwise intact. The aphasia is even more severe in the patient's writing. Severe agraphia is typical of the acute confusional state. In the confused patient nominal aphasia and agraphia should not be misconstrued as signs of focal disease. In contrast, Broca's, Wernicke's, or conduction aphasia can be taken as evidence of a coexistent focal brain lesion.[4] No elementary neurologic findings occur as an inherent part of the confused state.

Pathogenesis

While the level of attentiveness or arousal is a function of the brain stem reticular activating system, the prioritization and sequencing of stimuli appear to be a cortical function. This phasic, selective aspect of attention is essential to produce coherent thought and goal-oriented behavior.[9] Since the great majority of confusional states are due to generalized metabolic disturbances or intoxications the anatomic substrate for the acute confusional state is unknown. There are occasional reports of focal lesions of the undersurface of the occipital lobe and in the distribution of the right middle cerebral artery producing acute confusional states as their only manifestation. There are cortical areas in each lobe of the brain where multiple sensory modalities converge and these multimodal areas may have the role of sorting out the priority of sensory inputs and maintaining normal attentiveness and coherence.[11]

Differential Diagnosis

In Wernicke's aphasia the production of excessive well-articulated speech which may make no sense can be mistaken for confusion. The patient is also unaware of the deficit and often behaves in a suspicious or paranoid fashion. The intensity and frequency of aphasic errors with paraphasias and neologisms and the failure to comprehend spoken language are the key features which distinguish this patient with a dominant hemispheric posterior superior temporal gyrus lesion from the patient with an acute confusional state. The nominal aphasia which is often part of the confusional state is never very severe and is not associated with the failure of language comprehension.

In Korsakoff's syndrome the patient is disoriented but has an isolated inability to retain new memories for more than a minute or so. The confabulatory response is not essential to make the diagnosis of Korsakoff's syndrome. The patient with Korsakoff's syndrome can maintain a coherent stream of thought and appropriately utilize environmental clues to try to give correct answers. During the acute phase of Wernicke's encephalopathy due to thiamine deficiency, the patient is confused and the acute confusional state is often wrongly diagnosed as Korsakoff's syndrome. The diagnosis of Korsakoff's syndrome should not be made until the acute confusional state subsides, leaving the isolated defect in the formation of new memories. The amnestic syndrome is also seen in closed head trauma and infarction of the dominant mesial temporal lobe.

Denial syndromes should also be separated from acute confusion.

These consist of an active denial or inattentiveness to a specific focal, usually acute neurologic deficit. These are most common with left hemiplegias and cortical blindness due to vascular disease. These failures to perceive acute neurological defects are enhanced if the patient is also confused but do occur in nonconfused patients. Confused patients are not only unaware of their mental dysfunction but they tend to deny other obvious neurologic defects so that the phenomenon of denial does not have localizing significance in the confused patient.

Ganser's syndrome is usually precipitated by an acute life stress. The patient presents with a preconceived notion about how a "crazy person" would act and therefore considerable variation in the sophistication of this "pseudoinsanity" is found. Questions are answered in ways that belie a knowledge of the intention of the question but the answer is always, to some extent, wrong. For example, the patient may state that there are 8 days in the week, that it is night time when it is daytime, or that it is Winter when it is Spring. If a patient can be coaxed to talk spontaneously, normal thought sequencing may be evident. This "syndrome of approximate answers" promptly remits when the patient is confronted with the correct diagnosis. Once aphasia, Korsakoff's syndrome, denial syndromes, and Ganser's syndrome have been excluded, then the distinction must be made among a primary central nervous system etiology, a toxic or metabolic derangement, or a psychiatric process to account for the acute confusional state.

Central Nervous System Causes of Confusion

The common central nervous system disorders associated with acute confusion are trauma, seizure disorder, infections, dementing disease, nutritional problems, and mass lesions. In head trauma there is usually a period of loss of consciousness acutely, i.e., concussion which may be followed by agitated confusional state even in the absence of obvious focal deficit. The amnestic syndrome becomes evident only when the confusion subsides and then may persist for several months.

A variable period of confusion may follow a seizure. In most instances the duration of this confusion is so short as to allow the emergency room physician to ascertain that the patient is improving during a brief period of observation. Occasionally continuous psychomotor seizures will manifest as an acute behavioral syndrome with profound confusion. Some of these patients may show a state of intermittent pathologic laughter (gelastic epilepsy) or may appear to be hallucinating. Close observation of the patient may reveal some clonic twitches, mouthing or lipsmacking movements, but an electroencephalogram may be necessary to elucidate the diagnosis.

Encephalitis, especially due to herpes simplex and purulent meningitis are important infectious causes of the acute confusional syndrome and one of the reasons for lumbar puncture in all cases of acute confusion in which no clear contraindication exists.

Elderly patients or patients with dementia seem particularly prone to episodes of acute confusion. A relatively trivial non-neurologic illness such as pyelonephritis or pneumonia may present with an acute

confusion. If the management of such patients is aimed primarily at the
confusional state, then the possibility of diagnosing and treating some
other simple underlying medical illness will be tragically overlooked.

At the Boston City Hospital emergency floor, the most common
situation in which acute confusion occurs is in the elderly patient who
has drifted into congestive heart failure, a slight electrolyte imbalance,
mild carbon dioxide retention, or other usually treatable general medical
disease.

Nutritional disorders also remain a major problem in this country.
Certainly at a place where many alcoholic patients are treated, Wernicke
Korsakoff encephalopathy is not rare. These confused patients have
ataxia, bilateral sixth nerve palsies, and nystagmus. The disease is most
common in alcoholics, but food fadists and recluses may also develop
thiamine deficiency. The policy of discharging increasing numbers of
patients from state mental institutions has resulted in an increased
incidence of Wernicke-Korsakoff encephalopathy in nonalcoholic patients. Some of these patients become recluses and severely neglect their
nutrition. Pellagra caused by niacin deficiency is much rarer in our
society, but mental confusion, irritability, insomnia, and photosensitive
rash with diarrhea would suggest this diagnosis.

Intracranial space-occupying lesions may cause confusional states
as a nonfocal manifestation of distortion of the intracranial contents.
The mass may be tumor, blood, clot, cyst, or granuloma. In all of these
instances computer-assisted tomography is the major diagnostic maneuver to most immediately sort out these possibilities.

As previously discussed an occasional patient with an acute agitated
confusional state will be found to have only a small area of infarction
presumably in one of the multimodal cortical areas. This diagnosis is
usually made only after the acute phase of the illness has passed.

Toxic-Metabolic Derangements

Drug intoxication is the most common cause of the acute confusional state in late adolescence and young adults. While alcohol continues to
be the most abused drug, simple drunkenness is rarely the only problem
in persons brought to the accident floor because of confusion. The
physician should search for signs of trauma, infection, deficiency states,
and liver disease in a patient who is intoxicated. Amphetamines, lysergic
acid, cocaine, and phencyclidine (Angel Dust) often produce an excited
hyperalert confusion with hallucinations. The belladonna alkaloids can
cause a rather dramatic acute confusion in the elderly patient being
treated for parkinsonism. There may be a suppression of sweating, the
pupils are somewhat enlarged, and there is widespread cutaneous
vasodilatation. The accident room physician should be aware that this
syndrome can be immediately reversed by intravenous administration of
1 mg of physostigmine. This cholinergic agent crosses the blood brain
barrier and the response is of diagnostic significance. Many of the
prescription drugs in common use can cause acute confusional states
and this should be a prime consideration in any individual recently
started on medical treatment. Cimetadine has been found to be a fairly

common cause of confusion in recent years but other commonly used drugs such as propranolol also seem capable of rarely producing acute confusion. Every year some new agent is introduced into the medical practice or is abused as a street drug. The emergency room physician must remain alert to the pattern of drug use and abuse in his community.

The paradigm of the hyperalert acute confusional state is that associated with alcohol withdrawal. In alcohol withdrawal, confusion, tremulousness, illusions, and hallucinations with restlessness appear within 12 to 72 hours after cessation of drinking. Withdrawal seizures consistently occur before the onset of the mental symptoms. Any seizure occurring after that time should be considered a sign of another central nervous system process.

The range of alcohol withdrawal syndromes is wide. The most severe form is delirium tremens where simultaneous mental, motor and autonomic abnormalities occur. This is a life-threatening disorder with a significant mortality rate. The patient appears hyperalert, his attention being cast transiently from one object to another. He misconstrues sounds or appearances with delusions or frank hallucinations. The patient is unable to sleep, and the state of mental hyperalertness has a motor counterpart manifested by nearly continuous restless motor activity. There is often a coarse, distal irregular tremor. This motor hyperactivity must be taken into account in calculating the fluid, electrolyte, and nutritional needs of the patient. The autonomic features of delirium tremens include fever, diaphoresis, and tachycardia. The onset of the syndrome may be quite abrupt and it usually persists for 1 to 5 days. The state is terminated after a prolonged sleep. When the patient awakens there is no memory of the episode. Major withdrawal syndromes and seizures with confusion develop 2 to 8 days after withdrawal from chronic use of many sedatives and tranquilizers including the barbiturates, glutethimide, and paraldehyde.

The metabolic encephalopathies are partially listed in Table 1. The clinical appearance of the mental syndrome in nearly all of these disorders may be indistinguishable one from the other. The distinction must be based on a careful general medical evaluation and appropriate laboratory investigation for these disorders. The encephalopathy caused by endogenous derangements in metabolism usually cause a hypoalert or sleepy confusion with progression to coma. Some interesting exceptions to this rule include the hyperalert agitated mental syndromes which may be seen in acute porphyria and hyperthyroidism. The finding of asterixis (metabolic flap) or widespread small amplitude myoclonic jerks are characteristic of the metabolic encephalopathies.

A full discussion of the psychiatric disorders which may be associated with acute confusional states is beyond the scope of this article. Acute schizophrenia and manic depressive illness in the manic phase would be the two most common problems. Emergency room physicians should be very wary of making the diagnosis of a psychiatric disorder in a somnolent or obtunded confused patient. The first episode of acute schizophrenia is rare after age 30.

Laboratory Investigations

The work-up of the acutely confused patient is similar to that for the patient in coma: routine chest x-ray, complete blood count, sedimentation rate along with determination of serum glucose, electrolytes, calcium, blood urea nitrogen, and a toxic screen serve as a minimal core laboratory evaluation. Arterial blood gases, serum ammonia, liver function studies, serum cortisol, thyroxines, transaminase level, antinuclear factor, serum protein electrophoresis, lipid analysis, or urine test for porphyria and heavy metals may be required in certain instances. An electroencephalogram may offer important evidence of the seizure disorder or the widespread symmetric slowing with triphasic activity that characterizes metabolic encephalopathies. There is also a rapid frontally distributed electroencephalographic activity which signifies the presence of sedative drugs.

A lumbar puncture should be done on every patient who is acutely confused unless there is a distinct reason not to proceed with one. This reason might consist of two possibilities: one is that the patient may be seen at a phase when there is extremely rapid improvement going on as in a treated bout of hypoglycemia. If the diagnosis seems clear and the patient is rapidly improving the lumbar puncture may safely be deferred. If on the other hand the diagnosis seems clear but immediate improvement is not anticipated, the patient should still have a lumbar puncture. Many patients with obvious alcohol withdrawal syndrome have been found on lumbar puncture to have evidence of a primary intracranial process such as a subdural hematoma or meningitis which was the cause for the cessation of alcohol intake. The second circumstance when a lumbar puncture may be deferred arises from a patient with signs of markedly increased intracranial pressure due to a mass lesion. When this situation occurs it is not simply satisfactory to defer a lumbar puncture but there should be an urgent active substitution or an alternative diagnostic measure.

At the present time, CT scanning of the brain will clearly be the method of choice for the initial evaluation of confused and obtunded patients. Neurologic and neurosurgical consultation should be obtained for advice and guidance regarding the selection of procedures such as angiography or ventriculography. The role of other noninvasive examinations such as isotope brain scanning, flow scans, as well as the electroencephalogram will remain a matter of judgment which must take into account both the rate of progression of the patient's clinical status and the likelihood of diagnostic yield. Both electroencephalographic and rectilinear scanning may be quite difficult if the patient is restless or combative.

The treatment of the acute confusional state is basically the treatment of the underlying disorders. Consideration of the variety of disturbances listed in Table 1 suggests why it is preferable for the initial evaluation and treatment of acute confusion to be carried out in a general medical rather than a psychiatric facility. Certain therapeutic maneuvers should be carried out and the same concerns of circulation, respiration, substrate, and cofactor (thiamine) as discussed with coma should be urgently attended. Gastric lavage is often carried out during this early phase in appropriate cases. These preliminary maneuvers can usually be accomplished in 15 minutes by a trained emergency room staff.

The patient can often be quieted down and made tractable if approached with firmness and given simple clear explanations of various procedures that are being undertaken in his behalf. The environment should be well lighted. If restraints are necessary they should be applied with precautions so that the patient is positioned on his side to prevent aspiration in case he vomits. Proper padding and positioning of the restraints should avoid nerve compression palsies or brachial plexus traction. The unfortunate practice of tying a patient's limbs to the four corners of the bed promotes struggling and exposes the patients to risks of aspiration as well as brachial plexus palsies. Sedation is best avoided until a diagnosis is established which includes sedation as an appropriate part of the treatment. In these circumstances the goals of sedation are simply to calm the patient and reduce the nursing problem and prevent the patient from injuring himself.

Good management of the confused patient does not include adding the hazards of drug-induced coma to the patient's primary illness. Orders for sedative medication should therefore be written as each dose is needed.

Diazepam, chloral hydrate and paraldehyde, phenothiazines, and haloperidol are agents for the delirious patient. Paraldehyde is extremely effective in the treatment of patients with delirium tremens, but tends to be unpopular because of the odor which emanates throughout the ward. Eight to 10 ml of paraldehyde by the rectal or the oral route is still amont the most effective and safe agents for delerium tremens. Intramuscular paraldehyde is complicated by the development of sterile abscesses. The patient should not receive more than 10 ml every 2 hours and the dosage can be significantly reduced after the first 8 to 12 hours of treatment. The single most important aspect of the treatment of delerium tremens, however, is probably the meticulous maintenance of fluid and electrolyte balance. The restlessness, tremor, fever, and diaphoresis may raise fluid requirements to 4 to 7 liters per day. Sponge baths, cooling blankets, and salicylates may be required to suppress the fever associated with delirium tremens. Each patient with delirium tremens or other alcohol withdrawal syndrome requires a systematic search for head trauma, intracranial hematomas, meningitis, pneumonia, or other infections with or without liver failure, hypoglycemia, pancreatitis, anemia, and gastrointestinal bleeding which are the usual reasons why the patients might have stopped drinking.

REFERENCES

1. Adams, R. D., and Victor, M.: Delirium and other confusional states and Korsakoff's amnestic syndrome. Chap. 30., In Wintrobe, M. M., et al., eds.: Harrison's Principles of Internal Medicine. New York, McGraw Hill, 6th ed., 1970, pp. 184–193.

2. Chedru, F., and Geschwind, N.: Disorders of higher cortical functions in acute confusional states. Cortex, 8:395–411, 1972.
3. Fisher, C. M.: The pathologic and clinical aspects of thalamic hemorrhage. Trans. Amer. Neurol. Assoc., 1959.
4. Geschwind, N.: The aphasias. New Eng. J. Med., 284:654–656, 1971.
5. Gooddy, W.: Orientation. In Vinken, P. J., and Bruyn, G. M., eds.: Handbook of Clinical Neurology. New York, Elsevier, 1969, pp. 202–211.
6. Kemper, T. L., and Romanual, F. C. A.: State resembling akinetic mutism in basilar artery thrombosis. Neurology, 17:74–80, 1967.
7. Lipowski, Z. J.: Delirium clouding of consciousness and confusion. J. Nerv. Ment. Dis., 145:227–255, 1967.
8. Magoun, H. W.: The Waking Brain. Springfield, Illinois, Charles C Thomas, 1963.
9. McGhie, A.: Psychological apsects of attention and its disorders. In Vinken, P. J., and Bruyn, G. W., eds.: Handbook of Clinical Neurology. New York, Elsevier, 1969, pp. 137–154.
10. McNealy, D. E., and Plum, F.: Brain stem dysfunction with supratentorial mass lesions. Arch. Neurol., 7:32, 1962.
11. Mesulam, M. M., et al.: Acute confusional states with right middle cerebral artery infarctions. J. Neurol. Neurosurg. Psychiat., 39:84, 1976.
12. Ott, K. H., et al.: Cerebellar hemorrhage: Diagnosis and treatment. A review of 56 cases. Arch. Neurol., 31:160–167, 1974.
13. Plum, F., and Posner, J. B.: The Diagnosis of Stupor and Coma. Philadelphia, FA Davis Co., 2nd ed., 1972.
14. Sabin, T. D.: The differential diagnosis of coma. New Engl. J. Med., 290:1062–1064, 1974.
15. Segarra, J. M.: Cerebral vascular disease and behavior. Arch. Neurol., 22:408–418, 1970.

Boston City Hospital
818 Harrison Avenue
Boston, Massachusetts 02118

Adult Respiratory Distress Syndrome

Physiologic Basis of Treatment

Adam Hurewitz, M.D.,*
and Edward H. Bergofsky, M.D.**

A healthy 20 year old woman sustains multiple traumatic injuries during an automobile accident and requires an emergency splenectomy and blood transfusions. She is initially stable, but 12 hours postoperatively she becomes agitated and dyspneic. Tachycardia and tachypnea are prominent and her arterial Po_2 falls from 90 to 48 mm Hg. Breathing an enriched oxygen mixture raises her Po_2 to only 52 mm Hg. The chest radiogram demonstrates bilateral, diffuse interstitial and alveolar infiltrates and a heart of normal size. Immediate intubation and initiation of mechanical ventilation with positive end-expiratory pressures improve the arterial Po_2 to 64 mm Hg. However, after 48 hours the course is complicated by pneumonia caused by *Pseudomonas aeruginosa*, and progressive renal failure; on the fourth postoperative day the patient expires.

This case history exemplifies some of the cardinal clinical features of the adult respiratory distress syndrome: onset within 48 hours after the initiating incident, tachypnea followed by respiratory distress, falling arterial Po_2 without elevation of Pco_2, and bilateral pulmonary infiltrates.[33] This syndrome is now sufficiently common, not only in large medical centers, but in every community hospital, to warrant an extensive laboratory and clinical investigative program to elucidate its pathogenesis. Such studies have implicated a growing number of etiologic entities and an equally long list of pathogenetic mechanisms; but they have also yielded an accurate picture of the pathophysiology of adult respiratory distress syndrome which has led to improved application of the principles of respiratory physiology to treatment of this disorder. The following review will discuss the proposed mechanisms, the pathophysiology, and the clinical management of such patients.

*Assistant Professor of Medicine, SUNY, Stony Brook School of Medicine, Stony Brook, New York
**Professor of Medicine, SUNY, Stony Brook School of Medicine, Stony Brook, New York

Supported by Grants No. HL-00439, No. HL-23210, NHLBI, Department Health and Human Resources, and the Veterans Administration, Washington, D.C.

Table 1.   *Causes of Adult Respiratory Distress Syndrome*

I. Airway Source
   A. Direct pulmonary injury and inflammatory response
      1. Gastric acid aspiration[41, 48]
      2. Respiratory burns[30]
      3. Oxidant gas inhalation[73, 88]
      4. Pneumonias[26, 28]
   B. Inflammatory response with little direct injury
      1. Oxygen toxicity[23]
   C. Uncertain
      1. Near drowning[27, 77]
      2. War gases

II. Vascular Source
   A. Direct pulmonary injury and inflammatory response
      1. Paraquat ingestion[43]
      2. Pancreatitis[38]
      3. Drug-induced[42]
   B. Inflammatory response with little direct injury
      1. Endotoxemia[20, 45]
      2. Hemorrhagic shock[9]
      3. White cell transfusions (leukoagglutinins)[68]
      4. Fat embolism[3, 17, 60]
   C. Uncertain
      1. Nonthoracic trauma[8, 64]
      2. Disseminated intravascular coagulation[11, 36, 79]
      3. Cerebral injury[13, 87]

PATHOGENESIS

Inciting Agents

The disorders which most frequently predispose to adult respiratory distress syndrome include trauma, shock, toxins, and infections (Table 1). Although it may be useful to distinguish those causative agents which are inhaled from those which are bloodborne, the clinical expression is remarkably similar for all etiologies. Both routes may be associated with direct damage to the initial cell surface contacted; this direct injury is occasionally sufficient to explain acute respiratory failure. In many instances, however, an intense inflammatory response evoked by the initial injury predominates.[10] This response greatly amplifies the extent of lung injury and is the common pathogenetic mechanism of adult respiratory distress syndrome. This example of a "protective" biologic response participating as the major source of tissue injury is analogous to anaphylactic shock; the inciting agent itself may be innocuous, yet the response it elicits may be devastating.

The type I pneumocyte is highly susceptible to damage by a variety of inhaled substances. Destruction of this cell, which constitutes about 95 per cent of the alveolar surface,[45] severely compromises the integrity of the alveolar-capillary barrier. The aspiration of gastric acid[28] or certain microorganisms[14] has been demonstrated to produce initial extensive alveolar epithelial injury as well as a subsequent vascular permeability. Other agents, such as oxygen, appear to injure primarily the endothelial cells despite their mode of entry via the airways. Exceedingly large alveolar oxygen concentrations are believed to promote adult respiratory distress syndrome by stimulating the production of unstable oxygen derivatives by circulating granulocytes.[12] These oxidizing free radicals, which normally assist phagocytosis, participate in the secondary inflammatory response and injure pulmonary vascular endothelium.[15]

Intravascular causes of adult respiratory distress syndrome include gram-negative septicemia, fat emboli, and hemorrhagic shock. These disorders all seem to provoke, at most, minimal direct vascular damage, yet their capacity to initiate a fatal inflammatory response is well established.[7, 34] The initiators of this inflammatory response are endotoxins (septicemia), free fatty acids (fat emboli), and unknown factors in hemorrhagic shock (perhaps microthrombi). By contrast, the ingestion of paraquat (an herbicide)[24] or the release of proteolytic and lipolytic pancreatic enzymes[20] can cause direct endothelial injury as well as an indirect inflammatory response. Because direct endothelial injury is so unusual in adult respiratory distress syndrome, histologic documentation of endothelial damage is rarely detected.[2] An inflammatory mechanism permitting temporary widening of interendothelial junctions is not accessible to direct visualization but has been inferred from the residual signs of permeability edema.

The Amplification Response

Several mechanisms have been proposed to explain the occurrence of extensive pulmonary damage which is often out of proportion to the apparent initial injury. Investigation has focused upon the role of (1) the release of intracellular inflammatory agents, (2) freely circulating inflammatory agents, (3) microvascular stasis or thrombosis, and (4) altered surfactant synthesis. Despite some uncertainties, considerable data exist to support the role of each of these factors in amplifying the original lung injury.

Circulating granulocytes and platelets, as well as tissue macrophages, all contain a variety of mediators of inflammation.[17, 44] Granulocyte release of lysosomal hydrolases or phospholipases into the pulmonary circulation can produce extensive cell membrane damage.[46] Other mediators, such as the oxidant free radicals (i.e. superoxide, singlet oxygen, and hydroxyl radicals) synthesized by granulocytes, have also been demonstrated experimentally to damage structural lipids and proteins.[15] This mechanism may be particularly relevant to pulmonary oxygen toxicity, although its role in the pathogenesis of adult respiratory distress syndrome is not restricted to oxygen therapy.

A similar explanation is applicable for the role of platelets in adult respiratory distress syndrome. Their secretion of histamine, serotonin, or kinins could stimulate contraction of endothelial cells with subsequent widening of intercellular pores and an increased protein permeability. The observation that platelets[47] and granulocytes[17] aggregate in pulmonary capillaries during experimental adult respiratory distress syndrome has stimulated support for the mediator-release theory, since such microaggregates would permit high concentrations of inflammatory mediators to accumulate in the lungs. Investigation of experimental adult respiratory distress syndrome during granulocytopenia or thrombocytopenia may shed more light on this controversial theory.

The prostaglandins are inflammatory mediators of particular interest because of their metabolism in the lungs. Their role, if any, in adult respiratory distress syndrome is uncertain but they represent a potentially powerful and specifically reversible source of the amplification response.

Controversy persists regarding the role of microvascular stasis or thrombosis as a primary or secondary event in adult respiratory distress syndrome. Three lines of evidence support such a role: physiologic monitoring of a decreased pulmonary capillary volume[34] and an increased dead space;[1] microscopic visualization of vascular thromboses;[18] and clinical laboratory data compatable with intravascular coagulation (DIC).[3] Additional animal studies have demonstrated that the intravenous injection of fibrinogen degradation products is capable of causing a syndrome similar to adult respiratory distress syndrome.[30] The clinically significant aspect of microvascular aggregates in adult respiratory distress syndrome probably lies in their relation to the mediator-release response, and lesser significance should be attributed to increased alveolar dead space.

Altered surfactant function is also a fundamental though not fully understood mechanism in adult respiratory distress syndrome.[22] Unlike neonatal respiratory distress syndrome where abnormal production of surfactant is an initiating event, in adults such a primary pathogenetic role is less certain. Three possible routes by which surfactant dysfunction may occur are: (1) decreased synthesis; (2) increased destruction; and (3) production of normal amounts of a qualitatively abnormal surfactant. The transformation of type II pneumocytes to replace destroyed type I cells could result in quantitative or qualitative alterations of surfactant synthesis. Lipolytic substances released during the amplification response, or a clearance effect induced by large volumes of alveolar edema might explain an increased destruction of surfactant.

The Role of Permeability Pulmonary Edema

Experimentally induced adult respiratory distress syndrome in animals (i.e., infusions of endotoxin, fibrinogen degradation products, or fatty acids[6, 30, 32]) documents permeability pulmonary edema as being at least a major pathogenetic mechanism. Since the experimental model, at least superficially, resembles the clinical entity, permeability edema is

$$\dot{Q}_{NET \atop FILTRATION} = KA \left[(P_{MV} - P_{PMV}) - \sigma (\Pi_{MV} - \Pi_{PMV}) \right]$$

Figure 1.   The Starling Principles of Transmicrovascular Fluid Exchange. The net volume of liquid movement into the perimicrovascular space (interstitium) is related to a fluid conductance factor (K = membrane permeability constant, A = vascular surface area) and a pressure factor (composed of both hydrostatic (P_{mv}–P_{pmv}) and osmotic (π_{mv}–π_{pmv}) pressure gradients between the microvascular and perimicrovascular spaces. σ is the reflection coefficient describing the protein permeability of the endothelium. It varies between totally permeable ($\sigma = 0$) and totally impermeable ($\sigma = 1$).

also assumed to occur with clinical adult respiratory distress syndrome. The important physiologic characteristics of permeability edema include: (1) normal microvascular pressures; (2) elevated interstitial protein concentrations; and (3) increased transcapillary fluid flux.

In the healthy lung, the alveolar epithelium is impermeable to fluids and protein, while the vascular endothelium has a restricted permeability to both.[39] The net transcapillary exchange of liquid and solutes obeys

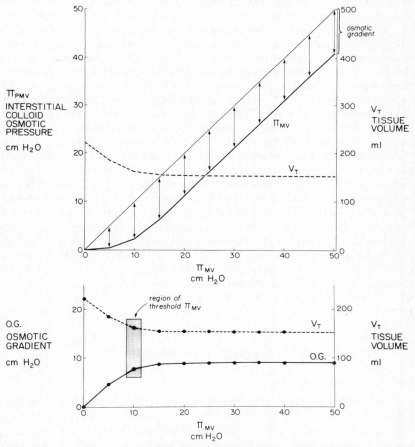

HOW PLASMA PROTEINS AFFECT OSMOTIC GRADIENT
AND LUNG WATER

Figure 2. Importance of the Colloid Osmotic Gradient in Regulating Pulmonary Fluid Balance. Upper panel shows microprocessor prediction of relationship between capillary osmotic pressure (π_{mv}) on the abscissa and interstitial osmotic pressure (π_{pmv}) on the ordinate; the curve is the line of deviation of corresponding points of π_{mv} and π_{pmv} from a line of identity. The difference between these lines is the osmotic gradient (arrows) at any π_{mv}. As indicated, when π_{mv} drops below 12 cm H_2O, the osmotic gradient narrows from the normal value of 10 cm H_2O, and as shown on the right ordinate, lung tissue water and volumes begin to increase. In the bottom panel, the two variables, osmotic gradient and the resulting tissue water volume are plotted against varying π_{mv} and the critical region of decreasing osmotic gradient and rising lung water volume is shown for the situation of normal microvascular pressure and permeability.

Starling's principles (Fig. 1). An osmotic gradient $(\pi_{mv} - \pi_{pmv})$ is thus established by the unequal protein concentrations in the vascular and interstitial compartments. This osmotic gradient is essential to the maintenance of an edema-free state in the lungs (Fig. 2). Any process which increases vascular permeability to proteins will tend to diminish the osmotic gradient;[23] the unopposed hydrostatic gradient $(P_{mv} - P_{pmv})$ will then permit significant edema to fill the interstital spaces initially and subsequently the alveolar spaces.[40] In the presence of increased vascular permeability, then, elevations of pulmonary vascular hydrostatic pressure will exacerbate the interstitial and alveolar edema; the narrowed osmotic gradient which results from permeability injury permits the hydrostatic gradient to exert a much more potent effect upon lung water distribution.

The resultant accumulation of lung water depends not only upon the hydraulic forces and permeability factors mentioned, but also upon the reabsorption capacity of the lymph vessels. In the steady state condition, the net extravascular accumulation of fluid and protein is removed by the lymphatics. Modest increases of fluid filtration are accommodated by increased lymph flow; recent evidence suggests it can increase 10-fold above baseline values.[39] Clinically important pulmonary edema thus possibly represents striking increments of transcapillary fluid filtration through increases of permeability or hydrostatic pressures.

The clinical confirmation of altered vascular permeability depends heavily upon indirect signs. The combination of the nonspecific signs of pulmonary edema (i.e., intrapulmonary shunt, reduced compliance, and radiographic signs of interstitial fluid accumulation) and the measurement of normal microvascular (pulmonary capillary wedge) pressures suggests a clinical diagnosis of noncardiogenic, or permeability, pulmonary edema. No methods are routinely employed to directly measure either the protein concentration or the accumulated volume of extravascular fluids in the lungs. Only by histologic observation of hyaline membranes does the clinician obtain direct evidence of permeability edema; even then, the source of these inspissated intra-alveolar proteins remains uncertain.

PATHOPHYSIOLOGY

Defect in Oxygenation

The hallmark of adult respiratory distress syndrome is severe hypoxemia. The hypoxemia, moreover, responds poorly to high inspired oxygen mixtures. In almost every instance, the low arterial Po_2 is associated with a normal to low Pco_2, indicative of adequate overall ventilation. As a result, widened alveolo-arterial Po_2 differences $(A-a\ Do_2)$ are calculated which may reach and exceed 50 to 60 mm Hg in patients with adult respiratory distress syndrome breathing room air. Thus, with normal or even supranormal alveolar oxygen tensions (90 to 110 mm Hg), arterial Po_2 is usually found below 50 mm Hg by the time the patient evinces the restlessness, tachypnea and dyspnea which clinically herald the onset of the syndrome.

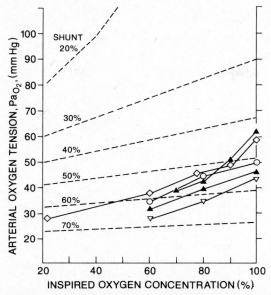

Figure 3.   The Effect of Variations in Inspired O_2 Concentration on the Arterial Po_2 When Different Degrees of Venous Admixture are Present. Dashed lines represent calculated values of arterial Po_2 which exist when venous admixture is fixed; i.e., it represents anatomic shunt. The solid lines represent values from 4 patients with adult respiratory distress syndrome; as inspired O_2 concentration rises, corresponding values for arterial Po_2 cut across the lines calculated for individual values for venous admixture, suggesting that venous admixture is decreasing with increased inspired O_2 concentrations. In one subject (open diamonds), the venous admixture decreases from a value of 65 per cent while breathing 21 per cent oxygen to 45 per cent while breathing 100 per cent oxygen. (*From* Briscoe, W., et al.: Catastrophic pulmonary failure. Amer. J. Med., *60*:248, 1976.)

Of the three possible explanations for a widened $A-a Do_2$, all have been invoked at one time or another to explain hypoxemia in adult respiratory distress syndrome. Of these, the first and foremost appears to be a ventilation-perfusion imbalance.[11] The anatomic basis of this defect may be the presence of noncompliant air spaces with a tremendous variety of ventilation to volume ratios throughout the lung. Either interstitial edema from an endothelial cell defect or partial alveolar atelectasis from damage to type I or II alveolar cells could account for this defect. A second mechanism to explain hypoxemia is the arteriovenous shunt; this concept implies that pulmonary blood flow through such defective areas can never have access to alveolar gas, no matter how high the inspired oxygen mixture is raised. The anatomic basis for this defect would be persistence of perfusion through micro-areas which are completely atelectatic or the alveoli of which are filled by exudate or edema.[45] A third mechanism is a defect of alveolo-capillary diffusion;[5] the anatomic basis of this physiologic defect would be expected to be either an interstitium thickened by fluid and exudate or alveoli partially filled with fluid. From the physiological standpoint, however, a diffusion defect very much resembles a ventilation-perfusion defect in that progressive increases in inspired oxygen produce predictably large rises in arterial Po_2. In a similar manner, from the anatomic standpoint, a

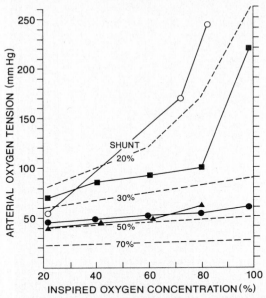

Figure 4.   Effect of Variations in Inspired O_2 Concentration on Arterial Po_2 in Dogs with Experimental Adult Respiratory Distress Syndrome and in One Subject With Chronic Obstructive Lung Disease. Same display of values for arterial Po_2 during alterations in inspired O_2 concentrations at various, but constant values for venous admixture, as shown in Figure 3. The three solid lines (solid symbols) demonstrate the relatively constant venous admixture in oleic acid–induced ARDS in the dog despite changes in inspired O_2 concentration. By contrast, the patient with obstructive lung disease (open circles) shows a very marked reduction in venous admixture with high inspired O_2 mixture. Patients with ARDS fall somewhere in between these two extremes with venous admixture representing a combination of anatomic shunt and ventilation-perfusion imbalance. (Modified from Briscoe, W., et al.: Amer. J. Med., 60:248, 1976.)

diffusion defect caused by alveolar edema may often be only a lesser version of the anatomic shunt resulting from alveolar filling.

Nonetheless, even though the anatomic bases for the three types of physiologic lesions possible in adult respiratory distress syndrome are uncertain, it makes clinical sense to distinguish just two types of defects of gas exchange: those with meager responses (anatomic shunts) and those with satisfactory responses ($\dot{V}/\dot{Q}$ imbalance or diffusion defects) to high inspired oxygen mixtures. Figure 3 demonstrates the partitioning of these two types of lesions in several patients with adult respiratory distress syndrome, by means of serial increments in inspired oxygen. The slope of increase in arterial Po_2 with increasing inspired oxygen in the group with adult respiratory distress syndrome clearly does not follow the prediction lines for a unique anatomic shunt-like lesion, but rather cuts across these lines, indicating a combination of both shunt-like and ventilation-perfusion-like defects. As shown in Figure 4, a group of dogs with lung damage induced by oleic acid have a much more pure form of anatomic shunt, while 6 patients with obstructive lung disease have a slope which reflects a predominant ventilation-perfusion de-

Table 2. *Oxygenation Parameters in Adult Respiratory Distress Syndrome (ARDS)*

PARAMETER	COMMON NAME	INDEX OF	NORMAL VALUE	TENDENCY IN ARDS*
PAO_2-PaO_2	A-a gradient	Ventilation-perfusion or diffusion	10 mm Hg	↑
PaO_2	Arterial O_2 tension	Effect of lung on arterial blood	90 mm Hg	↓
$\dot{Q}_s/\dot{Q}_T$	(1) Venous admixture	Ventilation-perfusion	6%	↑
	(2) Venous admixture breathing 100% O_2	Anatomic shunt	1%	↑
PaO_2/F_{IO_2}	Ventilation-perfusion index	Ventilation-perfusion or diffusion	500	↓
CaO_2-$C\bar{v}O_2$	A-V difference, O_2	Tissue perfusion	4 ml/dl	0
$P\bar{v}O_2$	Mixed venous O_2 Tension	Tissue oxygenation	40-45 mm Hg	↓

* ↓ = decreased, ↑ = increased, 0 = unchanged

rangement.[5] As indicated below, one goal of therapy in adult respiratory distress syndrome is the conversion of the anatomic shunt into a ventilation-perfusion derangement which permits the alleviation of the hypoxemia by moderately high inspired oxygen mixtures.

Appraisal of Oxygenation

Three areas of this appraisal are pertinent for adult respiratory distress syndrome: (1) the diagnosis of the mechanism of the hypoxemia; (2) the estimation of oxygen delivery by arterial blood; and (3) the assessment of tissue oxygenation (Table 2).

The *diagnosis* of *mechanisms* of *hypoxemia* usually begins with the assessment of A–a Do_2; this requires a calculation of alveolar oxygen tension which uses the empirical relationship.

$$P_AO_2 = F_IO_2 \cdot (P_B - 47) - \frac{P_aCO_2}{RQ}$$

where P_AO_2 = alveolar Po_2; F_IO_2 = inspired oxygen fraction; P_B = prevailing barometric pressure; and RQ = a constant equal to a respiratory quotient of 0.8. The A–a Do_2 is useful during room air breathing in estimating the severity of the syndrome (5 to 15 mm Hg is within normal limits and 50 to 60 mm Hg is a severe defect), but with increasing inspired oxygen levels, the A–a Do_2 widens increasingly, even though the physiologic defect need not change. The most accurate technique of measuring the defect is in the formal calculation of venous admixture by the relationship:

$$\dot{Q}_s/\dot{Q}_T = (C_cO_2 - C_aO_2) \div (Cco_2 - Cvo_2)$$

$\dot{Q}_s$ = shunt flow, $\dot{Q}_T$ = total pulmonary blood flow, and Cco_2, Cao_2 and Cvo_2 = capillary, arterial and mixed venous oxygen contents respectively. This relationship requires calculation of blood oxygen contents from Po_2, pH, and oxygen-carrying capacity of hemoglobin.

For simplicity, therefore, a ratio is often used relating the arterial Po_2 to the fraction of inspired oxygen (F_1o_2). Its advocates hope that this ratio tends to remain constant in a given case, even through increasing levels of inspired oxygen. For instance, a typical patient with severe adult respiratory distress syndrome may have the following relationships breathing 60 per cent oxygen ($F_1o_2 = 0.6$): $P_ao_2 \div F_1o_2 = k$ or $60 \div 0.6 = 100$. Thus, when this patient's alveolar Po_2 is 380 mm Hg as a result of breathing an F_1o_2 of 0.6 (see above alveolar gas equation), a typical arterial Po_2 of 60 mm Hg will yield a ratio or k of 100. When his F_1o_2 is raised to 1.0, the values could be $100 \div 1.0 = 100$, i.e., the same or similar ratio, suggesting that in this case shunt values and ventilation-perfusion ratios were constant despite changes in the fraction of inspired oxygen. Typical values in the normal individual would be $100 \div 0.21 = 500$, when the arterial Po_2 is 100 mm Hg while breathing 21 per cent oxygen and $600 \div 1.0 = 600$, the arterial Po_2 typical of 100 per cent oxygen breathing; these values, rising from 500 to 600, reflect the small decrease in ventilation-perfusion ratios expected in the normal when 21 per cent oxygen is replaced by 100 per cent oxygen in the inspired mixture. This ratio is useful as a rough index of the homogeneity of gas exchange, but when gross changes in either cardiac output or hemoglobin content occur, calculation of venous admixture by the more formal method is more accurate.

The *appraisal* of the *oxygen delivery capability* of arterial blood utilizes the product of arterial oxyhemoglobin saturation and oxyhemoglobin capacity (hemoglobin concentration × 1.34), which is the oxygen-carrying capability, and multiplies this value by cardiac output ($S_ao_2 \times$ [Hb] × 1.34 × CO). An equal reduction in any of the major variables reduces the oxygen delivery capability to the same degree. Thus, reductions in arterial oxygen saturation by a low arterial Po_2, low pH, or abnormal oxyhemoglobin dissociation curve are no worse than equivalent reductions in hemoglobin concentration or blood flow.

Although the oxygen delivery capability includes practically all the variables required to predict the *adequacy* of *tissue oxygenation*, the best practical parameter for this function is the mixed venous Po_2. This value is the final integration of oxygen delivery and tissue utilization and is considered a reasonable index of body tissue Po_2 levels.[29]

Lung Mechanics in Adult Respiratory Distress Syndrome

Adult respiratory distress syndrome consistently reduces the compliance of the lung. When dynamic lung compliances (relating the change in lung volume to the change in transpulmonary pressure during breathing) are measured during assisted ventilation, values as low as 20 ml per cm H_2O or even less are recorded. The inflation of such a lung to a tidal volume of 600 ml requires as much as 30 cm H_2O or more. When ventilated by a volume-cycled respirator, such a lung may require 40 to

Table 3. *Lung Mechanical and Hemodynamic Parameters in Adult Respiratory Distress Syndrome (ARDS)*

PARAMETER	COMMON NAME	INDEX OF	NORMAL VALUE	TENDENCY IN ARDS*
LUNG MECHANICS				
P_{insp}	Peak inspiratory pressure	Pressure against elastic recoil and airway resistance	7 cm H_2O for $V_T = 600$ ml	↑
P_{plat}	Plateau inspiratory pressure	Pressure against elastic recoil	6 cm H_2O for $V_T = 600$ ml	↑
$C_T°$	Respiratory system compliance	Elastic recoil of lung	100 ml/cm H_2O	↓
HEMODYNAMICS				
P_{PA}	Pulmonary arterial pressure	Right ventricular afterload	15 mm Hg mean	↑
P_W	Pulmonary wedge pressure	Pulmonary venous pressure	9 mm Hg	0
P_{PA}-P_W	Pulmonary vascular pressure gradient	Pulmonary driving pressure	6 mm Hg	↑
C.O.	Cardiac output	Adequacy of blood flow	6.0 L/min+	0
$\dfrac{P_{PA}-P_W}{C.O.}$	Pulmonary vascular resistance	Vasoconstriction, vascular obliteration	1.0 mm Hg/L/min	↑

* ↓ = decreased, ↑ = increased, 0 = unchanged
+ = 2.5 to 3.4 L/min/M²
° = Because C_T is related to its components, lung compliance (C_L) and chest compliance (C_{CW}) reciprocally, i.e., $1/CT = 1/C_L - 1/C_{CW}$, when C_L is greatly reduced, C_T closely approximates C_L.

60 cm H_2O of pressure at peak inflation to overcome the resistance of the endotracheal tube and of airways and the impedance of the chest and abdomen. Some of the reasons for this increase in elastic recoil may be inferred from histologic observations: they show turgidity of capillaries, diapedesis of cells into the interstitium, remnants of protein and fluid in alveoli, multiplication of Type II alveolar cells and microatelectasis.[2, 45]

From the physiological standpoint, reductions in compliance could be due to some combination of (1) increased elastic recoil of all air spaces and/or (2) dropping out of air spaces as a result of atelectasis, so that remaining, even fairly normal air spaces either are overexpanded or provide too small an expansible volume. Which of these mechanisms predominates will determine the relative success of positive end expiratory pressure.

Although only a few measurements have been made, lung volumes are generally severely reduced in adult respiratory distress syndrome.[33] The functional residual capacity, in particular, has been measured most frequently, because it requires little cooperation from the gravely ill

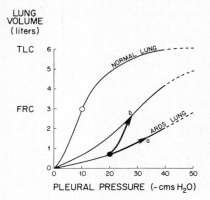

LUNG
VOLUME
(liters)

Figure 5. Pressure Volume Diagrams of Lung in Normal and ARDS States. The slope relating the pleural pressure required at any given lung volume, i.e., lung compliance is markedly reduced for the ARDS curve, compared with the normal. Since pleural pressures of only 60 to 80 cm H_2O are available, this curve clearly indicates that the vital capacity could not exceed 1 to 2 liters in this case. The effects of PEEP on the lung volumes and compliance is discussed in the text under management.

patient. Reductions of up to 50 per cent of the predicted value occur, attributable in part to spotty atelectasis of alveoli and in part to generalized decreases in the compliances of the remaining patent alveoli. Few measurements of voluntary forced expiratory volumes or vital capacity are available. But values below 50 per cent of predicted values can be inferred from the transpulmonary pressures measured during assisted ventilation at peak inspiration or from the pressure-volume diagrams of the lung in adult respiratory distress syndrome (Fig. 5).

MANAGEMENT OF ADULT RESPIRATORY DISTRESS SYNDROME

Two therapeutic directions are available for the management of adult respiratory distress syndrome. The first is the alleviation of the effects of acute respiratory failure through assisted oxygenation and mechanical ventilation. The second approach is the suppression of the amplification response which remains the source of continuing lung injury. Significant progress has been achieved in developing techniques to assist gas exchange in the failing lung; these include technical advances in supplementing oxygen delivery, mechanical ventilation of the lungs, and physiologic methods of reducing the intrapulmonary shunt. More recently, goals of therapy have focused not only on improvement of gas exchange in the lung, but also on delivery of oxygen to critical organs. Advances in methods of eliminating the amplification response are less impressive and primarily involve the use of corticosteroids; investigation of other, perhaps more specific anti-inflammatory agents is presently underway.

Oxygenation

Although correction of tissue hypoxia is the ultimate goal of treatment, initial measures are directed toward improvement in arterial hypoxemia. Since an arterial Po_2 of 60 mm Hg will saturate 90 per cent of hemoglobin with oxygen when the oxyhemoglobin dissociation curve is normal, this value, with an additional buffer of 5 or 10 mm Hg, is usually sought.

During the early phase of adult respiratory distress syndrome, when interstitial edema predominates, arterial hypoxemia is due to ventilation-perfusion abnormalities and an increased diffusion barrier. Alveolar ventilation is usually normal or elevated. The use of supplemental oxygen by nasal cannula or face mask will generally be sufficient to elevate the arterial Po_2 to > 60 mm Hg. As a result, endotracheal intubation and mechanical ventilation are not required at this stage. Most examples of adult respiratory distress syndrome, however, progress rapidly to a second phase, characterized clinically by progressive hypoxemia that no longer improves sufficiently with supplemental oxygen. This phase correlates with progressive alveolar edema and microatelectasis and a parallel increase in intrapulmonary shunt.[45] Typically, 60 per cent inspired oxygen cannot bring the arterial Po_2 above 60 mm Hg. In this circumstance, therapy is directed toward reduction of the venous admixture-like effect. Occasionally, 60 to 100 per cent oxygen by mask may be used for brief periods of time in the hope that the process will be self-limited. Usually, however, this approach cannot correct the hypoxemia and adds the risk of oxygen toxicity as well as uncontrolled tissue hypoxia.

Certain generalizations may be made regarding the effect of various concentrations and duration of supplemental oxygen. Inspired oxygen concentrations of 40 to 55 per cent are believed to represent the threshold of oxygen toxicity independent of the resulting arterial Po_2.[31, 35] Increased concentrations and duration of the use of supplemental oxygen are directly correlated with reductions in the vital capacity and the single breath carbon monoxide diffusing capacity.[8] In some instances, oxygen therapy itself contributes to the genesis of adult respiratory distress syndrome. Because this latter response may be related to oxygen-induced production of toxic-free-radicals (such as superoxide and hydroxyl radical)[12] anti-oxidants may prove to be of benefit in reducing oxygen toxicity. Present investigation is exploring the role of superoxide dismutase and vitamin E in preventing oxygen toxicity.[4, 50] When no alternatives exist to maintain oxygenation, even potentially toxic concentrations of oxygen should be used to maintain a minimal $P_{\bar{v}}O_2$ of 35 torr and Po_2 of 60 torr. If a Po_2 of more than 60 torr can be obtained, an attempt can be made to lower the F_IO_2 to 0.4 or less.

When the above inspired oxygen concentrations of 40 to 55 per cent are no longer able to maintain an arterial Po_2 of 60 ± 5 mm Hg, or in the uncommon case where alveolar hypoventilation in the form of arterial Pco_2 values in excess of 44 mm Hg occur, intubation and mechanical assistance are indicated (Fig. 6).

The use of a mechanical ventilator can yield two benefits: (1) assistance to ventilation, and (2) maintenance or restoration of lung inflation. Assisted ventilation is necessary for those cases with fatigue and alveolar hypoventilation evidenced by elevated Pco_2. The increased work of breathing of adult respiratory distress syndrome may also be alleviated by assisted ventilation but the clinical benefit from this effect has not been studied.

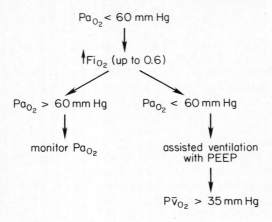

Figure 6. The Initial Management of Hypoxemia in Adult Respiratory Distress Syndrome. The reduction of arterial Po_2 below 60 mm Hg (90 per cent saturation of hemoglobin) requires therapeutic intervention. If supplemental oxygen (up to 0.6 F_IO_2) is sufficient to restore P_aO_2 to >60 mm Hg, the patient need only be monitored for further changes in oxygenation. When supplemental oxygen is not sufficient to restore an adequate P_aO_2, mechanical ventilation with PEEP is required (see Figure 8).

A more frequent benefit of mechanical ventilation is the maintenance of lung expansion. When supplemental oxygen can no longer ameliorate the severe hypoxemia of adult respiratory distress syndrome, lung expansion can reduce the amount of venous admixture by (1) restoration of a normal resting pulmonary mid-position (FRC, functional residual capacity) and (2) improvement of lung compliance.[13] In some instances the use of large tidal volumes of 15 ml per kg is sufficient to effect these changes. More frequently, the addition of airway pressures of 5 to 30 cm of water at the end of expiration (PEEP, positive end expiratory pressure) is required. Although the mechanisms whereby PEEP produces improved lung function are uncertain, possible explanations include the inflation of collapsed air spaces[25] and an improvement of alveolar surfactant production or function.[48]

The two possible mechanical effects of positive end expiratory pressure on lung volume and compliance are shown in Figure 5. A lung existing at a reduced volume in the presence of decreased compliance (right sided curve) may simply be inflated by PEEP to a higher position on the same curve; this position has two advantages: (1) this portion of the compliance curve is steeper in slope and, as shown, for the same volume change, less inflation pressure, i.e., transpulmonary pressure is needed; and (2) the increase in FRC can improve the degree of venous admixture and hence the arterial Po_2. In favorable cases, PEEP shifts the lung to the left to a curve of higher compliance with considerable augmentation of the above two advantages.

In the clinical setting, a reasonable estimate of compliance may be obtained by dividing the delivered tidal volume by the inspiratory plateau pressure ($C_L = V_T/P_{plat}$). The latter is obtained from the airway pressure manometer of the mechanical ventilation during temporary occlusion of expiratory flow at the height of inspiration. The "optimal" PEEP is established as that value of expiratory pressure at which compliance is maximal.[42] Although "optimal" PEEP, using maximally improvable lung compliance, is often a useful guide to the adjustment of PEEP, an even more important index may be the maximally obtainable

Figure 7. Improvement of Arterial P_{O_2} by Reduction of Shunt ($\dot{Q}_S/\dot{Q}_T$). At 40% shunt, increasing $P_{A}O_2$ from 100 mm Hg ($F_IO_2 = 0.21$) to 680 mm Hg ($R_IO_2 = 1.0$) hardly effects any increase in arterial P_{O_2}. Reduction of $\dot{Q}_S/\dot{Q}_T$ (see text) permits significant elevations of P_aO_2 to result with supplemental oxygen. At 25% shunt, the P_aO_2 can be rasied to 100 mm Hg at $F_IO_2 = 1.0$, and even an F_IO_2 of 0.4 can raise that P_aO_2 to 60 mm Hg.

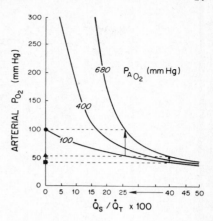

reduction in venous admixture.[16] Fortunately, venous admixture, whether it is composed of ventilation-perfusion defects of various degrees or absolute intrapulmonary shunts, appears to respond to progressive increments in PEEP. The enormous effect on arterial blood oxygenation which PEEP may bring about by reducing venous admixture, and particularly its shunt component, is shown in Figure 7. Here, little or no increase in arterial P_{O_2} could be obtained when the shunt fraction was 50 per cent, despite increases in inspired oxygen concentration to virtually 100 per cent. A reduction of only 15 per cent in shunt fraction restores the ability to raise arterial P_{O_2} with even moderate increments in inspired oxygen. Although some authors suggest a goal of <15 per cent shunt, this probably is not necessary. When the shunt is reduced to 25 per cent, an F_IO_2 should be sufficient to raise the P_aO_2 to 60 mm Hg.

The third index for the use of PEEP is the value of the mixed venous P_{O_2}. This level, as indicated above, is far more integrative than other indices; it represents the tissue level of oxygenation and as such is the balance between the amount of oxygen delivered to the tissues and their oxygen utilization. It thus serves as a suitable index of the efficacy of virtually the entire therapeutic regimen used in adult respiratory distress syndrome. However, the mixed venous P_{O_2}, because it reflects oxygen delivery to tissues and, hence, cardiac output, is particularly pertinent for the use of PEEP.[25] The importance of this correlation stems from recent observations that PEEP may have produced significant alterations of cardiac output. These may be due to (1) reduced venous return to the heart, induced by the elevated pressures imposed upon the pleural space; (2) raised pulmonary vascular resistance following compression of perialveolar capillaries during lung inflation; and (3) depressed myocardial contractility, probably resulting from a reflex response to inflation of the noncompliant lung.[9, 36] On the other hand, PEEP may raise cardiac output if pleural pressure is sufficiently raised so as to produce a net reduction in ventricular afterload. A generalized approach to selecting the most beneficial PEEP is illustrated in Figure 8.

In actual practice, the lung is so stiff in true adult respiratory

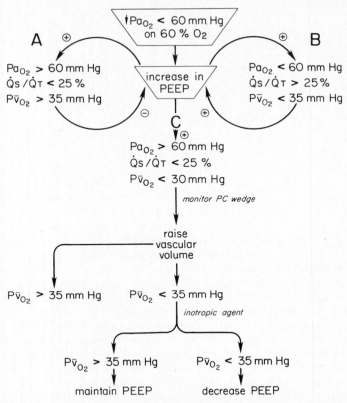

Figure 8.   Guidelines for the Use of PEEP in ARDS: PEEP is instituted when supplemental oxygen of 60 per cent cannot restore the arterial Po_2 to 60 mm Hg. Three general responses may follow an increase of PEEP: A, Significant improvement of both arterial (P_aO_2) and mixed venous ($P_{\bar{v}}O_2$) oxygen tensions to acceptable values. No further increase of PEEP is necessary. B, Partial or absent improvement of P_aO_2 and $P_{\bar{v}}O_2$ (but no fall in either) warrants a trial of higher PEEP. C, Worsening $P_{\bar{v}}O_2$, secondary to a fall in cardiac output, despite improvements of shunt ($\dot{Q}_S/\dot{Q}_T$) and thus P_aO_2. In this case, attempts to improve cardiac output through fluid replacement or the use of inotropic agents may permit a normalization of $P_{\bar{v}}O_2$ and further increments of PEEP if needed. If such efforts to avert a fall of $P_{\bar{v}}O_2$ cannot be overcome, PEEP must be decreased.

distress syndrome that very high levels of PEEP barely restore the functional residual capacity to normal. Under these circumstances, it can be predicted that the chief effect would be compression of some small pulmonary vessels by high alveolar pressures, increases in pulmonary vascular resistance and right ventricular (and perhaps left ventricular) dysfunction sufficient to decrease cardiac output.[25] Thus, a fall in mixed venous Po_2 while raising PEEP indicates that the decrease in cardiac output more than offsets any increase in arterial Po_2 and that tissue oxygenation has deteriorated. The measurement, of course, requires the insertion of a flow-directed, right heart, cardiac catheter,[43] but this approach, though invasive, yields three additional pieces of information: (1) actual cardiac output (usually by a thermal indicator-dilution method for which the cardiac catheter may be designed), (2) arteriovenous oxygen concentration difference which is inversely proportional to cardiac output and may usually be used to confirm or substitute for that value (see above), and (3) the pulmonary wedge pressure, as an index of left atrial pressure.

Management of Pulmonary Edema

Although less effective than PEEP in reducing intrapulmonary shunt, efforts to limit or lessen the interstitial and alveolar edema are an important aspect of managing adult respiratory distress syndrome. The Starling principles predict that a reduced intravascular pressure will minimize lung water accumulation; hence, the lowest wedge pressure compatible with a normal cardiac output is desirable. Diuretics may be of benefit both by reducing intravascular pressure and by raising intravascular oncotic pressure during free-water clearance. The latter effect is minimized by the presence of increased vascular permeability to protein. By the same principles, even the correction of hypoalbuminemia may not enhance the osmotic gradient ($\pi_{mv} - \pi_{pmv}$), since the administered albumin will rapidly distribute into the lung interstitium.

Efforts to Inhibit the Amplification Response

Corticosteroids are the only agent presently used to combat the amplification response. Animal models of adult respiratory distress syndrome seem to demonstrate a role for steroids when given prior to exposure to the inducing agent.[26, 28, 46, 48] Most clinical evidence, however, does not document benefit from these agents. However, the proven anti-inflammatory potential of corticosteroids and the probable role of inflammation in adult respiratory distress syndrome continue to encourage further study of the therapeutic utility of these agents.[19, 35, 37, 72] With presently available data, it is difficult to argue either for or against the often used regimen of methylprednisolone, 30 mg per kg per day for 48 hours,[38] if given at the onset of the disease.

Other agents are being investigated as potential inhibitors of the amplification response. These include antiprostaglandins (Indomethacin) anti-oxidants (vitamin E,[30, 41, 50] superoxide dismutase, catalase) and anticoagulants. There is no indication for their use at this time.

Prognosis

The mortality of adult respiratory distress syndrome remains as high as 40 to 60 per cent despite improvements in methods of maintaining oxygenation. The ability to oxygenate the lungs (i.e., with PEEP) if achieved at the expense of other organ systems (i.e., low output renal failure)[21] will not improve mortality. Greater attention to cardiac output and tissue oxygenation ($P_{\bar{v}}O_2$) may avert the problems seen when overzealous efforts are applied to improving pulmonary function. The future development of effective means of suppressing the lung's response to inflammatory mediators may be the key to improving prognosis. Until such prophylactic measures become available, maintaining tissue oxygenation during the acute phase of respiratory failure is the essential goal of treating adult respiratory distress syndrome.

The long-term follow-up of patients who have recovered from adult respiratory distress syndrome offers two important perspectives to the clinician. First, those patients who survive often recover reasonable normal lung function when studied one year later.[27, 49] Second, many of the patients who achieved normal lung function after adult respiratory distress syndrome received 'toxic' concentrations of oxygen therapy (i.e., $F_IO_2 > 0.6$ for more than 5 days). These data reinforce the suggestion that supportive therapy in the acute phase of adult respiratory distress syndrome should be vigorous in maintaining oxygenation, even if potentially toxic levels of oxygen supplementation are required. If these severely ill patients can be brought through the acute phase of adult respiratory distress syndrome, their chances of survival with relatively normal lung function is excellent.

REFERENCES

1. Askenezi, J., Wax, S., Neville, J., et al.: Prevention of pulmonary insufficiency through prophylactic use of PEEP and rapid respiratory rates. J. Thorac. Cardiovasc. Surg., 75:267, 1978.
2. Bachofen, M., and Weibel, E.: Alteration of the gas exchange apparatus in adult respiratory insufficiency associated with septicemia. Amer. Rev. Resp. Dis., 116:589, 1977.
3. Bone, R., Francis, P., and Pierce, A.: Intravascular coagulation associated with the adult respiratory distress syndrome. Amer. J. Med., 61:585, 1976.
4. Boyd, M., Catignani, G., Sasame, H., et al.: Acute pulmonary injury in rats by nitrofurantoin and modification by vitamin-E, dietary fat and oxygen. Amer. Rev. Resp. Dis., 120:93, 1979.
5. Briscoe, W., Smith, J., Bergofsky, E. H., et al.: Catastrophic pulmonary failure. Amer. J. Med., 60:248, 1976.
6. Brigham, K., Woolverton, W., Blake, L., et al.: Increased sheep lung vascular permeability caused by Pseudomonas bacteremia. J. Clin. Invest., 54:792, 1974.
7. Burgher, L., Dines, D., Linscheid, R., et al.: Fat embolism and the adult respiratory distress syndrome. Mayo Clin. Proc., 49:107, 1974.
8. Caldwell, P., Lee, W., Jr., Schildkraut, H., et al.: Change in lung volume, diffusing capacity and blood gases in man breathing oxygen. J. Appl. Physiol., 21:1477, 1966.
9. Cassidy, S.: Indirect mechanisms that reduce cardiac output during positive pressure ventilation and lung inflation. Prac. Cardiol., 6:110, 1980.
10. Cross, C., and Hyde, R.: Treatment of pulmonary edema, In Staub, N., ed.: Lung Water and Solute Exchange. New York, Marcel Dekker, Inc., 1978, p. 471.
11. Dantzker, D., Brook, C., Dehart, P., et al.: Ventilation-perfusion distribution in the adult respiratory distress syndrome. Amer. Rev. Resp. Dis., 120:1039, 1979.
12. Deneke, S., and Fanburg, B.: Normobaric oxygen toxicity of the lung. New Engl. J. Med., 303:76, 1980.
13. Falke, K., Pontoppidan, H., Kumar, A., et al.: Ventilation with end-expiratory pressure in active lung disease. J. Clin. Invest., 51:231S, 1972.
14. Ferstenfeld, J., Schluetor, D., Rytel, M., et al.: Recognition and management of adult respiratory distress syndrome secondary to viral interstitial pneumonia. Amer. J. Med., 58:709, 1975.
15. Fisher, A., Bassett, D., Forman, H.: Oxygen toxicity of the lung. Biochemical aspects. In Fishman, A., and Renkin, E., eds.: Pulmonary Edema. Amer. Physiol. Soc., Bethesda, Maryland, 1979.
16. Gallagher, T., Civetta, J., and Kirby, R.: Terminology update: Optimal PEEP, Crit. Care Med., 6:323, 1978.
17. Goldstein, D.: Polymorphonuclear leukocyte lysosomes and immune tissue injury. Prog. Allergy, 20:301, 1976.
18. Goodman, J., Lim, R., Jr., Blaisdell, F., et al.: Pulmonary microembolism in experimental shock. Amer. J. Path., 52:391, 1968.
19. Hammerschmidt, D., White, J., Craddock, P., et al.: Corticosteroids inhibit complement-induced granulocyte aggregation. J. Clin. Invest., 63:798, 1979.

20. Hayes, M., Rosenbaum, R., Zibelman, M., et al.: Adult respiratory distress syndrome in association with acute pancreatitis. Amer. J. Surg., 127:317, 1974.
21. Hedley-Whyte, Jr., Burgess, G., Feeley, T., et al.: Effect of pattern of ventilation on hepatic, renal and splanchnic function. In Applied Physiology of Respiratory Care. Boston, Little, Brown & Co., 1976.
22. Henry, J.: The effect of shock on pulmonary alveolar surfactant: Its role in refractory respiratory insufficiency of the critically ill or severely injured patient. J. Trauma, 8:756, 1968.
23. Hurewitz, A., Bicker, A., and Bergofsky, E. H.: Hypoalbuminemia aggravates hydrostatic, not permeability, pulmonary edema. Amer. Rev. Resp. Dis., 1218:149, 1980 (abstract).
24. Kimbrough, R.: Toxic effects of the herbicide paraquat. Chest, 65s:65s, 1974.
25. King, E., Jones, R., and Patakas, D.: Evaluation of positive end-expiratory pressure therapy in the adult respiratory distress syndrome. J. Canad. Anesthes. Soc., 20:546, 1973.
26. Kusajima, K., Wax, S., and Webb, W.: Effects of Methylprednisolone on pulmonary microcirculation. Surg. Gynec. Obstet., 139:1, 1974.
27. Lakskminalayan, S., R. Stanford, and T. Petty: Prognosis after recovery from adult respiratory distress syndrome. Am. Rev. Resp. Dis., 113:7, 1976.
28. Lawson, D., DeFalco, A., Phelps, J., et al.: Corticosteroids as treatment for aspiration of gastric controls: An experimental study. Surgery, 59:845, 1966.
29. Lutch, J., and Murray, J.: Continuous positive pressure ventilation-effects on systemic oxygen transport and tissue oxygenation. Ann. Intern. Med., 76:193, 1972.
30. Luterman, A., Manwaring, D., Curreri, P.: The role of fibrinogen degradation products in the pathogenesis of the respiratory distress syndrome. Surgery, 82:703, 1977.
31. Michel, E., Langevin, R., and Gell, C.: Effect of continuous human exposure to oxygen tension of 418 mm Hg for 168 hours. Aerospace Medicine, Feb. 1960, p. 138.
32. Parker, F., Jr., Wax, S., Kusajima, K., et al.: Hemodynamic and pathologic findings in experimental fat embolism. Arch. Surg., 108:70, 1974.
33. Pontoppidan, H., Geffin, B., and Lowenstein, E.: Acute respiratory failure in adults. New Engl. J. Med., 287:690, 743, 799, 1972.
34. Porcelli, R., Foster, W., Bergofsky, E., et al.: Pulmonary circulatory changes in pathogenesis of shock lung. Amer. J. Med. Sci., 268:250, 1974.
35. Robertson, W., Hargreaves, J., Herlocker, J., et al.: Physiologic response to increased oxygen partial pressure II, respiratory studies. Aerospace Med., 35:618, 1964.
36. Robotham, J., Lixfeld, W., Holland, L., et al.: The effects of positive end-expiratory pressure on right and left ventricular performance. Amer. Rev. Resp. Dis., 121:677, 1980.
37. Schumer, W., and Nyhus, L.: The role of corticoids in the management of shock. Surg. Clin. N. Amer., 49:147, 1969.
38. Sladen, A.: Methylprednisolone: Pharmacologic doses in shock lung syndrome. J. Thorac. Cardiovasc. Surg., 71:800, 1976.
39. Staub, N.: Pulmonary edema. Physiol. Rev., 54:678, 1974.
40. Staub, N., Nagano, H., and Pearce, M.: Pulmonary edema in dogs, especially the sequence of fluid accumulation in lungs. J. Appl. Physiol., 22:227, 1967.
41. Steiner, M., and Anastasi, J.: Vitamin E, an inhibitor of the platelet release reaction. J. Clin. Invest., 57:732, 1976.
42. Suter, P., Fairley, B., and Isenberg, M.: Optimum end-expiratory pressure in patients with acute pulmonary failure. New Engl. J. Med., 292:284, 1975.
43. Swan, H., Ganze, W., Forrester, J., et al.: Catheterization of the heart in man with use of a flow-directed balloon-tipped catheter. New Engl. J. Med., 283:447, 1970.
44. Swank, R.: Platelet aggregation: Its role and cause in surgical shock. J. Trauma, 8:872, 1968.
45. Teplitz, C.: The core pathobiology and integrated medical sciences of adult respiratory insufficiency. Surg. Clin. N. Amer., 56:1091, 1976.
46. Turino, G., Rodriguez, J., Greenbaum, L., et al.: Mechanisms of pulmonary injury. Amer. J. Med., 57:493, 1974.
47. White, M., Shepro, D., and Hechtman, H.: Pulmonary function and platelet-lung interaction. J. Appl. Physiol., 34(S):697, 1973.
48. Wyszogrodski, I., Kyei-Aboagye, K., Taeusch, H., Jr., et al.: Surfactant inactivation by hyperventilation: Conservation by end-expiratory pressure. J. Appl. Physiol., 38:461, 1975.
49. Yahav, J., Lieberman, P., and Molho, M.: Pulmonary function following the adult respiratory distress syndrome. Chest, 74:247, 1978.
50. Yam, J., and Roberts, R.: Pharmacological alteration of oxygen-induced lung toxicity. Toxicol. Appl. Pharmacol., 47:367, 1979.

HSC, T17 Room 040
SUNY Stony Brook
Stony Brook, New York 11794

Evaluation of Acute Chest Pain

Richard R. Schneider, M.D.,*
and Stanley G. Seckler, M.D.†

Acute chest pain probably compels more people to see a physician than any other pain. Most people are concerned that their chest pain connotes serious heart disease. Unfortunately for the physician consulted, evaluation of chest pain is not a simple matter. The causes of chest discomfort are many, and pain may be a manifestation of diseases — both grave and benign — of one or more of the organ systems. The potentially life-threatening implications of the pain, coupled with the psychological make-up of the patient, can greatly influence the perception of the pain and the manner in which it is described to the physician. Evaluation of chest pain is made even more difficult since its distribution and severity is often not related to the seriousness or origin of the disease process. The physical examination and laboratory findings may be entirely normal or may demonstrate profound abnormalities — again without necessarily correlating with the prognostic implications. Matters may be further complicated by the presence of two or more kinds of pain in the same patient or by a confirmed pathologic diagnosis which may be causally unrelated to the discomfort.

Possible causes of chest pain are listed in Table 1, and the more common etiologies are discussed below in some detail. Even with an exhaustive set of guidelines, however, evaluation of acute chest pain may remain a challenge to the most astute physician.

CHEST PAIN OF CARDIAC ORIGIN

Although difficult to determine, the presence or absence of myocardial ischemia or necrosis as the cause of a patient's chest pain has important implications for the patient's physical and mental well being. The diagnosis of coronary artery disease may have profound effects on a

*Instructor in Medicine, Mount Sinai School of Medicine, City University of New York; Director, Cardiac Invasive Laboratory, Mount Sinai Hospital Services–City Hospital Center, Elmhurst, New York

†Professor of Clinical Medicine, Mount Sinai School of Medicine, City University of New York; Chief, Department of Medicine, Mount Sinai Hospital Services–City Hospital Center, Elmhurst, New York

Table 1. *Causes of Chest Pain*

CARDIAC ORIGIN

Coronary artery disease
   Atherosclerotic
      Angina pectoris
      Coronary insufficiency
      Intermediate coronary syndrome
      Unstable angina
      Variant angina or Prinzmetal's angina
      Myocardial infarction
   Syphilitic aortitis
   Coronary emboli
   Progressive systemic sclerosis
   Periarteritis nodosa
   Takayasu's disease
   Kawasaki's disease
   Nitroglycerin withdrawal
   Ergot ingestion
   Spontaneous vasospasm with normal
     coronaries
Aortic valvular disease
Right ventricular hypertrophy
Idiopathic hypertrophic subaortic stenosis
Mitral valve prolapse

PERICARDIAL ORIGIN

Viral
Bacterial
Tuberculosis
Acute myocardial infarction
Post-infarction (Dresslers)
Trauma
Uremia
Neoplasm
Connective tissue disease
Post radiation

AORTIC ORIGIN

Dissecting aneurysm
   Hypertension
   Pregnancy
   Coarctation
   Marfan's syndrome
   Cystic medial necrosis
   Blunt trauma

INTRATHORACIC NONCARDIAC

Pulmonary embolism
Pulmonary hypertension, primary or
  secondary

Tracheobronchitis
   Viral
   Irritant inhalation
Pleurisy
   Lobar pneumonia
   Pulmonary infarction
   Viral
   Neoplasm
   Connective tissue diseases
Subphrenic abscess
Pneumothorax
Pneumomediastinum
Mediastinal tumors

GASTROINTESTINAL ORIGIN

Esophageal
   Esophageal reflux
   Disordered motility
   Esophagitis
   Rupture (Boerhaave)
   Tear (Mallory-Weiss)
   Neoplasm
Peptic ulcer
Pancreatitis
Biliary colic
Cholecystitis
Gaseous distention
Paraesophageal hernia

MUSCULOSKELETAL

Muscle strain
Rib fractures
Arthritis
Teitze's syndrome
Tumors
Bornholm's disease
Xyphodynia

NEUROLOGIC

Herpetic neuralgia
Radiculitis
Thoracic outlet syndrome
Pancoast's syndrome
Traumatic neuropathy
Vertebral and spinal disease

FUNCTIONAL

Narcotic
Psychological

person's economic, social, and personal functioning. The physician must not be cavalier in arriving at such a diagnosis but should insist on an in depth appraisal, including history, physical examination, routine electrocardiogram, chest roentgenogram, and use of the various newer diagnostic modalities now available. The physician must be equally careful when he rules out coronary artery disease since failure to recognize and treat the disorder may lead to a false sense of security and possible catastrophe.

Myocardial ischemia typically occurs in the setting of fixed atherosclerotic obstructions in the proximal portions of one or more of the coronary arteries. Ischemia of the subtended myocardium occurs when oxygen demand outstrips the maximum that can be supplied by the limited blood flow through the stenotic vessel. Flow may be adequate in the basal state, but may fall short when oxygen demand is heightened by increased heart rate or wall tension caused by exercise, emotional upset, exposure to cold, ingestion of large meals, or intercurrent pathologic processes such as infection, hypertension, pulmonary congestion, or tachydysrhythmia.[26] Ischemia may also be precipitated by decrease in coronary blood flow or loss of oxygen-delivering capacity. Diminished coronary flow may occur with hypotension or a sudden narrowing or occlusion at the stenotic site caused by coronary vasospasm which may occur spontaneously or in response to exercise, REM sleep, or exposure to cold.[39, 40, 46, 58, 75] Oxygen-delivering capacity will diminish with anemia of any etiology or with alterations of the normal oxygen-hemoglobin relationship caused by either toxins, such as carbon monoxide, or by genetic or acquired molecular hemoglobin defects.[57, 71] A careful history, should, therefore, consider the precipitation or exacerbation of pain by the factors mentioned above and the effect of the removal of the noxious stimulus.

The ischemic myocardium stimulates afferent visceral nerve fibers. The cerebral cortex cannot localize these signals as myocardial in origin. Myocardial afferents may enter the spinal cord at various levels from T1-T4 and stimulate sensory pathways from somatic sites. Typically, myocardial ischemia produces a pressure sensation deep to the sternum that is commonly associated with a perception of pain from the left chest and shoulder and the medial aspect of the left upper extremity. The patient may respond with the classic position of the clenched fist over the chest (the Levine sign). Pain in the right chest, shoulder, and upper extremity, in the epigastrium, neck, jaw, teeth, hands, thumb, or mastoid, may also occur in the presence or absence of substernal discomfort. The common substernal chest pain initiated by exertion and relieved by rest was originally described by Heberden[29] in 1768 as "angina pectoris." The other forms of discomfort associated with myocardial ischemia may be termed an "anginal equivalent" for a given individual. While "typical angina pectoris" may occur in a person with normal coronary arteries and presumably in the absence of myocardial ischemia,[16, 20, 71] atypical or mild pain may be a manifestation of severe coronary obstruction and myocardial ischemia.[16]

Although the pattern of symptoms may be highly suggestive, more objective data are necessary to confirm the diagnosis. Relief of symptoms by nitroglycerin is suggestive of ischemia. The presence of abnormal Q-waves on the standard resting twelve lead electrocardiogram indicates the possibility of coronary artery disease having caused a previous myocardial infarction but does not confirm the present symptoms as being caused by myocardial ischemia. During spontaneous pain the electrocardiogram will almost always reveal ST segment changes if the pain is caused by myocardial ischemia. The absence of electrocardiographic changes during pain is strong evidence against the diagnosis of coronary disease. It cannot be overemphasized, however, that the electrocardiogram may be entirely normal within seconds after the disappearance of pain. Ambulatory electrocardiographic monitoring may detect significant ST segment changes in patients with coronary artery disease even in the absence of an episode of pain.[56] Electrocardiographic monitoring, thallium-201 myocardial scintigraphy, and radionuclide cineangiography at rest and with maximal or submaximal exercise offer relatively sensitive and specific means of detecting exercise-induced myocardial ischemia.[3, 8]

All the diagnostic information, including history and noninvasive testing, must be interpreted on an individual basis. According to Bayes' theorem, the specificity and sensitivity of a clinical finding depends on the prevalence of the disease in the group of patients under investigation. In practical terms, this means that a 55 year old man with one or more coronary risk factors (cigarette smoking, positive family history, hypertension, diabetes mellitus, hypercholesterolemia) and very atypical symptoms is still more likely to have significant coronary artery disease than a 22 year old woman with no risk factors who complains of classical angina pectoris.

If symptoms of myocardial ischemia begin to occur more frequently, with less exertion, or for prolonged periods up to 20 to 30 minutes, then terms such as intermediate coronary syndrome, crescendo angina, unstable angina, or coronary insufficiency are used.[23] While stable angina may be successfully managed on an outpatient basis, the more severe and unstable forms are probably best managed in hospital with electrocardiographic monitoring and therapy with nitrates and beta-blockers.[23] Angina occurring at rest with documented electrocardiographic changes is called variant or Prinzmetal's angina.[40, 51] It is caused by coronary vasospasm in normal or diseased coronary arteries.[46, 58] Treatment with nitrates and/or calcium channel blocking agents is indicated.[25, 49, 75] Recurrent ischemic episodes unrelieved by medical therapy may require intra-aortic balloon couterpulsation and possibly coronary angiography and coronary bypass surgery.[2, 72]

Myocardial ischemia lasting longer than 20 to 30 minutes may result in necrosis. If the oxygen supply-demand balance is restored by relief of vasospasm or decrease in myocardial oxygen demand, necrosis may be limited to the subendocardial fibers since their blood supply is the most tenuous. If, however, blood supply is not restored because of coronary thrombus formation or prolonged vasospasm, transmural infarction may occur.[14, 38, 45, 61] The classical symptoms of myocardial infarction are prolonged substernal chest pain with radiation and associated dyspnea, diaphoresis, pallor, and palpitations. Electrocardiographic manifestations of abnormal Q-waves and/or marked ST segment elevation will be seen and the patient must be admitted to the coronary care unit. However, as many as 25 per cent of patients with acute myocardial infarction may present without chest pain.[69] Diminished chest pain may be present in diabetics with acute myocardial infarction.[9]

Myocardial ischemia and infarction may occur in the absence of atherosclerotic coronary disease.[32] Other causes of myocardial ischemia include right ventricular hypertrophy secondary to pulmonary hypertension. Occlusion of the coronary orifice may occur in syphilitic aortitis[17] or dissecting aortic aneursym.[64] Coronary occlusion may be caused by emboli from intracardiac thrombi or vegetations of infective endocarditis. Coronary vasospasm may occur as a withdrawal phenomenon in workers in nitroglycerin factories who are absent from work for more than two or three days.[34] Vasospasm may also be precipitated by ingestion of drugs containing ergot derivatives such as those used to treat migraine headaches. Progressive systemic sclerosis,[12] periarteritis nodosa, Takayasu's disease, and Kawasaki's disease may be associated with coronary artery abnormalities. Patients with significant aortic stenosis may have typical angina pectoris in the presence of normal coronary arteries.[48] Severe aortic regurgitation may exacerbate ischemia by lowering diastolic coronary perfusion pressure further compromising flow through a stenotic vessel.[22] Aortic valvular disease may be diagnosed by physical examination and noninvasive studies including echocardiography[21] and external carotid pulse recordings.[68]

Idiopathic hypertrophic subaortic stenosis may be associated with ischemic symptoms in the presence of normal coronary arteries.[15, 54] However, patients with idiopathic hypertrophic subaortic stenosis are not immune to coronary atherosclerosis. The diagnosis is suspected by finding a systolic ejection murmur that is intensified with the Valsalva maneuver and markedly diminished with squatting.[68] The electrocardiogram may reveal abnormal Q-waves and high voltage QRS with ST segment and T-wave abnormalities that may be confused with myocardial infarction or the ischemic changes of coronary disease. Echocardiographic findings of asymmetric septal hypertrophy and systolic anterior motion of the anterior leaflet of mitral valve confirms the diagnosis.[21] Treatment with propranolol[54] or verapamil[13] may be effective. Nitrates may be ineffective as they cause a decrease in left ventricular chamber size and an increase in the subaortic obstruction. Diagnosis does not warrant hospitalization but the possibility of sudden death in this disorder makes treatment mandatory for the symptomatic patient.[13]

Mitral valve prolapse is associated with various types of chest pain. It is usually ill defined, precordial or substernal, fleeting or of long duration.[31] The diagnosis is suspected by the presence of the typical late systolic murmur and/or mid-systolic click which moves closer to S_1 during the Valsalva maneuver.[68] Echocardiographic evidence of prolapse is usually, but not always, found in patients with the typical physical findings.[37] The presence of an increased number of fingerprint arches[67] and skeletal chest abnormalities has been described with this disorder. The electrocardiogram may be normal or display repolarization abnormalities in the inferior and lateral leads. Response to therapy with propranolol is variable. Because of the prevalence of ill-defined benign chest discomfort and mitral valve prolapse in the general population, the presence of both in a given individual does not necessarily imply a cause and effect relationship. Although ventricular fibrillation and sudden death have been reported, it is extremely rare and hospitalization is not indicated. Antibiotic prophylaxis against infective endocarditis is indicated, as is medical follow-up to detect development of hemodynamically significant mitral regurgitation which occurs in a small percentage of patients, especially those with a late systolic murmur.[41]

CHEST PAIN OF PERICARDIAL ORIGIN

The pericardium has few pain fibers except in the parietal pericardium adjoining the diaphragm. Pain from other areas of pericardium may be secondary to inflammation of the adjacent pleura. Pericardial pain most frequently is sharp or burning and is typically precordial. Pain from the medial diaphragmatic pericardium may radiate via C3–C5 to the left shoulder and trapezius. Anterior chest, upper abdominal, and back pain simulating pancreatitis or cholecystitis may occur with lateral diaphragmatic pericardial inflammation. Classically, the pain is worse in the recumbent and left lateral position and is partially or completely relieved by sitting, leaning forward, or lying in the right lateral decubitus position. Swallowing and coughing may exacerbate the pain. Severe crushing substernal pain mimicking myocardial infarction or pain that is exacerbated by each heartbeat may occur, but such patterns are rare. Pericardial inflammation can result from acute idiopathic or viral pericarditis. In the first few days after acute transmural myocardial infarction, mild pericardial inflammation often causes typical pericardial pain even prior to the appearance of a friction rub or pericardial effusion. Post-myocardial infarction and post-pericardiotomy pericarditis may occur 10 days to three months after the acute event. A diagnosis of bacterial, tuberculous, uremic, traumatic, neoplastic, collagen vascular, and post-radiation pericarditis depends upon identification of the underlying disorder.

Physical examination may reveal a scratchy friction rub with a presystolic, systolic and/or diastolic component. In cases with associated cardiac tamponade, jugular venous distention, systemic hypotension, and a greater than 10 per cent fall in systolic blood pressure during normal inspiration (paradoxic pulse) may occur.[43] Large effusions may cause signs of pulmonary consolidation near the inferior left scapula (Ewart's sign). The electrocardiogram may display diffuse ST segment elevations that are distinguishable from myocardial ischemia by upward concavity and from early repolarization by associated P-R depression in both limb and precordial leads, ST depression in V_1, and ST elevation in

V_6.[65] Chest x-ray may be normal or may reveal a "water bottle" heart with loss of hilar markings. When there is pericardial effusion echocardiography will often reveal an echo-free space posterior to the left ventricular free wall that is not present behind the left atrium. An anterior echo-free space is commonly seen in association.[21]

CHEST PAIN OF AORTIC ORIGIN

Sudden severe anterior chest or interscapular pain should alert the physician to aortic dissection. Prompt diagnosis, which depends upon a high index of suspicion, is mandatory because immediate medical and surgical intervention may be life-saving. Dissection usually occurs in patients with known or suspected hypertension (82 per cent in one series),[64] but also occurs in pregnancy, aortic coarctation, Marfan's syndrome, cystic medial necrosis, and secondary to blunt chest trauma. Proximal dissection is usually associated with anterior pain, and distal dissection with back pain.[29] The pain may be, but is not necessarily, tearing in quality. It is usually migratory and occurs less commonly in the low back, epigastrium, midabdomen, or suprapubic areas. Proximal dissection is more frequent in younger patients, especially in association with Marfan's syndrome and cystic medial necrosis. Patients with distal dissection tend to be older and hypertensive. Physical examination of patients with proximal dissection may reveal the diastolic blowing murmur of aortic regurgitation, signs of pericardial tamponade, pulse deficits of the upper extremities, or signs of cerebral vascular accident or ischemic peripheral neuropathy. A pulsatile sternoclavicular joint is rarely seen. Associated or isolated distal dissection may present with lower extremity pulse deficits and signs of ischemia or infarction of the kidneys, spinal cord, mesentery, or peripheral nerves.

The electrocardiogram is nondiagnostic and may be normal, but usually reveals changes of left ventricular hypertrophy or nonspecific repolarization abnormalities. Signs of previous myocardial infarction may be present; rarely signs of acute myocardial infarction may be seen when a coronary artery has been compromised. Chest x-ray commonly displays an abnormally wide mediastinum or aortic contour and occasionally a left hemothorax caused by aortic bleeding. Intimal calcification separated from the outer aortic margin is a useful sign of distal dissection. M-mode echocardiographic findings of proximal dissection include widened aortic walls with parallel motion of the separated wall margins, a dilated aortic root, and possibly signs of pericardial effusion or diastolic fluttering of the anterior leaflet of the mitral valve if aortic regurgitation is present.[43] These findings, however, also occur in patients without dissection.[11] Distal dissection may be represented on two dimensional echocardiography as a dilated or double lumen descending thoracic aorta.[42] Definitive diagnosis reqires contrast aortography.[60] Management of proximal dissection requires surgical intervention. Dissections arising beyond the left subclavian artery, however, may be managed initially with hypotensive agents including sodium nitroprusside and propranolol, with subsequent surgery if there is vital organ compromise or impending rupture, or if medical therapy fails.[63]

CHEST PAIN OF INTRATHORACIC NONCARDIAC ORIGIN

Massive acute pulmonary embolism may cause acute pulmonary hypertension resulting in crushing central chest pain that resembles myocardial infarction. Submassive embolism may present with signs of pulmonary infarction with associated pleural inflammtion causing typical sharp chest pain exacerbated by inspiration. Symptoms commonly associated with pulmonary emboli are dyspnea, apprehension, cough, and hemoptysis. Physical examination may reveal tachycardia, tachypnea, fever, and increased intensity of the pulmonic component of the second heart sound. Less common are gallops, wheezing, diaphoresis, cyanosis, and signs of phlebitis.[55] Patients at high risk are those with a history of heart disease, thrombophlebitis, recent surgery, long periods of immobilization, chronic obstructive pulmonary disease, previous pulmonary embolus, malignancies, ingestion of oral contraceptives, or recent pregnancy. Except for arterial blood oxygen tension, laboratory studies are of little value. Significant pulmonary embolism is almost never associated with a Po_2 greater than 90 mm Hg, and in only 11.5 per cent of patients is it greater than 80 mm Hg.[55] Electrocardiographic abnormalities are common but nonspecific. Sinus tachycardia, T-wave inversion, and ST segment elevations and depressions are the most common, but none occurs in more than 50 per cent of patients. Right or left axis deviation, complete or incomplete right bundle branch block, $S_1S_2S_3$ or $S_1Q_3T_3$ patterns, premature atrial or ventricular depolarizations, P-pulmonale, right ventricular hypertrophy, and paroxysmal supraventricular arrhythmias may be seen but are nonspecific, with none occurring in more than 12 per cent of patients.[66] The electrocardiographic findings are transient and usually revert to normal within one to two weeks. Chest x-ray in persons with no previous pulmonary or cardiac disease may be very useful since signs of consolidation or diaphragmatic elevation are present in about 40 per cent of cases. Other roentgenographic findings include pleural effusion, pulmonary hilar engorgement, plate-like atelectasis, focal hyperlucency, and right or left ventricular enlargement.[55]

A normal four-view perfusion lung scan virtually excludes the diagnosis,[4] but a positive scan is relatively nonspecific. An abnormal perfusion scan in association with a normal ventilation scan or abnormal impedance phlebogram is much more specific for pulmonary embolism.[59] When the diagnosis remains in doubt, contrast pulmonary angiography may be necessary.[53] Patients with massive and submassive pulmonary emboli require immediate hospitalization and treatment with intravenous heparin or thrombolytic agents.[59] Pulmonary embolectomy is reserved for patients with cardiovascular collapse unresponsive to medical treatment.

Other intrathoracic causes of chest pain do not always require immediate hospitalization and treatment. Primary pulmonary hypertension and pulmonary hypertension caused by chronic lung or mitral valve disease are serious disorders that may cause chest pain but do not necessarily demand immediate hospitalization. Common viral upper respiratory infections may cause tracheobronchitis and anterior chest pain which is exacerbated by coughing. Inhalation of toxic substance such as ammonia, chlorine, polluted or superheated air, sulfur, or nitrous dioxide may cause similar symptoms.

Pleural inflammation causes severe stabbing chest pain which is aggravated by inspiration and coughing and is sometimes associated with pleural effusion on chest x-ray. Pleuritis may result from lobar pneumonia, pulmonary infarction, viral infection, pericarditis, primary or secondary neoplasms, connective tissue diseases, and infradiaphragmatic processes such as subphrenic abscess or pancreatitis.[36] A pleural friction rub is occasionally heard.

The sudden onset at rest of sharp lateralized pleuritic pain radiating to the shoulder or back associated with dyspnea in an otherwise healthy young person is characteristic of spontaneous pneumothorax.[30] Diagnosis is confirmed by chest x-ray. Complete resolution without specific therapy is the rule but a chest tube may be necessary in patients with significant respiratory compromise. Pneumomediastinum, which infrequently occurs with pneumothorax, more often occurs independently in healthy persons with transient acute airway obstruction caused by coughing, vomiting, bronchial asthma, Valsalva maneuver during parturition, or straining when lifting. Increased intra-alveolar pressure causes rupture of a peripheral alveolus and dissection of air into the mediastinum. The pain, substernal or precordial and radiating to the back, neck, and shoulders, is frequently associated with dyspnea.[44] Physical examination reveals a crunching sound over the precordium (Hamman's sign)[27] and subcutaneous crepitation in the neck, face, mouth, axilla, chest wall, abdominal wall, scrotum, or back. Air in the mediastinum and subcutaneous tissues is seen on the chest x-ray film. Resolution is usually spontaneous but decompression of subcutaneous tension may be necessary. Esophageal rupture (Boerhaave syndrome) and other forms of acute mediastinitis cause severe substernal chest pain. Chronic mediastinitis and mediastinal tumors[59] cause vague deep chest pain. These conditions are seldom suspected until mediastinal abnormalities are seen in the chest x-ray. Chest pain precipitated by ingestion of alcohol is characteristic of mediastinal Hodgkin's disease.

CHEST PAIN OF GASTROINTESTINAL ORIGIN

Substernal chest pain mimicking myocardial ischemic pain is commonly esophageal in origin. Esophageal pain may be caused by reflux esophagitis, disordered motility, progressive systemic sclerosis, neoplasm, or infection.[10, 19, 70] Typical "heartburn" type pain, pain worse while recumbent and relieved by antacids, and pain associated with dysphagia or regurgitation suggests the esophagus as the source.

Squeezing chest pain upon straining or lifting, which is relieved by nitroglycerin, may be caused by esophageal spasm or reflux, and yet mimic typical angina pectoris.[10, 47] Differential diagnosis is aided by several tests, none of which is definitive. A standard upper gastrointestinal series and esophagogram may reveal hiatus hernia and, occasionally, associated reflux. Although gross motility abnormalities such as achalasia will be diagnosed, other motility disorders can be documented only if the study is performed during an episode and recorded cinegraphically.[50] Other causes, such as peptic or gastric ulcer or malignant disease may be excluded.

An acid perfusion test (Bernstein test)[7] is helpful if pain is exactly reproduced, but results are often equivocal. Measurement of intraesophageal pH with indwelling probes can document reflux but is definitive only if typical pain occurs during a fall in pH, or if the pain is reproduced in the absence of a fall in pH thereby excluding reflux as the etiology.[64] Exclusion of reflux, however, does not exclude various motility disorders any of which may cause chest pain.[50] Esophageal manometric studies are diagnostic if pain occurs during the study. However, finding normal or abnormal motility in the absence of pain still leaves the diagnosis in doubt.[50] Ergonovine maleate may be used to provoke esophageal spasm in some patients.[33] Endoscopy may disclose candida esophagitis, neoplasms, strictures, chronic inflammatory changes, or ulcers but is of little value in diagnosing motility disorders.[73] Radioisotopic gastroesophageal scintiscanning, a new technique, may prove useful in detecting and quantifying esophageal reflux.[24]

Biliary colic and acute cholecystitis usually produce pain that is most severe in the right upper quadrant or epigastrum, but occasionally the pain may be predominantly substernal and mimic myocardial ischemia.[28] Disorders of intestinal motility may cause gaseous viscous distention;[35] if this occurs in the stomach, or in the hepatic or splenic flexures of the colon, pain may be referred to the adjacent chest (splenic flexure syndrome). The pain of acute pancreatitis may radiate to the epigastrium and substernal area. Electrocardiographic repolarization abnormalities may accompany acute pancreatitis and thus further complicate the diagnosis. Duodenal ulcer pain may radiate to the xyphoid, and gastric ulcers or tumors near the gastroesophageal junction may cause low substernal chest pain, but ulcers and tumors located more caudally rarely produce significant chest pain. Hepatic or splenic swelling or inflammation may cause capsular pain that radiates to the adjacent diaphragmatic pleura. Paraesophageal hernia is a rare disorder which may cause chest pain in the absence of reflux.

CHEST PAIN OF MUSCULOSKELETAL ORIGIN

Inflammation or trauma of the muscles, bones, cartilage, or joints of the thoracic cage is a frequent cause of chest pain. Rib fractures are not uncommon, especially in alcoholics, and are readily diagnosed by the history of trauma, presence of joint tenderness, localization of pain to the fracture site during manual chest compression and typical roentgeno-graphic findings.[36] Strains of the accessory thoracic muscles are common and the pain, which frequently radiates to the left shoulder or arm, may be exacerbated by movement or lifting, causing confusion with angina pectoris. Pain and tenderness of the costochondral cartilage is also quite common but should not be confused with Tietze's syndrome which is rare and requires true cartilaginous swelling for the diagnosis. While pain from these conditions can be quite severe and may gain the patient admission to the coronary care unit, specific maneuvers have been described which will reproduce and localize the cause of the pain as noncardiac.[20, 36] These patients, however, may occasionally be subjected to coronary angiography to clarify the diagnosis.[1] Intercostal muscle strain caused by persistent coughing, epidemic pleurodynia (Bornholm disease — coxsackie B), influenza, acute or chronic inflammation of the xyphoid process (xyphodynia),[62] and superficial phlebitis of the chest wall (Mondor's syndrome) may also cause chest pain. Still open to speculation is the etiology of the benign sharp stabbing pleuritic pain lasting seconds to minutes so frequently experienced by healthy young persons.

CHEST PAIN OF NEUROLOGIC AND FUNCTIONAL ORIGIN

Herpes zoster infection of the thoracic pleural nerves causes chest wall pain that is recognized by its distribution along one or more adjacent thoracic dermatomes, and the subsequent appearance, several days to three weeks later, of a vesicular rash in the distribution of the nerve. The pain is sharp and severe with a superficial burning quality. The pain usually resolves in weeks but in an unfortunate few may persist as post herpetic neuralgia.

Osteoarthritis of the cervical spine may cause nerve root compression with pain radiating down the arm and occasionally the anterior chest.[18] Patients may be concerned because of the common belief that left arm pain is cardiac in origin. The distribution of the pain and exacerbation with neck movement, coughing, or sneezing in association with narrowing of the vertebral foramina, noted on oblique roentgenographic views of the cervical spine, suggests the diagnosis.[74]

Compression of the nerves of the arm and anterior chest may also occur with thoracic outlet syndrome, scalenus anticus compression, or cervical ribs. Diagnosis is made when coexistent motor, sensory, and vascular deficits are present or can be elicited by upper extremity maneuvers which further compromise the nerves or blood vessels. Nerve compression also occurs when carcinoma of the superior aspect of the lung extends to involve the lower cords of the brachial plexus (Pancoast's syndrome). Other disorders that may cause chest pain include traumatic intercostal neuropathy and lesions of the thoracic vertebrae or spinal cord.

In some patients chest pain may be solely psychological in origin, but the physician should keep in mind that no psychological state, regardless of severity, affords immunity to the more serious etiologies of chest discomfort. Narcotic addicts may present with a complaint of chest pain to obtain drugs; however, chest pain may also be a manifestation of the withdrawal syndrome. De Costa's syndrome, soldier's heart, and neuro-circulatory asthenia are terms which have been used to describe patients with complaints of anxiety, palpitations, restlessness, and vague chest discomfort. With newer diagnostic techniques many of these patients are found to have specific organic disorders such as mitral valve prolapse.[74] These advances in diagnosis are helpful to the clinician, but it would certainly be presumptuous for modern medicine to assume that all causes of human chest pain have already been identified.

REFERENCES

1. Amsterdam, E. A., Lee, G., De Maria, A. N., et al.: Prognosis in patients with chest pain and normal coronary arteries: Absence of cardiac mortality and morbidity. Circulation, 56(Suppl. 3):34, 1977.
2. Aroesty, J. M., Weintraub, R. M., Paulin, S., et al.: Medically refractory unstable angina pectoris II. Hemodynamic and angiographic effects of intraaortic balloon counterpulsation. Amer. J. Cardiol., 43:883–888, 1979.
3. Bailey, I. K., Griffith, L. S. C., Rouleau, J., et al.: Thallium — 201 myocardial perfusion imaging at rest and during exercise. Comparative sensitivity to electrocardiography in coronary artery disease. Circulation, 55:79–87, 1977.
4. Bell, W. R., and Simon T. L.: A comparative analysis of pulmonary perfusion scans with pulmonary angiograms, Amer. Heart J., 92:700–706, 1976.
5. Benjamin, S. P., McCormack, L. J., Effler, D. B., et al.: Primary tumors of the mediastinum. Chest, 62:297–303, 1972.
6. Bennett, J. R., and Hendrix, T. R.: Diffuse esophageal spasm: A disorder with more than one cause. Gastroenterology, 59:273–279, 1970.
7. Bernstein, L. M., and Baker, L. A.: A clinical test for esophagitis. Gastroenterology, 34:760–781, 1958.
8. Borer, J. S., Kent, K. M., Bacharach, S. L., et al.: Sensitivity, specificity and predictive accuracy of radionuclide cineangiography during exercise in patients with coronary artery disease: comparison with exercise electrocardiography. Circulation, 60:572–580, 1979.
9. Bradley, R. F., and Schonfeld, A.: Diminished pain in diabetic patients with acute myocardial infarction. Geriatrics, 17:322–326, 1962.
10. Brand, D. L., Martin, D., and Pope, C. E.: Esophageal manometrics in patients with angina-like chest pain. Amer. J. Dig. Dis., 22:300–304, 1977.
11. Brown, O. W., Popp, R. L., and Kloster, F. E.: Echocardiographic criteria for aortic root dissection. Amer. J. Cardiol., 36:17–20, 1975.
12. Bulkley, B. H., Klacsmann, P. G., and Hutchins, G. M.: Angina pectoris, myocardial infarction and sudden cardiac death with normal coronary arteries: a clinicopathologic study of 9 patients with progressive systemic sclerosis. Amer. Heart J., 95:563–569, 1978.
13. Canedo, M. I., Frank, M. J., and Abdulla, A. M.: Rhythm disturbances in hypertrophic cardiomyopathy: prevalence, relation to symptoms and management. Amer. J. Cardiol., 45:848–855, 1980.
14. Chapman, I.: The cause-effect relationship between recent coronary artery occlusion and acute myocardial infarction. Amer. Heart J., 87:267–271, 1974.
15. Cohen, L. S., and Braunwald, E.: Amelioration of angina pectoris in idiopathic hypertrophic subaortic stenosis with beta-adrenergic blockade. Circulation, 35:847–851, 1967.
16. Cohn, P. F.: Silent myocardial ischemia in patients with a defective anginal warning system. Amer. J. Cardiol., 45:697–702, 1980.
17. Connolly, J. E., Eldridge, F. L., Calvin, J. W., et al.: Proximal coronary artery obstruction. New Eng. J. Med., 271:213–219, 1964.
18. Davis, D., and Ritvo, M.: Osteoarthritis of the cervicodorsal spine (radiculitis) simulating coronary-artery disease. Clinical and roentgenologic findings. New Eng. J. Med., 238:857–866, 1948.

19. Dodds, W. J., Hogan, W. J., and Miller, W. N.: Reflux esophagitis. Amer. J. Dig. Dis., 21:49–67, 1976.
20. Epstein, S. E., Gerber, L. H., and Borer, J. S.: Chest wall syndrome. A common cause of unexplained cardiac pain. J.A.M.A., 241:2793–2797, 1979.
21. Feigenbaum, H.: Echocardiography. Philadelphia, Lea & Febiger, 2nd ed., 1976.
22. Feldman, R. L., Nichols, W. W., Pepine, C. J., et al.: Influence of aortic insufficiency on the hemodynamic significance of a coronary artery narrowing. Circulation, 60:259–268, 1979.
23. Fischl, S. J., Herman, M. V., and Gorlin, R.: The intermediate coronary syndrome —clinical, angiographic and therapeutic aspects. New Eng. J. Med., 288:1193–1198, 1973.
24. Fisher, R. S., Malmud, L. S., Roberts, G. S., et al.: Gastroesophageal (GE) scintiscanning to detect and quantitate GE reflux. Gastroenterology, 70:301–308, 1976.
25. Goldberg, A., Reichek, N., Wilson, J., et al.: Nifedipine in the treatment of Prinzmetal's (Variant) Angina. Amer. J. Cardiol., 44:804–810, 1979.
26. Gorlin, R.: Pathophysiology of cardiac pain. Circulation, 32:138–148, 1965.
27. Green, J. A.: Unusual sounds emanating from the chest. Arch. Intern. Med., 71:410–414, 1943.
28. Gunn, A., and Keddie, N.: Some clinical observations on patients with gallstones. Lancet, 2:239–241, 1972.
29. Heberden, W.: Commentarii de Morborum, Historia et Curatione. A. Londini, T. Payne, 1802.
30. Hyde, L.: Benign spontaneous pneumothorax. Ann. Intern. Med., 56:746–751, 1962.
31. Jeresaty, R. M.: Mitral valve prolapse — click syndrome. Prog. Cardiovas. Dis., 15(6):623–652, 1973.
32. Khan, A. H., and Haywood, L. J.: Myocardial infarction in nine patients with radiologically patent coronary arteries. New Eng. J. Med., 291:427–431, 1974.
33. Koch, K., Carlson, G., Long, A., et al.: The ergonovine stress test: a provocative test for diffuse esophageal spasm or variant angina? Clin. Res., 28(2):279A, 1980.
34. Lange, R. L., Reid, M. S., Tresch, D. D., et al.: Nonatheromatous ischemic heart disease following withdrawal from chronic industrial nitroglycerin exposure. Circulation, 46:666–678, 1972.
35. Lasser, R. B., Bond, J. H., and Levitt, M. D.: The role of intestinal gas in functional abdominal pain. New Eng. J. Med., 293:524–526, 1975.
36. Levene, D. L.: Chest Pain: An Integrated Diagnostic Approach. Philadelphia, Lea & Febiger, 1977.
37. Markiewicz, W., Stoner, J., London, E., et al.: Mitral valve prolapse in one hundred presumably healthy young females. Circulation, 53:464–473, 1976.
38. Maseri, A., L'Abbate, A., Baroldi, G., et al.: Coronary vasospasm as a possible cause of myocardial infarction. A conclusion derived from the study of "preinfarction" angina. New Eng. J. Med., 299:1271–1277, 1978.
39. Maseri, A., Parodi, O., Severi, S., et al.: Transient transmural reduction of myocardial blood flow, demonstrated by thallium-201 scintigraphy, as a cause of variant angina. Circulation, 54:280–288, 1976.
40. Maseri, A., Silva, S., Maurizio, D. N., et al.: "Variant" angina: one aspect of a continuous spectrum of vasospastic myocardial ischemia. Amer. J. Cardiol., 42:1019–1035, 1978.
41. Mills, P., Rose, J., Hollingsworth, J., et al.: Long-term prognosis of mitral-valve prolapse. New Eng. J. Med., 297:13–18, 1977.
42. Mintz, G. S., Kotler, M. N., Segal, B. L., et al.: Two dimensional echocardiographic recognition of the descending thoracic aorta. Amer. J. Cardiol., 44:232–238, 1979.
43. Moothart, R. W., Spangler, R. D., and Blount, S. G.: Echocardiography in aortic root dissection and dilatation. Amer. J. Cardiol., 36:11–16, 1975.
44. Munsell, W. P.: Pneumomediastinum. A report of 28 cases and review of the literature. J.A.M.A., 202:689–693, 1967.
45. Oliva, P. B., and Breckinridge, J. C.: Arteriographic evidence of coronary arterial spasm in acute myocardial infarction. Circulation, 56:366–374, 1977.
46. Oliva, P. B., Potts, D. E., and Pluss, R. G.: Coronary arterial spasm in Prinzmetal angina — documentation by coronary arteriography. New Eng. J. Med., 288:745–751, 1973.
47. Orlando, R. C., and Bozymski, E. M.: Clinical and manometric effects of nitroglycerin in diffuse esophageal spasm. New Eng. J. Med., 289:23–25, 1973.
48. Paquay, P. A., Anderson, G., Diefenthal, H., et al.: Chest pain as a predictor of coronary artery disease in patients with obstructive aortic valve disease. Amer. J. Cardiol., 38:863–869, 1976.
49. Parodi, O., Maseri, A., and Simonetti, I.: Management of unstable angina at rest by verapamil. A double-blind cross-over study in coronary care unit. Brit. Heart J., 41:167–174, 1979.

50. Pope, C. E.: Esophageal function tests in the differential diagnosis of chest pain. *In* Chest Pain: Diagnostic Testing. 1980, pp. 15–21.

51. Prinzmetal, M., Kennamer, R., Merliss, R., et al.: Angina pectoris I. A variant form of angina pectoris: Preliminary report. Amer. J. Med., 27:375–388, 1959.

52. Reddy, P. S., Curtiss, E. I., O'Toole, J. D., et al.: Cardiac tamponade: hemodynamic observations in man. Circulation, 58:265–272, 1978.

53. Robin, E. D.: Overdiagnosis and overtreatment of pulmonary embolism: The emperor may have no clothes. Ann. Intern. Med., 87:775–781, 1977.

54. Rosing, D. R., Kent, K. M., Maron, B. J., et al.: Verapamil therapy: A new approach to the pharmacologic treatment of hypertrophic cardiomyopathy. Circulation, 60:1208–1213, 1979.

55. Sasahara, A. A.: Current problems in pulmonary embolism: Introduction. Progr. Cardiovasc. Dis., 17(3):161–165, 1974.

56. Schang, S. J. Jr., and Pepine, C. J.: Transient asymptomatic ST segment depression during daily activity. Amer. J. Cardiol., 39:396–402, 1977.

57. Scharf, S. M., Thames, M. D., and Sargent, R. K.: Transmural myocardial infarction after exposure to carbon monoxide in coronary artery disease. New Eng. J. Med., 291:85–86, 1974.

58. Selzer, A., Langston, M., Ruggeroli, C., et al.: Clinical syndrome of variant angina with normal coronary arteriogram. New Eng. J. Med., 295:1343–1347, 1976.

59. Sharma, G. V., and Sasahara, A. A.: Diagnosis and treatment of pulmonary embolism. Med. Clin. N. Amer., 63:239–250, 1979.

60. Shuford, W. H., Sybers, R. G., and Weens, H. S.: Problems in the aortographic diagnosis of dissecting aneurysm of the aorta. New Eng. J. Med., 280:225–231, 1969.

61. Silver, M. D., Baroldi, G., and Mariani, F.: The relationship between acute occlusive coronary thrombi and myocardial infarction studied in 100 consecutive patients. Circulation, 61:219–227, 1980.

62. Sklaroff, H. J.: Xiphodynia — another cause of atypical chest pain: six case reports. Mt. Sinai J. Med., 46:546–548, 1979.

63. Slater, E. E., and De Sanctis, R. W.: Dissection of the aorta. Med. Clin. N. Amer., 63:141–154, 1979.

64. Slater, E. E., and De Sanctis, R. W.: The clinical recognition of dissecting aortic aneurysm. Amer. J. Med., 60:625–633, 1976.

65. Spodick, D. H.: Differential characteristics of the electrocardiogram in early repolarization and acute pericarditis. New Engl. J. Med., 295:523–526, 1976.

66. Stein, P. D., Dalen, J. E., McIntyre, K. M., et al.: The electrocardiogram in acute pulmonary embolism. Progr. Cardiovasc. Dis., 17(4):247–257, 1975.

67. Swartz, M. H., Herman, M. V., and Teichholz, L. E.: Dermatoglyphic patterns in patients with mitral valve prolapse: A clue to pathogenesis. Amer. J. Cardiol., 38:588–593, 1976.

68. Tavel, M. E.: Clinical Phonocardiography and External Pulse Recording. Chicago, Year Book Medical Publishers, Inc., 3rd ed., 1978.

69. Uretsky, B. F., Farquhar, D. S., Berezin, A. F., et al.: Symptomatic myocardial infarction without chest pain: prevalence and clinical course. Amer. J. Cardiol. 40:498–503, 1977.

70. Vantrappen, G., Janssens, J., Hellemans, J., et al.: Achalasia, diffuse esophageal spasm and related motility disorders. Gastroenterology, 76:450–457, 1979.

71. Vokonas, P. S., Cohn, P. F., Klein,M. D., et al.: Hemoglobin affinity for oxygen in the anginal syndrome with normal coronary arteriograms. J. Clin. Invest., 54:409–415, 1974.

72. Weintraub, R. M., Aroesty, J. M., Paulin, S., et al.: Medically refractory unstable angina pectoris I. Long-term follow up of patients undergoing intraaortic balloon counterpulsation and operation. Amer. J. Cardiol., 43:877–882, 1979.

73. Winans, C. S.: The role of endoscopy in the diagnosis of esophageal pain. *In* Chest Pain: Diagnostic Testing. 1980, pp.27–33.

74. Wooley, C. F.: Where are the diseases of yesteryear? Da Costa's syndrome, soldiers heart, the effort syndrome, neurocirculatory asthenia and the mitral valve prolapse syndrome. Circulation, 53:749–751,1976.

75. Yasue, H., Omote, S., Takizawa, A., et al.: Exertional angina pectoris caused by coronary arterial spasm: effects of various drugs. Amer. J. Cardiol., 43:647–652, 1979.

City Hospital Center at Elmhurst
79–01 Broadway
Elmhurst, New York 11373

Cardiac Procedures in Acute Care Situations

Gerald F. Fletcher, M.D.,* and Patrick Murphy, M.D.†

Acute care situations today involve many areas of patient care: the emergency setting in the "field" (mobile intensive care units, stadiums, shopping malls, restaurants), hospital emergency rooms, intensive care units, operating and recovery rooms, and in the diagnostic or ambulatory areas of hospitals where emergency or "Code 99" teams are activated for management of cardiopulmonary arrest. Of late, other areas have evolved as settings for acute cardiac care — namely, exercise and cardiac catheterization laboratories and cardiac exercise rehabilitation programs. Patients in any of these areas may have problems that justify the use of certain cardiac procedures.

Cardiac procedures discussed here will include electrical cardioversion (defibrillation), intravenous insertion of Swan-Ganz catheter, intravenous insertion of a pacemaker for control of bradycardia (usually complete atrioventricular block), pericardiocentesis, and intra-aortic counterpulsation. Central venous pressure monitoring, titration of specific drugs such as nitroprusside and dopamine, and other specific pharmacological interventions will not be discussed.

At the onset it is important to emphasize that specific cardiac procedures should be utilized judiciously, only after proper subjective and objective assessment. Data are often limited in the acute setting; however, such assessment of need is important in order to avoid loss of time, patient discomfort, and needless cost. The reader should consider these points as the procedures are discussed.

ELECTRICAL CARDIOVERSION

Direct current cardioversion (DCC) has assumed a prominent role in the therapy of a wide range of atrial and ventricular arrhythmias. Since its introduction in 1962 by Lown,[24] it has been used both independently

---

*Director of Internal Medicine, Georgia Baptist Medical Center, and Professor in Medicine (Cardiology) Emory University School of Medicine
†Fellow in Medicine (Cardiology) Emory University School of Medicine

and in conjunction with pharmacologic antiarrhythmic intervention. Of the two basic mechanisms of arrhythmogenesis, DCC is most effective against those caused by continuous circuit re-entry phenomena. These include atrial fibrillation, atrial flutter, paroxysmal supraventricular tachycardia, ventricular tachycardia, or ventricular fibrillation.

The mechanism of action of DCC is thought to be interruption of the continuous circuit re-entry pathways, thereby allowing the patient's own intrinsic sinus mechanism to become manifest.

Indications for direct current cardioversion include rapid atrial tachyarrhythmias causing hemodynamic compromise (atrial fibrillation with a rapid ventricular response, atrial flutter with 1:1 or 2:1 conduction, paroxysmal supraventricular tachycardia with rapid rate); ventricular tachycardia; or ventricular fibrillation.

This section will deal with the use of emergency DCC for supraventricular tachyarrhythmias resulting in hemodynamic compromise and for life-threatening ventricular arrhythmias. In the case of the former, the patients are often conscious and well oriented despite hemodynamic impairment. To use DCC in such patients without sedation or limited anesthesia is not warranted; therefore, "elective" cardioversion will be discussed in this context.

Methods

Emergency DCC for sustained ventricular tachycardia and ventricular fibrillation should be done as quickly as possible. One electrode is placed in the second right intercostal space and the other in the fifth intercostal space in the left mid axillary line. Electrode paste should be used to lower electrical impedance. An anteroposterior paddle apparatus is preferable to the above if available, because the energy requirement may be reduced by as much as 50 per cent.[25] A charge of 200 to 400 watt/seconds should be delivered and repeated if not initially successful.

Elective cardioversion as described by Lown[24] and Resnekov[31] requires an oscilloscopic display of the electrocardiogram circuitry to synchronize the electrical shock and the patient's QRS complex, an electrocardiographic recording for arrhythmias (usually on lead V_2), and a capacitor capable of delivering shocks up to 400 watt/seconds. Ideally, the clinician should work in conjunction with an anesthesiologist during the procedure. An intravenous infusion is advantageous for administration of the anesthetic.

Prior to the actual cardioversion, the synchronizer (to time electrical shock away from points of cardiac vulnerability, i.e. the T wave) should be tested. If this is functioning appropriately, the patient should then receive either a short-acting barbiturate (pentothal or brevital) or diazepam, 5 to 10 mg, given intravenously as the amnestic drug. The paddles are then positioned as described above for emergency DCC. After a brief period of hyperventilation with face mask for oxygen supplementation, the electrical shock should be applied.

The amount of current the clinician chooses to deliver will vary depending on the specific arrhythmias being treated, the patient's hemodynamic status, and body size.[8] Usually, DCC for supraventricular arrhythmias should begin at 50 to 100 watt/seconds, and increased in increments of 50 watt/seconds until conversion or a level of 400 watt/seconds is reached.

Comments

In most reviews, the immediate results of DCC are excellent. Sinus rhythm can be obtained after cardioversion in approximately 85 per cent of patients with atrial fibrillation,[31] and in about 95 per cent of patients with atrial flutter, paroxysmal supraventricular tachycardia, and ventricular tachycardia.[29] DC cardioversion has greatly enhanced our ability to effectively treat hemodynamically significant and life-threatening atrial and ventricular arrhythmias.

Complications

Although very few complications follow DCC, several must be addressed. Most of the rhythm disturbances encountered post cardioversion are secondary to enhanced vagal tone (due to thoracic parasympathetic stimulation with the electrical shock). This enhanced vagal activity may manifest as transient sino-atrial block or even atrioventricular block. Atropine may be used if the above persists.[25]

Sinus arrest is occasionally seen post cardioversion, especially in patients with undetected sinus node dysfunction. Atropine or isoproterenol should be administered, and if no response is elicited, a temporary transvenous pacemaker should be inserted.

SWAN-GANZ CATHETER HEMODYNAMIC MONITORING

The role of the cadiac care unit includes prevention and treatment of arrhythmias associated with myocardial infarction as well as chronic rhythm disturbances. In addition, the current cardiac intensive care approach to treatment of accute myocardial infarction attempts to prevent or detect and effectively treat the mechanical and electrical sequelae of regional myocardial ischemia or infarction. Another evolving concept involves aggressive approaches of preserving jeopardized ischemic myocardium.[23, 19]

In the past decade, hemodynamic monitoring has evolved to widespread clinical use.[34, 40] The development of this system has provided a new and important source of physiologic and pathophysiologic information aiding the clinician in assessing an acutely ill patient, his prognosis, and certain therapeutic manipulations.

Indications for hemodynamic monitoring include (1) assessment of ventricular function (both right and left); (2) determination of hemodynamic prognostic indices (hemodynamic subsets) (discussed later); (3) monitoring physiologic changes during the acute phase of myocardial infarction; (4) assessment of both beneficial and detrimental effect of pharmacological intervention in acute myocardial infarction; and (5) assessment of new interventions and methods which may salvage ischemic myocardial tissue and reduce the size of the infarction.[12, 34, 35]

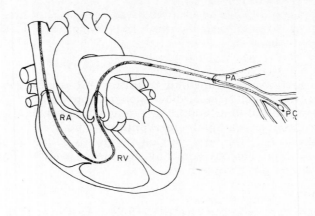

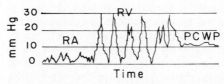

Figure 1. *Above*, Artist's representation of Swan-Ganz catheter balloon tip in pulmonary capillary wedge position (PC). RA, right atrium; RV, right ventricle; PA, pulmonary artery.

    Below, Simulated representative pressure tracing for consecutive chambers for various catheter positions. RA, right atrium; RV, right ventricle, PCWP, pulmonary capillary wedge pressure.

Methods

The Swan-Ganz catheter may be introduced into the venous system by an antecubital, subclavian, femoral, or jugular vein. Once the catheter has been introduced (by any of the above approaches — usually antecubital or subclavian veins), it is advanced into the superior vena cava.

The balloon is then inflated and the catheter advanced sequentially through the right atrium, the right ventricle, and the pulmonary artery while the appropriate contours appear on the monitoring oscilloscope (Fig. 1). In 10 to 15 per cent of the patients with severely reduced cardiac output, venous return may be insufficient to "float" the catheter into the pulmonary arterial system. In such cases, fluoroscopy may be needed to optimally position the catheter.

Comments

Acute myocardial infarction cannot be viewed as a single functional entity, rather a serious of hemodynamic subsets.[12] Forrester and associates have devised the concept of clinical subsets based on pulmonary congestion (as a consequence of increased pulmonary capillary wedge pressure, PCWP) and peripheral hypotension (as a manifestation of a depressed cardiac index, CI). Table 1 relates the therapeutic effects relative to the clinical and hemodynamic subsets.[34, 35]

Specific therapeutic modalities (Table 2) may be instituted once a patient's hemodynamic status has been assessed. The use of hemodynamic assessment has led to substantial short-term improvement of patients post infarction. However, there are as yet no conclusive data indicating that any therapeutic intervention reduces infarct size or results in improved long-term survival.[12] As therapeutic nuances emerge and/or earlier surgical intervention is utilized, the hemodynamic assessment of patients after myocardial infarction may reduce acute morbidity and possibly increase long-term survival by optimizing ventricular performance and limiting infarct size.

Complications

1. If a peripheral vein is used for insertion, venospasm is occasionally a problem. (Injection of a local anesthetic with dilute solutions of lidocaine may relieve the venospasm.)

2. The subclavian and internal jugular approaches have inherent potential complications: pneumothorax, hemothorax, subclavian artery laceration associated with the subclavian approach, and laceration to the common carotid artery and injury of the recurrent laryngeal nerve associated with the internal jugular approach.[12]

3. Ventricular ectopy may be induced while the catheter with the balloon inflated traverses the right ventricle.

4. The catheter may lodge in the wedged position because of distal migration of the tip during continuous monitoring. (This can be documented by fluoroscopy or routine portable chest x-ray examination). The catheter may then be withdrawn by 1 to 2 cm increments until the characteristic pulmonary arterial contour appears.

5. Repeated wedge determinations via balloon inflation during extended periods of monitoring may cause pulmonary infarction. Also, excessive inflation of the balloon can result in balloon fracture. (In the absence of mitral stenosis or pulmonary hypertension, the pulmonary

Table 1. *Clinical and Hemodynamic Subsets of Acute Myocardial Infarction*

CLINICAL SUBSETS

Class 1. No pulmonary congestion or peripheral hypoperfusion.
Class 2. Pulmonary congestion without hypoperfusion.
Class 3. Peripheral hypoperfusion without congestion.
Class 4. Both pulmonary congestion and peripheral hypoperfusion.

HEMODYNAMIC SUBSETS

H1: PCWP $\leq$ 18 mm Hg
    CI $>$ 2.2 L/min/m^2
H2: PCWP $>$ 18 mm Hg
    CI $>$ 2.2 L/min/m^2

H3: PCWP $\leq$ 18 mm Hg
    CI $\leq$ 2.2 L/min/m^2
H4: PCWP $>$ 18 mm Hg
    CI $\leq$ 2.2 L/min/m^2

Table 2. *Clinical and Hemodynamic Subsets of Swan-Ganz Monitoring with Therapeutic Correlations*[34,35]

CI	PCWP	AP	CLINICAL SUBSET	HEMODYNAMIC SUBSET	THERAPY	EFFECTS OF THERAPY		
						CI	PCWP	AP
5.2	13	135	Hyperfunction	–	Propranolol	3.8	12	120
2.4	12	92	Normal	H I	Conservative	2.9	4	84
2.8	23	120	LV failure	H II	Nitroprusside	2.8	12	100
1.5	26	72	Shock	H IV	IACP, nitroprusside Dopamine, dobutamine	2.3	18	67
1.5	6	79	Hypovolemia	H III	Volume replacement	1.9	15	85

Abbreviations: CI, Cardiac index in L/min/m²
AP, Arterial pressure (systolic)
H, Refers to hemodynamic subset noted in text
LV, Left ventricular
IACP, Intra-aortic counterpulsation
PCWP, Pulmonary capillary wedge pressure

artery end diastolic pressure may be used instead of the pulmonary capillary wedge pressure as a reflection of left ventricular end diastolic pressure with less risk to the patient.)

TEMPORARY TRANSVENOUS PACEMAKERS

Electrostimulation of the heart has progressed to treatment of a variety of cardiac arrhythmias and conduction abnormalities. Often such electrical abnormalities occur in the presence of a myocardium that is otherwise quite normal. Therefore, urgent and appropriate application of pacing techniques in such acute care settings must be available and the clinician must be alert to the indications and capabilities of the techniques.

Indications

A partial list of the indications for temporary pacing is outlined in Table 3. The optimal use of pacemakers for rhythm control depends on the site of the origin of the arrhythmias, the status of atrioventricular

Table 3. *Indications for Temporary Pacing in Acute Care Settings*

I. Hemodynamically compromising arrhythmias
   A. Sinus node dysfunction[28, 32, 7]
      1. Bradycardia-tachycardia syndrome
      2. Sinus arrest
      3. Sinus bradycardia (profound)
   B. Supraventricular arrhythmias[11]
      1. Override pacing in atrial flutter and paroxysmal atrial tachycardia
      2. Atrial fibrillation with slow ventricular response
   C. Disturbance of atrioventricular conduction[27]
      1. Acquired third degree heart block and symptomatic second degree heart block
      2. Pre-excitation syndrome with rapid supraventricular tachyarrhythmias[11]

II. Prophylaxis for standby emergency
   A. Arrhythmias associated with acute myocardial infarction[5, 30, 15]
      1. Symptomatic bradycardia, sinoatrial block, and sick sinus syndrome
      2. Drug-resistant tachyarrhythmias
      3. Right bundle branch block with either left anterior fascicular block or left posterior fascicular block
      4. Acute onset of Mobitz II second degree arterioventricular block with anterior myocardial infarction
   B. Arrhythmias associated with cardiac catheterization[20]
   C. In surgery[18]
   D. Miscellaneous
      1. Threatened bradycardia in drug trial for tachycardia treatment[9]
      2. Digitalization with failure of arterioventricular conduction and resultant bradycardia[26]
      3. Prior to therapy for tachyarrhythmias with concomitant heart block or fascicular block

III. Malfunction of implanted pacemaker[13]

IV. Postoperative control of rhythm and cardiac output after open heart surgery[16] conduction, the presence or absence of hemodynamic compromise, and concomitant effects of electrolytes and drugs on cardiac conduction. For the purposes of this discussion, we will concentrate on the use of endocardial right ventricular pacing, which is by far the most often utilized of the pacing techniques in acute care.

Methods

The pacing electrode for temporary atrial or ventricular pacing may be inserted by a number of techniques. The choice of a particular technique depends on the expertise of the clinician performing the procedure.

The majority of temporary right ventricular pacing is accomplished by transvenous endocardial stimulation.[9] The transvenous routes most commonly used are the subclavian, supraclavicular, jugular (both internal and external), femoral, and brachial. Cutdown approaches utilizing the brachial vein are rarely used, as the catheter may be displaced secondary to arm movement.

The subclavian approach[9,33] is most commonly used today. This is best accomplished by placing the patient in slight Trendelenberg position (to increase filling of the major superior veins). The patient's face should be rotated away from the side of the puncture and a soft towel placed under the patient's scapula with the neck in slight hyperextension.

Aseptic technique is used to prepare the skin. Local anesthetic is applied subcutaneously and along the path to be taken by the venous puncture needle. Direct needle puncture using an external plastic sheath or positioning of a plastic introducer sheath via the Seldinger technique may be used. The needle is inserted at the junction of the proximal and middle thirds of the clavicle and directed infraclavicularly toward the jugular notch (the triangle formed by the sternal and clavicular heads of the sternocleidomastoid muscle).

As the needle is advanced, slight negative pressure should be kept on the syringe plunger. The needle/sheath apparatus should enter the subclavian vein shortly after clearing the clavicle. The syringe and needle can then be removed, leaving the plastic sheath in the lumen of the subclavian vein. The pacing electrode catheter can then be inserted. Three basic types of pacing electrodes are available: nondisposable, bipolar disposable, and semifloating with balloon assist.[6]

If inserted under fluoroscopic control, the catheter may be observed as it passes through the superior vena cava, right atrium, and right ventricle. Optimal positioning in the apex of the right ventricle can thus be accomplished. If portable fluoroscopy is not available or the patient is unable to be transported to remote fluoroscopy, the catheter may be positoned at the bedside utilizing electrocardiographic control.

In this latter technique, the pacing catheter is connected to the V lead of a well grounded EKG machine and the pacing catheter advanced while observing the configuration of the P wave and QRS complex. Upon entering the right atrium, two large atrial complexes will be observed. The pacing catheter is advanced through the tricuspid valve into the right ventricle. Here the EKG will show a decreasing amplitude of the P wave and a large amplitude QRS complex once the right ventricle has been entered.

The electrical thresholds to pacing and sensing are then determined immediately after positioning of the pacing catheter. For optimum temporary pacing, the pacing threshold should be below 1.0 milliamp, preferably 0.6 milliamp. Usually for continuous maintenance pacing, the output is left at 5.0 milliamp.

A myocardial signal of at least twice the triggering requirement of the pulse generator should be available for demand pacing. If either the sensing or pacing threshold is too high for effective function, the catheter should be repositioned. The desired rate is then set and the catheter secured by suture at its skin insertion site.

Complications

The risk of the subclavian approach includes subclavian artery puncture, pneumothorax, laceration of the subclavian vein with hemothorax, air embolus, and venous thrombosis. Once the transvenous pacing catheter is inserted, malplacement (e.g., coronary sinus instead of right ventricular pacing), malposition (i.e., apex versus outflow tract of right ventricle) may be encountered.

PERICARDIOCENTESIS

Needle aspiration of the pericardial space has diagnostic and therapeutic usefulness. However, the procedure still remains somewhat controversial. In the acute care situation, pericardiocentesis is utilized to relieve acute cardiac tamponade.

Controversy surrounds the selection of the direct surgical approach versus "blind" needle aspiration. The indirect method has the obvious advantages of immediate bedside use without transfer of the patient to the operating room. The direct surgical approach has the advantages of direct visualization of the pericardium and epicardium, thus avoiding most of the complications of the indirect method (as outlined later).

For the purposes of this discussion, only the indirect procedure will be addressed. Assuming that the clinician has made the diagnosis of acute cardiac tamponade in a hemodynamically compromised patient, minutes count and time is of the essence. A delay may result in death and immediate intervention may be lifesaving.

Method

Indirect needle aspiration of the pericardial space is a major procedure, preferably performed by a physician with expertise in its accomplishment. The patient should be optimally positioned at 60 degrees elevation from the horizontal and the needle inserted via one of the two approaches using standard techniques.[3, 37]

The first method involves insertion of the needle near the cardiac apex, approximately 1 cm inside the left border of cardiac dullness. The needle is then directed toward the fourth dorsal vertabra.

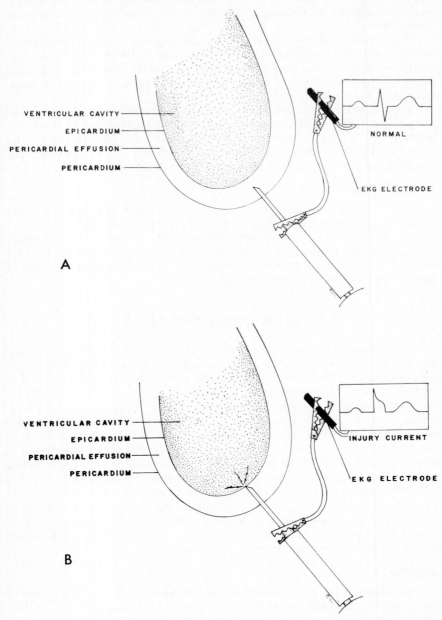

Figure 2.   A, Artist's representation of needle in proper position in pericardial space for aspiration of fluid. Electrocardiographic S-T segments are normal as recorded by monitoring V lead electrode.

B, Artist's representation of needle in contact with epicardium causing "injury current" (S-T segment elevation) on electrocardiogram recorded through monitoring electrode.

The second method (favored by more), utilizes the subxiphoid approach. With aseptic technique, a 16 to 18 gauge intracatheter is inserted in the angle between the left costal margin of the xiphoid and directed toward the right shoulder. Prior to advancement of the needle, sterile alligator clamps should be attached to the base of the needle and the EKG chest lead electrode. This allows for continuous monitoring of the procedure (Fig. 2 displays the technique for safe electrocardigraphic monitoring).

The needle is then advanced slowly, while slight negative pressure is applied to an attached syringe. Once the pericardial space has been entered and pericardial fluid obtained, the needle is withdrawn, leaving the polyurethane catheter in place for aspiration. Pericardial fluid is withdrawn until the patient's hemodynamically unstable state has been reversed or until fluid can no longer be aspirated.

If grossly bloody fluid is obtained, an immediate hematocrit of the fluid should be compared with the patient's venous blood hematocrit to be certain that the needle is not in one of the cardiac chambers. Also, failure of the blood to clot offers further assurance that the bloody fluid was not obtained from a cardiac chamber.

While advancing the needle, if the recording electrocardiogram (usually utilizing V_1) shows an abrupt acute injury pattern of ST segment elevation, the needle should be withdrawn since this probably indicates epimyocardial puncture (Fig. 2). The physician should then retract the needle apparatus 1 to 2 cm, reassess his anatomic landmarks, then proceed again with a slightly more medial approach directed toward the right shoulder.

Comments

Occasionally, recurrent cardiac tamponade or a very large pericardial effusion requires repeated aspirations and the patient must be considered for pericardiotomy or pericardiectomy. However, in severely ill patients, repeated pericardiocentesis or surgical intervention requiring general anesthesia may lead to increased morbidity and mortality. In general, the technique is quite effective initially in relieving tamponade and is often lifesaving.

Complications

Mortality and morbidity associated with indirect, percutaneous pericardiocentesis remain low, but may be underestimated in frequency.[21] Even in experienced hands, clinicians who utilize the indirect method can expect, sooner or later, to perforate or tear an atrial or a ventricular wall, or lacerate a coronary artery. For the above reasons, a thoracic surgery team should be readily available in the event one of the above life-threatening complications occur.

INTRA-AORTIC COUNTERPULSATION

Intra-aortic balloon (AB) counterpulsation (IACP) has been established both in the experimental laboratory and clinically as an effective means of supplying assistance to the compromised myocardium.[1] IACP is thought to exhibit its beneficial effects by augmenting diastolic blood pressure and reducing left ventricular ejection impedance, thereby enhancing coronary flow and reducing cardiac work. Thus, the ratio of myocardial oxygen supply to demand is favorably affected.[4, 41, 44]

Indications

1. Post infarction angina and cardiogenic shock.
2. "Weaning" patients from cardiopulmonary bypass.
3. Post cardiotomy low cardiac output state.
4. Preoperative support in the presence of severe left ventricular dysfunction.
5. Management of recurrent life-threatening arrhythmias associated with low cardiac output states.
6. Experimentally and clinically to reduce infarct size.

Only those indications associated with states of potentially reversible myocardial decompensation will be addressed in this section.

Methods

One of the major disadvantages of most currently used AB systems is that they must be inserted by surgical cutdown. Usually, the patient is taken to the operating room where the common femoral artery is isolated and a vascular graft or other prosthesis is attached. The techniques of surgical cutdown for balloon insertion results in considerable delay in the application of IACP very early in situations in which it is indicated.

Bergman and Casanella[2] and Subrammian[38] have recently described their experience with percutaneous AB placement. This technique utilizes the Seldinger technique for percutaneous femoral artery catheter placement.[36] The femoral artery is percutaneously punctured and a 12 French sheath is utilized to pass the intra-aortic balloon assembly (usually a 30 to 40 cc single-chamber 12 French catheter which has been carefully wrapped with guide wire) to a position just below the left subclavian artery.

The catheter placement is documented via fluoroscopy or X-ray. When IACP begins, the balloon immediately unwraps and functions as a conventional AB. This procedure, in contrast to surgically placed AB, requires a total insertion time of only 4 to 5 minutes.

Comments

Gold and associates[14] were among the first to demonstrate the beneficial effects of IACP on medically refractory rest angina in pre-infarction and post-infarction states. The beneficial effects of IACP were later verified by Weintrub and co-workers[43] who showed abolition or lessening of chest pain and/or electrocardiographic changes in 10 of 16 patients with refractory preinfarction angina. Weintrub and associates[42] have recently reported a series of 60 patients with medically refractory unstable angina pectoris who underwent a combination of AB assist, cardiac catheterization, and coronary revascularization. Of their series, one perioperative and one late death occurred, with a 25 per cent perioperative infarction rate.

Utilizing the above triad, the survivors did exceptionally well (mean of 31 months follow-up): 77 per cent were considered "employable" and more than 90 per cent were in New York Heart Association functional class I or II. Thus, in patients with unstable angina, IACP seems to be an effective palliative procedure that will allow time for diagnostic angiographic and conservative surgical procedures to be instituted if indicated.

Complications

Clinical studies have generally estimated that less than 20 per cent of patients receiving the AB have complications related to its insertion or use. Until recently, no systemic necropsy examination of patients undergoing IABP insertion has been performed. Isner and co-workers[17] examined 45 patients at necropsy who had undergone IACP prior to their death. They found that 36 per cent of the patients had one or more complications (total of 20 complications). The complications consisted of aortic dissection, arterial perforation, arterial thrombi or emboli, limb ischemia and local wound infection.

Of the entire 20 complications, only 4 (20 per cent) were suspected prior to death, and 12 of the 20 complications were the direct result of balloon insertion. Thus, most of the complications of the IACP were related to balloon insertion, and clinical evaluation usually underestimates their frequency.

SUMMARY

In this discussion we have included cardiac procedures which in general require the expertise of a cardiologist or other physicians trained explicitly in the fundamentals of the procedure. At times, such individuals may be qualified nurses or physicians assistants. This is true especially in the use of electrical cardioversion and Swan-Ganz catheters. In such circumstances, however, the procedures should be performed only under the close supervision of the cardiologist.

The procedures herein considered are all invasive with exception of electrical conversion which, to the conscious patient, is often more "traumatic" than the invasive aspect of the other procedures. It must, therefore, again be emphasized that these cardiac procedures are to be used only after careful bedside evaluation of the patient.

Before cardioversion is undertaken, for example, the decision must be made as to whether or not the patient is hemodynamically compromised by a dysrhythmia. For Swan-Ganz catheter consideration one might wish to try a fluid challenge in a hypotensive patient before the catheter is inserted. In a "thirsty" patient with flat neck veins and clear lung fields to auscultation, the fluid challenge may be of diagnostic and therapeutic benefit.

With regard to pacemakers, for example, one might benefit from use of a vagolytic drug (atropine) for sinus bradycardia in the setting of acute myocardial infarction before initiating the procedure. Before pericardiocentesis, the clinician must be sure that the venous engorgement, decreased heart sounds, increased heart rate and decreased blood pressure are not all due only to severe myocardial failure. In the latter setting, pericardiocentesis could be of extreme danger to the patient.

Lastly, the indication for counterpulsation must be considered carefully. Unless it is an early intervention for the coronary patient whose management involves plans for catheterization and bypass surgery, this procedure could be only palliative for a severely jeopardized myocardium. In this event, the procedure may serve only as a mechanism of prolonging inevitable death.

With the above noted reservations considered, the cardiac procedures herein described may be of the utmost importance in patient management and are often life saving. The skill and wisdom of the physician and health team in the use of their intervention provides the groundwork for success or failure. Only with proper utilization of patient data and other associated management regimens will cardiac procedures in acute care be utilized to their maximal capacity.

REFERENCES

1. Austin, W. G.: Intra-aortic balloon counterpulsation — current applications. Cardiovasc. Clin., 7:285–290, 1970.
2. Bergman, D., and Casanella, W. J.: Percutaneous intra-aortic balloon pulsation: Initial clinical experience. Ann. Thorac. Surg., 29:153–155, 1980.
3. Bishop, L. H., Jr., Estes, E. H., Jr., and McIntosh, H. D.: Electrocardiogram as a safeguard in pericardiocentesis. J.A.M.A., 162:264–265, 1956.
4. Braunwald, E.: Effects of drugs and of counterpulsation on myocardial oxygen consumption: Observations on the ischemic heart. Circulation, 39–40 (Suppl):220–228, 1969.
5. Chatterjee, K., Harris, A., Leatham, A.: The risk of pacing after infarction, and current recommendations. Lancet, 2:1061–1063, 1969.
6. Chatterjee, K., Swan, H. J. C., Ganz, W., et al,: Use of a balloon-tipped flotation electrode catheter for cardiac monitoring. Amer. J. Cardiol., 36:56–61, 1975.
7. Conde, C. A., Leppo, J., Lipski, J., et al.: Effectiveness of pacemaker treatment in the bradycardia-tachycardia syndrome. Amer. J. Cardiol., 32:209–214, 1973.
8. Connell, P. N., Ewy, G. A., Dahl, C. F., et al.: Transthoracic impedance to defibrillator discharge. Effect of electrode size and electrode chest wall interface. J. Electrocardiog., 6:313M, 1973.
9. Escher, D. J., and Furman, S.: Emergency treatment of cardiac arrhythmias: Emphasis on the use of electrical pacing. J.A.M.A., 214:2028–2034, 1970.
10. Escher, D. J., Furman, S., and Solomon, N.: Cardiovascular dynamics in paced patients. Clin. Res., 16:228, 1968.
11. Fisher, J. D., Cohen, H. L., Mehra, R., et al.: Cardiac pacing and pacemakers. II. Serial electrophysiologic-pharmacologic testing for control of recurrent tachyarrhythmias. Amer. Heart J., 93(5):658–668, 1977.
12. Forester, J. S., Diamond, G., Chatterjee, K., et al.: Medical therapy of acute myocardial infarction by application of hemodynamic subsets. New Engl. J. Med., 295:1356–1362, 1976.
13. Furman, S.: Cardiac pacing and pacemakers. I. Indications for pacing bradyarrhythmias. Amer. Heart J., 93:523–530, 1977.
14. Gold, H. K., Leinbach, R. C., Sanders, C. A., et al.: Intra-aortic balloon pumping for control of recurrent myocardial ischemia. Circulation, 47:1197–1203, 1973.
15. Hindman, M. C., Wagner, G. S., JaRo, M., et al.: The clinical significance of bundle branch block complicating acute myocardial infarction. 2. Indications for temporary and permanent pacemaker insertion. Circulation, 58:679–688, 1978.

16. Hofshire, P. J., Nicoloff, D. M., Moller, J. H.: Postoperative complete heart block in 64 children treated with and without cardiac pacing. Amer. J. Cardiol., 56:235, 1977.
17. Isner, J. R.: Complications of the intra-aortic balloon device: Clinical and morphologic obstructions in 45 necropsy patients. Amer. J. Cardiol., 45:260–280, 1980.
18. Kastor, J. A.: Cardiac electrophysiology: Hemiblocks and stopped hearts. Editorial. New Eng. J. Med., 294:244–251, 1978.
19. Killip, T., and Kimball, J. T.: Treatment of myocardial infarction in a coronary care unit. A two year experience with 250 patients. Amer. J. Cardiol., 20:457–464, 1967.
20. Kimbiris, D., Dreifus, L. S., Linhart, J. W.: Complete heart block occurring during cardiac catheterization in patients with preexisting bundle branch block. Chest, 65:95–97, 1974.
21. Kirkpatrick, Z. M.: On pericardiocentesis. Amer. J. Cardiol., 16:722–728, 1965.
22. Kotte, J. H., and McGuire, J.: Pericardial paracentesis, modern concepts. Cardiovasc. Dis., 20(7):102–103, 1951.
23. Lown, B., Fakhro, A. M., Hood, W. B., Jr., et al.: The coronary care unit — new perspectives and directions. J.A.M.A., 199:188–198, 1967.
24. Lown, B., Amarasingham, R., and Newman, J.: New method for terminating cardiac arrhthymias. Use of synchronized capacitor discharge. J.A.M.A., 182:548–555, 1962.
25. Lown, B., Kleiger, R., and Wolff, G.: The technique of cardioversion. Amer. Heart J., 67:282–284, 1964.
26. Mason, D. T., Zelis, R., Lee, G., et al.: Current concepts and treatment of digitalis toxicity. Amer. J. Cardiol., 27:546–559, 1971.
27. Michaelsson, G., and Engle, M. A.: Congenital complete heart block: An international study of the natural history. Cardiovasc. Clin., 4:85–101, 1972.
28. Narula, O. S.: Artrioventricular conduction defects in patients with sinus bradycardia. Analysis of His bundle recordings. Circulation, 44:1096–1110, 1971.
29. Razavi, M., Duarte, E. P., and Tahmooressi, P.: Cardioversion: Ten-year Cleveland Clinic experience. Cleve. Clin. Quart., 43:175–180, 1976.
30. Resnekov, L., and Lipp, H.: Pacemaking and acute myocardial infarction. Progr. Cardiovasc. Dis., 14:475–499, 1972.
31. Resnekov, L., and McDonald, L.: Appraisal of electrocardioversion in treatment of cardiac dysrhythmias. Brit. Heart J., 30:786–811, 1968.
32. Rosen, K. M., Loeb, H. S., Sinno, M. Z., et al.: Cardiac conduction in patients with symptomatic sinus node disease. Circulation, 43:836–844, 1971.
33. Rosenberg, A. S., Grossman, J. I., Escher, D. J., et al.: Bedside transvenous cardiac pacing. Amer. Heart J., 22:699–703, 1969.
34. Rotshin, R. A.: Hemodynamic evaluation of left ventricular function in shock complicating myocardial infarction. Circulation, 45:127–139, 1972.
35. Russell, R. O., and Rackley, C. E.: Hemodynamic Monitoring in a Coronary Intensive Care Unit. Mt. Kisco, New York, Futura Publishing Company, 1974.
36. Seldinger, S. I.: Catheter replacement of the needle in percutaneous arteriography: A new technique. Acta Radiol., 39:368–376, 1953.
37. Spodick, D. H.: Acute cardiac tamponade. Pathologic physiology, diagnosis and management. Prog. Cardiovasc. Dis., 10:64–96, 1967.
38. Subramian, V. A.: Preliminary clinical experience with percutaneous intra-aortic balloon pumping. Abstract. Circulation, 60:II–103, 1979.
39. Sulg, I. A., Cronqvist, S., Schuller, H., et al.: The effect of intracardial pacemaker therapy on cerebral blood flow and electroencephalogram in patients with complete atrioventricular block. Circulation, 39:487–494, 1969.
40. Swan, H. J. C., and Ganz, W.: Catheterization of the heart in man with use of a flow-directed balloon-tipped catheter. New Eng. J. Med., 283:447–451, 1970.
41. Weber, K. T., Janicki, J. S.: Intra-aortic balloon counterpulsation: A review of physiological principles, clinical results and device safety. Ann. Thorac. Surg., 17:602–626, 1974.
42. Weintraub, R. M., Aroesty, J. M., Paulin, S., et al.: Medically refractory unstable angina pectoris. I. Long-term follow up of patients undergoing intra-aortic balloon counterpulsations and operation. Amer. J. Cardiol., 43(5):877–881, 1979.
43. Weintraub, R. M., Voukydis, P. C., Aroesty, J. M., et al.: Treatment of preinfarction angina with intra-aortic balloon counterpulsation and surgery. Amer. J. Cardiol., 34:809–814, 1974.
44. Whittle, J. V., Feldman, R. L., Pepine, C. J., et al.: Mechanisms of the beneficial effect of intra-aortic balloon pumping in patients with refractory angina. Abstract, 29th Annual Scientific Session, American College of Cardiology, March 1980, p. 478.

Georgia Baptist Medical Center
Atlanta, Georgia 30312

The Evaluation and Treatment of Patients with Arterial Aneurysms

*Sandor A. Friedman, M.D.**

A true aneurysm is a segmental dilatation of an artery secondary to weakening and stretching of its wall. In most cases, the process of aneurysm formation is really an exaggeration in a local area of the aging process in which smooth muscle and elastic tissue in the media of the vessel are gradually replaced by collagen (arteriosclerosis). Stenoses and sharp bends in the arterial anatomy encourage this dilatation by decreasing laminar flow and increasing pressure against the wall.

Arterial aneurysms are quite common. Fomon et al.,[9] in a review of 7642 consecutive autopsy records, found evidence of 249 aneurysms of the aorta or its major branches (3.3 per cent). In subjects over age 25, the incidence was 4.5 per cent, and this figure does not include peripheral aneurysms. The abdominal aorta was the most frequent site (77 cases) followed by the ascending aorta (55 cases).

Once established, an aneurysm is subject to a vicious cycle. As blood flows through the ectatic segment, turbulence develops and forward velocity decreases. The results are thrombus formation and increased wall pressure, which in turn causes the aneurysm to dilate further. This process may continue until the aneurysm ruptures or serious thromboembolic episodes develop. Clinical manifestations depend very much on the location and shape of the aneurysm. Saccular aneurysms are subject to greater lateral pressure and, therefore, expand and rupture more quickly than fusiform lesions.

This report will review current concepts in diagnosis and management of the most common true aneurysms as well as dissecting aneurysms of the aorta. Congenital cerebral aneurysms, which are etiologically and clinically quite distinct from other aneurysms, will not be discussed.

ANEURYSMS OF THE THORACIC AORTA

With the decreasing prevalence of tertiary syphilis, arteriosclerosis has become the major cause of aneurysms in the thoracic aorta. In a

*Chief, Department of Medicine, Coney Island Hospital; Professor of Medicine, State University of New York, Downstate Medical Center, Brooklyn, New York

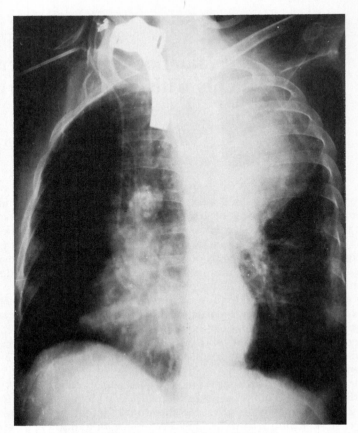

Figure 1.   An aneurysm of the transverse and descending aorta appears on the x-ray film as a mediastinal mass.

review from the Mayo Clinic, Joyce et al.[13] identified arteriosclerosis as the cause in 78 of 107 patients with thoracic aneurysms (73 per cent) and lues as the cause in 19 per cent. In the latter case aneurysms are almost always confined to the ascending aorta. Other causes included closed chest trauma (5 per cent), dilatation distal to aortic valvular stenosis and Marfan's syndrome. Occasional congenital aneurysms are usually near the ligamentum arteriosum.

The great majority of patients with thoracic aneurysms are asymptomatic, and the diagnosis is usually made incidentally from a routine chest roentgenogram. In the Mayo Clinic series, at the time of diagnosis 17 per cent had pain, which was quite nonspecific in character and involved either the upper back or the chest. When clinical signs and symptoms do occur, they vary significantly with the location of the aneurysm.

Lesions of the ascending aorta rarely cause symptoms but may produce a number of clinical signs. Careful palpation of the chest with the patient leaning forward and holding his breath in expiration may reveal a pulsation along the upper right sternal border. Percussion may even identify an area of dullness corresponding to the pulsation. Since aneurysms in this area often lead to stretching and dilatation of the aortic valve ring, an early diastolic murmur of aortic regurgitation can often be heard. In contrast to aortic valvular disease, the aortic closure sound is loud, and the murmur is generally heard best at the aortic area and along the right sternal border. In some cases, the only clinical clue to the presence of the aneurysm may be a loud aortic second sound. When regurgitation is present, a systolic ejection murmur may be present and is often more prominent than the diastolic murmur.

Aneurysms of the transverse aorta may produce many signs and symptoms because of their proximity to mediastinal structures. The patient may present with hoarseness due to recurrent laryngeal nerve compression; dyspnea with wheezing or stridor secondary to tracheo-bronchial compression; dysphagia, anemia, and weight loss because of esophageal involvement; and even superior vena cava syndrome. With the appearance on chest x-ray of a mediastinal mass (Fig. 1) and any of those syndromes, it is not surprising that these patients are generally first thought to have bronchogenic or esophageal carcinoma. Careful physical examination may reveal a pulsation along the upper chest just to the right or the left of the sternum. Aneurysms of the descending aorta are the most treacherous because they are almost always silent until they rupture. Even when they occasionally become large enough to erode into a vertebra, pain is often mild or absent.

Arteriosclerotic thoracic aneurysms are associated with diffuse arteriosclerosis. In the Mayo Clinic Series,[13] 11 patients had abdominal aneurysms, and coronary, cerebrovascular, and peripheral arterial diseases were also prevalent. Long-standing hypertension is a major etiologic factor in most of these patients.

The most important laboratory test is the chest roentgenogram, taken in several views. With lateral and oblique views one can often distinguish between a true aneurysm, generalized aortic ectasia, and a mediastinal tumor. However, serious mistakes are possible, so that further confirmation of the diagnosis is mandatory. Fluoroscopy can demonstrate the expansile nature of the mediastinal shadow, but one must be wary of a transmitted aortic pulse through a nonvascular tumor. Therefore, unless the fluoroscopic findings are classical, it is advisable to confirm the presence of an aneurysm with an angiographic procedure. If surgical repair is contemplated, aortic catheterization is required in order to delineate clearly the size and extent of the aneurysm and to visualize properly the brachiocephalic arteries.

If surgery is not under consideration, aortography after the intravenous injection of radiopaque material or a radionuclide such as technetium-99 will usually suffice. Whenever there is uncertainty in distinguishing between neoplasm and aneurysm, the angiogram should be done first, rather than procedures such as bronchoscopy and esophagoscopy, which might injure a dilated contiguous aorta.

Decisions concerning therapy are difficult, as medical treatment is limited. Lues can be treated with penicillin, and hypertension can be controlled, but the vicious cycle of aneurysmal expansion continues. A decision for or against surgical repair depends on adequate knowledge of surgical risks, natural history of the lesion, and likely longevity of the patient. The only modern prospective data on conservatively treated patients comes from the Mayo Clinic Series.[13] Of 98 patients traced, 49 (50 per cent) were still alive 5 years after initial diagnosis as compared to an expected rate of 90 per cent for the normal population of the same age; 30 per cent survived 10 years. Where the cause of death could be ascertained, 32 per cent died of ruptured aneurysm, and the remainder succumbed to other arteriosclerotic disease. Shape and location of the aneurysm had no effect on the outcome, but mortality was approximately twice as high for symptomatic lesions and those over 6 cm in diameter as for the smaller lesions. In the autopsy series of Fomon and associates, only one of 84 aneurysms under 5 cm in diameter was ruptured, whereas the rupture rate was 15 per cent for those between 5 and 10 cm and rose to 43 per cent for those over 10 cm.

Surgical techniques for handling the thoracic aorta and providing extracorporeal perfusion have improved, but replacement of the thoracic aorta with a prosthetic graft still carries a high mortality rate even for experienced cardiovascular surgeons in specialized centers. In resection of the ascending or transverse aorta, adequate circulation must be maintained through both carotid arteries, at least one vertebral artery, and arteries supplying the lower portion of the body (especially the kidneys and spinal cord). In the case of the ascending aorta, the aortic valve may also have to be replaced. In the transverse aorta, surgery is particularly hazardous because the origins of the brachiocephalic vessels must be inserted into the prosthesis. Recent published mortality rates for elective resection vary from 14 per cent to 20 per cent for this kind of surgery.[3] Repair of descending aortic aneurysms is less hazardous, but partial bypass (left atrium to femoral artery or femoral vein to femoral artery with a pump oxygenator) is still required. A surgical mortality of 11 per cent has been reported for repair of aneurysms in this location.[6]

It seems reasonable to treat patients with small aneurysms conservatively, following them with serial chest x-ray films at 3 to 6 month intervals. On the other hand, patients with large, symptomatic lesions, especially expanding ones and those in the descending aorta, should be considered for surgery if their general medical condition allows. One must remember, however, that patients with coronary artery and cerebrovascular disease tolerate poorly major vascular surgery with its attendant blood loss, hypotension, and manipulation of the extracranial cerebral arteries. The decision for or against surgical repair must take these risk factors into account.

ANEURYSMS OF THE ABDOMINAL AORTA

The terminal portion of the aorta is by far the most common site for aneurysm formation because of the sharp angulation of its bifurcation. These aneurysms are almost always of arteriosclerotic origin and often involve the entire bifurcation of the aorta including the proximal common iliac arteries. Fortunately, because the area of turbulent blood flow is rather long, most abdominal aortic aneurysms are fusiform rather than saccular.

In the entire field of public health and preventive medicine, there is no more neglected lesion than the abdominal aortic aneurysm. It is literally a time bomb, and yet relatively little emphasis is placed on its detection by physical examination in contrast to many other cardiovascular disorders of less importance or reversibility. In one study of 100 consecutive patients referred for surgical repair of abdominal aneurysms, 19 lesions had been found inadvertently during a radiologic examination performed for other reasons.[10] In each case, the aneurysm was easily palpable. Ninety-eight per cent of these aneurysms are entirely below the level of the renal arteries. Two retrospective studies have suggested that approximately one of every 250 people over the age of 50 succumbs from rupture of an abdominal aneurysm.[16]

Unfortunately, these aneurysms rarely cause symptoms until they are close to or at the point of rupture. Perhaps 10 per cent of patients will sense a chronic or intermittent pounding or abdominal palpitation, but abdominal or back pain almost always means rupture or impending rupture. When pain occurs, it is often quite nonspecific and may vary considerably in location. Although it is usually in the epigastrium or lower back and of a steady, sharp or gnawing quality, it may also occur in the lower abdomen and is even occasionally colicky.

The key to diagnosis is physical examination. Careful palpation of the abdominal aorta is one of the most important items in the routine health screening of healthy middle-aged people especially those with a history of hypertension or other arteriosclerotic disease. The pulsation of the abdominal aorta is palpable in the epigastric area in all but obese individuals. One must gain experience with this localized pulse in order to appreciate when it is abnormal. An aneurysm is usually a pulsatile mass. One feels a globular, hard tumor with an expansile quality. There is often lateral as well as anterior pulsation. Since the aneurysmal aorta is often tortuous and uncoiled, it may sometimes be located quite far from the epigastrium, particularly in the left upper quadrant and occasionally the right upper quadrant.

Not infrequently, it may be difficult to distinguish between generalized ectasia and tortuosity of the abdominal aorta and a true aneurysm. There may be a wide pulsation without a mass. In thin individuals a strong anterior pulsation in the epigastrium may be a normal finding. With age and uncoiling this pulsation may move laterally but still not represent an aneurysm. On the other hand, such a pulsation in a heavier patient may represent an aneurysm. In fact, palpation of any pulsation must raise the suspicion of an aneurysm in an obese individual. As a general rule, one should not be able to feel a normal aortic pulsation below the umbilicus except in very thin individuals.

In about two thirds of abdominal aneurysms, medial calcification is heavy enough to be detected with abdominal roentgenography. The aneurysm may be seen as a curvilinear calcification on an anteroposterior film of the abdomen and on a lateral view as calcification just in

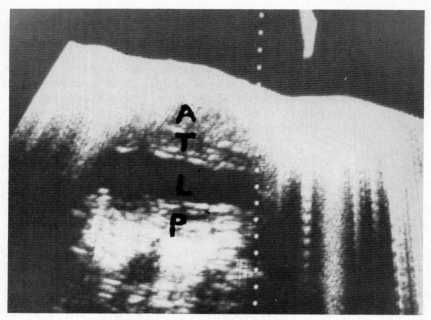

Figure 2.   Sonogram of abdominal aorta demonstrates an aneurysm. A thrombus close to the anterior wall encroaches on the lumen. A, anterior wall; T, thrombus; L, lumen; P, posterior wall.

front of the lumbar spine. A lateral x-ray taken with bone technique is most useful because one can often see calcification of both the anterior and the posterior walls and thus obtain a reasonable estimate of the size, shape and location of the aneurysm. Until recent years, the lateral film of the abdomen was the single best non-invasive laboratory test for detecting and confirming the presence of an abdominal aortic aneurysm.

The development of abdominal sonography has made the diagnosis of these aneurysms simple, painless, and extremely accurate. Ultrasound delineates the anatomy of the abdominal aorta in great detail (Figs. 2 and 3). With a series of transverse and longitudinal views, the sonographer can locate an aneurysm, distinguish it from generalized ectasia and estimate very carefully its width, depth, and length. The sonogram also detects clot within the lumen of the aneurysm.

With the advent of ultrasonography, aortography has been relegated to a minor role in the evaluation of patients with suspected abdominal aneurysms. In fact, aortography is far inferior to ultrasound as a diagnostic tool. Because of the frequent presence of mural thrombosis, which may sometimes form a thick layer along the walls of the aneurysm, an aortogram may grossly underestimate its size and even miss it completely (Fig. 2). Often the diagnosis is made through aortography on the basis of an asymmetric narrowing of the aortic lumen secondary to thrombosis rather than dilatation of its wall. The major role of aortography is visualization of the peripheral circulation beyond the aorta. If there is extensive peripheral arterial disease, it may be important to see the distal run-off in order to choose properly the site of distal anastomosis of the graft used in surgical repair. Some surgeons prefer to have a preoperative aortogram in every case because they are concerned about the mesenteric circulation. Since the inferior mesenteric artery is generally sacrificed at surgery, they want to make sure that there are no major stenoses in the celiac axis or superior mesenteric artery that may result in intestinal ischemia. In most cases, however, this is a moot point because the inferior mesenteric artery is usually occluded before surgery. Serious gastrointestinal problems are quite unusual after aneurysmal surgery.

Patients with abdominal aneurysms often have generalized cardiovascular disease. In one series, 47 per cent had definite coronary artery disease; 43 per cent had peripheral arterial obstruction; 8 per cent had cerebrovascular disease; and 34 per cent had hypertension.[10] Nevertheless the findings in longitudinal studies of patients with this lesion support an aggressive approach. The 5 year survival rate from the time of initial diagnosis for untreated patients has varied from 17.2 to 36.4 per cent.[1] Approximately half the deaths are caused by aneurysmal rupture. Several groups have shown that aneurysmectomy prolongs life. DeBakey et al. reported that 72 per cent of patients who had undergone resection were alive 3 years after surgery, and 58 per cent after 5 years. Szilagyi and co-workers[1] compared untreated and treated patients after excluding those with advanced age, hypertension and heart disease, and

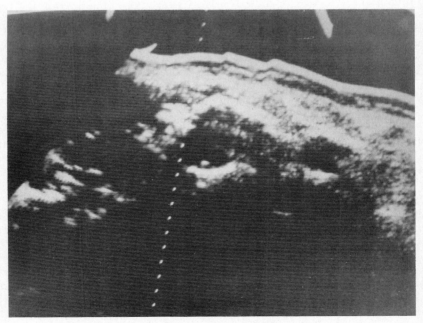

Figure 3.   Sonogram of abdominal aorta showing two aneurysms.

found a doubling of life expectancy in the operated group. Mortality rate for elective aneurysmectomy has fallen. DeBakey and co-workers[5] had a 9 per cent operative mortality rate in 1964; in 1966 a 4 per cent rate was reported in a group of patients of whom 88 per cent had other cardiovascular disease.[10]

Close attention should be paid to the blood pressure and urine output during and after surgery. Continuous electrocardiographic monitoring is advisable because arrhythmias and silent myocardial infarcts are common. In particular, one must watch for signs of acute arterial occlusion in the lower extremities. Embolism from the aneurysmal sac or an atheromatous plaque can occur during aortic manipulation, and an embolectomy may be necessary on occasion.

Although it is generally agreed that the great majority of patients, even those with occlusive arterial disease, should undergo elective repair, there are some whom it is still prudent to exclude. Surgery on lesions above the renal arteries is quite hazardous. Patients with severe angina, congestive heart failure, or frequent episodes of cerebral ischemia are poor candidates because of a higher surgical mortality rate and a relatively high probability of dying of occlusive disease before aneurysmal rupture can occur. Some patients with unstable angina may be candidates for aneurysm repair after successful coronary artery surgery. Aneurysms under 5 cm rarely rupture before expanding further and are best left untouched if the patient has other significant cardiovascular disease. On the other hand, tender aneurysms of any size and those associated with unexplained abdominal and back pain should be repaired as soon as possible.

Rupture of an abdominal aortic aneurysm is usually fatal, but some patients may be saved if they obtain prompt and competent care. An early leak may be temporarily tamponaded by retroperitoneal thrombus. Back or abdominal pain with or without hypotension may develop several hours before hemorrhage into the peritoneal cavity occurs. The sudden appearance of low back or abdominal pain in a patient with a palpable aneurysm warrants immediate laparotomy. In an obese patient over the age of 60, the constellation of severe unexplained pain and shock should suggest the strong possibility of a ruptured aneurysm even if none is palpable. If there is no electrocardiographic evidence of an acute myocardial infarction, surgical exploration should be performed immediately.

As long as the patient maintains a systolic blood pressure above 60 to 70 mm Hg, it is probably not advisable to replete blood volume rapidly until the aorta has been clamped above the site of perforation because a higher perfusing pressure can cause dislodgement of the tamponading thrombus. After aortic clamping, prompt restoration of effective blood volume is essential, using Swan-Ganz monitoring of pulmonary artery and pulmonary wedge pressure as a guide. Mannitol may be given intravenously to induce diuresis and protect against renal failure. Arterial pH must be determined, and metabolic acidosis should be corrected with sodium bicarbonate. The postoperative course is often turbulent. Because of increased permeability of the inflamed mesentery and peritoneum, vast amounts of fluid may be sequestered retroperitoneally during the first 24 to 36 hours. Abrupt declines in circulating blood volume lead quickly to shock and oliguria. Blood pressure, wedge pressure and urine output should be monitored continuously as fluids are rapidly replaced. The appearance of acute renal failure may necessitate dialysis (preferably hemodialysis) for several days. After the first 48 hours, the sequestered fluid begins to be reabsorbed, and congestive heart failure and sudden pulmonary edema may develop if the patient has underlying heart disease. For this reason, prophylactic digitalization soon after surgery is often advisable. Adequate oxygenation is important at all times. The patient may require the use of a respirator intermittently during the first few days because the large abdominal incision, the orthopneic position, and the presence of acute respiratory distress syndrome may impede ventilation. If the patient survives the first 5 days with good cardiopulmonary and renal function, he is likely to recover, provided that wound dehiscence or retroperitoneal infection does not supervene.

Several other less common complications of abdominal aortic aneurysms deserve mention. Because of the large amount of mural thrombus in the sac, peripheral embolization can occur and result in acute femoropopliteal arterial occlusion or small infarcts on the feet. A bleeding diathesis secondary to consumption coagulopathy has also been reported in association with abdominal aortic and occasionally other aneurysms.[21] Any patient with a syndrome of disseminated intravascular coagulation, in the absence of sepsis or neoplasm, should be investigated for an occult aneurysm.

A rare complication of arteriosclerotic aneurysms is bacterial infection, most commonly in aneurysms of the abdominal aorta. In one autopsy study, 6 of 178 arteriosclerotic aortic aneurysms were infected.[22] Salmonella has been the most frequent offender (35 per cent of cases), followed by Staphylococcus (12 per cent). Patients generally present with fever of unknown origin or prolonged, intractable sepsis. Rupture has occurred in 79 per cent. Early surgical intervention, after institution of adequate antibiotic therapy, is necessary.

ANEURYSMS OF THE EXTREMITIES

The popliteal artery is the second most common site for aneurysm formation. Although this lesion is almost always arteriosclerotic in origin, post-stenotic dilatation just distal to points of compression at Hunter's canal and the arcuate popliteal ligament increases the vulnerability of the artery. Continuous trauma with extension and flexion of the knee also contributes to the pathogenesis. Patients with popliteal aneurysms generally have multiple aneurysms. In a study of 152 patients with this lesion, 59 per cent had bilateral popliteal aneurysms, 35 per cent also had abdominal aortic aneurysms, and 29 per cent had femoral aneurysms.[24]

Diagnosis depends on careful palpation of the popliteal pulse behind the knee. A patent aneurysm is easily recognized as an expansile tumor, but a thrombosed aneurysm may appear cystic. Ultrasound examination

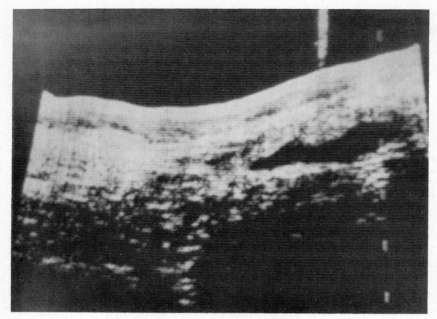

Figure 4. Sonogram of the knee area reveals a popliteal aneurysm. A large thrombus narrows the lumen.

accurately distinguishes an aneurysm from all other lesions and also delineates thrombi in the lumen[18] (Fig. 4). It should be employed in any patient with a prominent popliteal pulse or mass behind the knee. In many cases, plain roentgenograms will also confirm the diagnosis of aneurysm by outlining the calcified walls of the vessel.

Complications of popliteal aneurysm include thromboembolism, rupture, and compression. Rupture occurs in less than 10 per cent of patent lesions and almost never when they are occluded. Compression of the popliteal vein may lead to edema, venous thrombosis and pulmonary embolism. Occasional pressure on the posterior tibial nerve leads to pain and paresthesias along the calf and heel.

Thromboembolism is the most frequent complication. Gradual thrombosis of the aneurysmal lumen may cause intermittent claudication and progressive distal ischemia, while rapid occlusion may lead to rest pain and gangrene. In addition, showers of emboli into the tibial and digital arteries are quite common. One should always search for a popliteal aneurysm in a patient with one or more focal areas of gangrene on a foot. In two series, evidence of thromboembolism was found in approximately two thirds of the patients at the time of initial diagnosis of popliteal aneurysm.[4, 8]

A popliteal aneurysm is a serious threat to the viability of the limb. Of 70 cases managed conservatively, Gifford and co-workers[11] reported thromboembolism in 11 patients, venous compression in 5 and rupture in 4 during a mean observation period of 44 months. Eighteen limbs eventually required amputation. Of the 45 patients with previously uncomplicated aneurysms, 5 (11 per cent) had amputations. Wychulis et al.[24] reported complications in 29 per cent and amputation in 3 per cent of patients with initially asymptomatic aneurysms.

Surgical excision with replacement by a graft is recommended for all but the most debilitated patients. Arteriography should be performed first to outline the distal arterial run-off. There were only two operative deaths in 107 cases from three surgical series. Crichlow and Roberts[4] reported patency of distal vessels in 77 per cent and adequate blood flow in 81 per cent of patients after a mean postoperative period of 4.8 years. Wychulis et al.[24] reported a favorable surgical outcome in patients with asymptomatic aneurysms but an 11 per cent amputation rate in 64 patients who underwent surgery after suffering serious thromboembolism. Patients with already occluded aneurysms should be treated like others with peripheral arterial disease.

Femoral aneurysms are similar in clinical behavior to popliteal aneurysms. Thromboembolism occurred in 23 of 89 patients in one series, and 7 of 44 treated conservatively required limb amputation.[20] Surgical repair is indicated for all patent lesions.

Chronic compression from a thoracic outlet syndrome is the most common cause of aneurysmal dilatation of the subclavian artery.[7] This aneurysm is generally small, but it may be gradually occluded or shower emboli into the hand. One should think first of this lesion in any patient with upper extremity claudication or digital artery occlusion. Surgery must be directed at the aneurysm and the compressing structure in the thoracic outlet.

CAROTID ARTERY ANEURYSMS

Aneurysmal dilatation of the extracranial portion of the common and internal carotid arteries is quite rare. One surgical group found only 3 cases of carotid artery aneurysm during a 10 year period in which 300 aneurysms of the major arteries were identified.[2] A major diagnostic difficulty is the differentiation of this relatively rare lesion from the rather common kinking or looping of the extracranial carotid arteries. The latter was seen in 80 per cent of 114 carotid angiograms performed on patients between 60 and 80 years of age. This kinking is particularly common in the region of the lower part of the sternocleidomastoid muscle on the right side of the neck. In contrast, carotid aneurysms almost always occur further cephalad at the bifurcation of the common carotid artery.

When an aneurysm is present, physical examination usually reveals a fusiform pulsatile swelling in the upper neck. A bruit is often present. Transient ischemic attacks secondary to thromboembolism from the aneurysmal sac are quite common (perhaps 50 per cent of cases). Surgical repair after angiographic confirmation of the diagnosis is usually advisable.

VISCERAL ANEURYSMS

The most common visceral aneurysm occurs in the splenic artery, followed by the renal arteries (approximately 1 per cent of all aneurysms) (Table 1). Both of these lesions are generally discovered incidentally on abdominal x-ray films as round calcifications. Splenic aneurysms usually result from idiopathic medial degeneration. They are the only aneurysms with a predilection for females and are most likely to occur as a complication of portal hypertension.[23] Rupture rate is high, and surgical excision with splenectomy is always advisable. Pneumococcal vaccine should be administered postoperatively.

Renal aneurysms are more likely to rupture in pregnant women and when they are uncalcified.[12] They may also lead to renal infarction and renovascular hypertension. They are sometimes discovered during angiograms performed in evaluation of hypertensive patients (Table 1).

DISSECTING ANEURYSMS

A dissecting aneurysm is really a misnomer because it is not a true aneurysm but rather a propagating hematoma within the medial layer of the artery. The basic lesion is cystic necrosis of the media rather than generalized stretching of the wall. Because of the resulting lack of structural support, a tear in the intima eventually develops, and blood begins to leak through the cystic spaces of the media under systemic arterial pressure.

The pathogenesis of a dissecting hematoma lies in the gradual loss of elasticity of the media under the continuous lifelong impact of force generated by the left ventricle. It is for this reason that dissections almost always begin in the thoracic aorta, which is subject to the maximum strain from this impact. Isolated peripheral vessel dissections have been described in a number of locations, particularly the carotid and renal arteries, but they are very rare. The elastic nature of the thoracic aorta is a remarkable quality. By distending with each left ventricular systole, the elastic fibers store energy which is released to form the diastolic pressure when they recoil. This rubber-band effect partially protects the aortic wall from the impact of each heart beat, as it limits myocardial thrust to a glancing rather than direct blow. As the aortic wall ages and loses elastic tissue, it becomes stiffer and weaker. As a result, it is less able to withstand the impact of systole which is now a more direct blow. The increasing impact on the wall hastens the process of elastic fiber atrophy and fuels a vicious cycle that in some individuals ends in medial necrosis and dissection.

It is not surprising that the leading etiologic factor for dissection of the aorta is hypertension. Sustained systemic hypertension accelerates the aging of the aortic media so that many hypertensive patients have very stiff aortas by the time they reach the age of 50. Dissection can occur at any age, but most often in the sixth and seventh decades. About three fourths of all dissections are secondary to hypertension.

Table 1. *Peripheral Aneurysms*

LOCATION	USUAL ETIOLOGY	AGE AND SEX DISTRIBUTION	USUAL MODE OF PRESENTATION	COMPLICATIONS	INDICATIONS FOR SURGERY
Popliteal and femoral	Arteriosclerosis	Mostly males over 60	1. Pulsatile mass 2. Thromboembolism	1. Thromboembolism 2. Venous compression 3. Local expansion 4. Rupture occasionally	1. Patent lesions 2. Severe peripheral ischemia
Subclavian	1. Trauma of thoracic outlet syndrome 2. Arteriosclerosis	No predilection	1. Pulsatile mass 2. Thromboembolism	Thromboembolism	1. Patent lesions 2. Severe claudication
Splenic	Idiopathic medial degeneration (more common with portal hypertension, splenomegaly, and multiparity)	Mostly females, any age (mean in 50's)	1. Curvilinear calcification in left upper quadrant 2. Rarely palpable	Rupture in 6.6 to 9.2%	All lesions (excision with splenectomy)
Renal	Idiopathic	No sex predilection; mean age in 50's	1. Round calcification on X-ray 2. Hypertension (found on renal arteriogram)	1. Rupture in up to 15% (more likely in uncalcified lesions and during pregnancy) 2. Hypertension (probably due to renal thromboembolism) 3. Renal infarction	1. Uncalcified lesions and large calcified lesions 2. Women in childbearing age 3. Renal infarction
Carotid	Arteriosclerosis	Usually over age 60	1. Pulsatile mass under the angle of the jaw	1. Strokes 2. Transient ischemic attack	All lesions

There is a smaller incidence peak for dissection in the earlier decades because of the true connective diseases, principally Marfan's syndrome. In these cases, the basic connective tissue structure of the aorta is poor so that it cannot tolerate even normal systemic pressure. Not all patients with Marfan's syndrome have the characteristic arachnodactyly and ectopic lentis. In fact, many of the young patients with dissection or true aneurysm of the thoracic aorta represent a forme fruste of this syndrome and have no other identifying clinical features. Twenty-four hour urine collection for hydroxyproline may be of diagnostic aid.

Dissection is also a rare complication of pregnancy perhaps because of sudden changes in intrathoracic pressure. It is particularly common in coarctation of the aorta because of a combination of hypertension and prolonged impact on the thoracic aortic wall owing to distal obstruction to blood flow.

When dissection occurs, it is likely to begin either just distal to the aortic valves (proximal dissection) or distal to the origin of the left subclavian artery (distal dissection). Although the medical literature suggests that proximal dissection is more common than distal lesions, the truth is probably the reverse. Proximal dissections tend to produce more dramatic clinical findings and are therefore more likely to be detected, whereas distal lesions may be much more subtle. Aortography in recent years has frequently demonstrated the presence of distal dissections even when symptoms were quite evanescent or absent.

The clinical findings depend on the course of the dissecting hematoma. It may extend distally through the aortic wall and continue into any or all of the major branches of the aorta. Conversely, it may extend only a short distance and then clot or re-enter the main lumen of the aorta through a second, more distal intimal tear. It may immediately rupture through the adventitia at any point or form a saccular aneurysm. It may occlude the lumen of a branch artery of the aorta, not interfere with blood flow at all or actually form a false lumen that carries the bulk of blood flow through the artery.

With all of these pathologic possibilities, it is easy to understand why dissecting hematomas vary so much in their clinical manifestations. They can cause a syndrome of regional ischemia whenever an appropriate branch artery is involved. When multiple ischemic areas are involved, one tends to think quickly about the presence of dissection, but it is important to remember that evidence of proximal artery occlusion anywhere can be a sign of dissection. Many patients have presented only with signs of a stroke caused by carotid artery occlusion, mesenteric or renal infarction, or lower limb ischemia associated with absent femoral pulses.

It is helpful to remember that dissection involves the immediate branch of the aorta rather than distal vessels so that the most proximal pulse must be weak or missing if ischemia is due to dissection. For example, a stroke is associated with loss or diminution of a carotid pulse. If the stroke involves the right cerebral hemisphere (left hemiparesis), blood pressure in the right arm is likely to be diminished because the right carotid and subclavian arteries generally originate from one brachiocephalic vessel (innominate artery).

Proximal dissections can produce several complications that do not occur with distal lesions. Since dissecting hematomas always proceed in a distal direction, only proximal lesions can involve the extracranial arteries, causing serious neurologic sequelae. Secondly they often involve the area of the aortic ring and lead to aortic regurgitation. This valvular dysfunction may be asymptomatic or lead to acute and massive left ventricular failure. Clinically, this acute aortic regurgitation may appear quite different from chronic aortic insufficiency. Pulse pressure may not be elevated, hypotension may be present, and signs of hyperdynamic circulation conspicuously absent. Thirdly, proximal dissections may rupture into the pericardial or left pleural cavity. This is a frequent mode of demise for patients with this lesion.

Pain is not always a conspicuous symptom. Although the majority of patients experience chest and/or back pain at the time of dissection, it is usually not the classic textbook description of tearing chest pain radiating to the back, arms, and abdomen. The pain may be mild and may radiate in strange ways. Distal dissections often occur without pain, and when pain does occur, it is usually limited to the back. It is often mistakenly ascribed by both patient and physician to muscle strain or tension. Since many patients with hypertension also have coronary artery disease, dissections are often confused with myocardial infarctions.

It is apparent that a dissecting hematoma may be a great masquerader, often presenting in unexpected ways. The diagnosis of this treacherous lesion depends on an awareness of its vagaries and a high index of suspicion in dealing with acute cardiovascular events. One must always consider aortic dissection as a diagnostic possibility in the following clinical situations especially when there is a history of hypertension:

1. A patient with aortic regurgitation murmur who complains of chest or back pain.
2. Symptoms of acute regional ischemia such as hemiparesis or flank pain and hematuria when there is no obvious source for arterial embolism.
3. Multiple areas of acute ischemia.
4. Acute, unexplained left ventricular failure.
5. Atypical chest or back pain.
6. Disappearance and spontaneous reappearance of proximal pulses.

The most important noninvasive test in looking for aortic dissection is a chest roentgenogram, including posterior-anterior and lateral views. Almost all patients with dissection have at least a somewhat prominent thoracic aortic shadow. This shadow does not generally reach the sizes seen with true aortic aneurysms unless the false channel is massive or the weakened wall has stretched into a true saccular aneurysm, but a totally normal aortic shadow is strongly against the diagnosis of dissecting hematoma. Prominence of the ascending aorta to the right of the heart shadow or of the descending aorta along the left mediastinal border is strong evidence in favor of the diagnosis in the appropriate clinical situation (Fig. 5). Sometimes, one can see a fine radiolucent line running vertically through the aortic shadow, suggesting the presence of a double lumen.

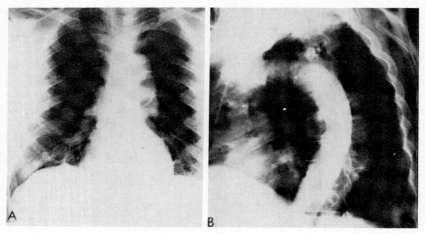

Figure 5.   *A*, Chest roentgenogram reveals prominence of descending aortic shadow. *B*, Aortogram shows false channel of a distal dissection in the same patient.

M-mode echocardiography of the aortic root may be extremely helpful in making a diagnosis of proximal aortic dissection.[17] Under normal conditions, the anterior and posterior walls of the aortic root produce parallel dominant echoes, which move anteriorly in systole and

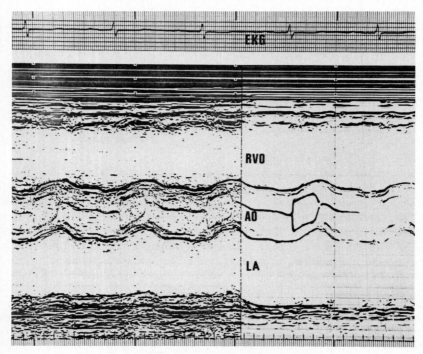

Figure 6.   Normal echocardiogram of the aortic root.

posteriorly in diastole. The aortic valve echoes occur within these two parallel echoes, separating in systole and joining together in diastole (Fig. 6).

When dissection occurs in the aortic root, the layers of the aortic wall may appear duplicated (Fig. 7). Two dominant echoes separated by a space are present in the anterior or posterior wall or both rather than one discrete echo. These echoes maintain parallelism during the motions of the aorta throughout the cardiac cycle. The space represents the false lumen and may be echo-free or filled with soft, diffuse echoes if clotting has occurred.

The echocardiogram may also reveal other abnormalities. Fluttering of the anterior mitral leaflet indicates the presence of aortic regurgitation. General widening of the aortic root suggests an aortic ring rather than valve leaflet cause for the regurgitation, and early closure of the

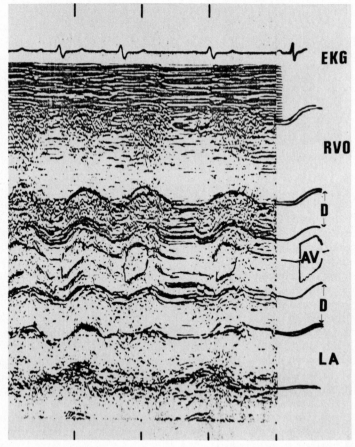

Figure 7.   Echocardiogram shows reduplication of the anterior and posterior walls of the aortic root in a patient with proximal aortic dissection. RVO, right ventricular outflow; D, false channel between reduplicated walls; AV, aortic valve; LA, left atrium.

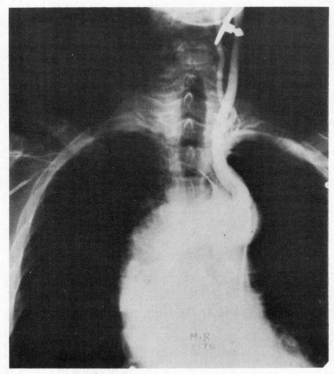

Figure 8. Aortogram shows a proximal aortic dissection. A large false channel has narrowed aortic lumen and occluded the innominate artery near its origin.

mitral valve points to an acute process. In cases of ruptured dissection, hemopericardium may be seen as an echo-free space between the layers of pericardium. It must be pointed out, however, that a normal one-dimensional echocardiogram does not rule out the diagnosis of proximal aortic dissection.

The only definitive test for dissection remains aortography, which is generally performed in retrograde fashion through a femoral artery. The purposes of aortography are two-fold: to make the diagnosis and to indicate the origin of the dissection by locating the intimal tear (Fig. 8). One must be extremely careful in performing this procedure because the catheter may pass inadvertently into the false channel if it is larger than the true lumen. If dye is then injected under pressure, the aorta may easily perforate. One should always inject first by hand in order to determine the exact position of the catheter. If the hematoma has clotted and obliterated the false channel, it may not be visualized. In fact, some dissections are difficult to delineate even with aortography and may be identified only by eccentric narrowing of the true lumen or a very faintly opacified false channel (Fig. 9).

Treatment of dissection depends to a large extent on location, but the first principle is to control hypertension. This must be achieved without using agents that increase cardiac contractility (the rate of rise of left ventricular pressure, dp/dt). If the patient is not in congestive heart failure, the goal is to decrease contractility in order to reduce its impact on the aortic wall. The drug of first choice in a hypertensive patient with an aortic dissection is a ganglionic-blocking agent, given by intravenous drip and titrated to bring the blood pressure abruptly to normal. This rapid lowering carries a risk of provoking cerebral ischemia or acute renal failure, but fortunately these complications are rare. Simultaneously, therapy with oral agents is begun and progressively increased until a ganglionic-blocking agent is no longer needed. One attempts to accomplish this goal within 48 hours before significant tachyphylaxis renders the patient resistant to the action of the ganglionic blocker.

Beta blockers such as propranolol are ideal agents because they decrease the ionotrophic force of the left ventricle. Diuretic agents, alpha

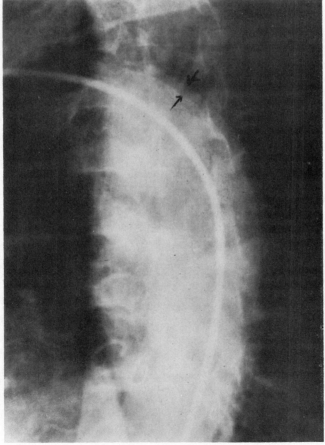

Figure 9. An aortogram reveals a faintly visualized, narrow false channel in a distal aortic dissection.

methyl dopa, clonidine, and guanethidine may also be added if necessary. On the other hand, one should avoid the direct vasodilator drugs such as hydralazine, diazoxide, and nitroprusside, which lead to an increase in cardiac output.

Differences of opinion exist about long-term care of patients after a distal dissection. Some believe that surgical repair is advisable perhaps a few months later, but many believe that continued vigorous control of blood pressure is adequate.[19] In one surgical series, the operative mortality for chronic distal dissections was 22 per cent, and actuarial 5-year survival was approximately 57 per cent.[15] A 52 per cent survival rate at 3½ years has been described with medical therapy alone.[14]

The development of a saccular aneurysm or regional ischemia is an unequivocal indication for surgery. In following these patients with medical therapy, one should obtain chest x-ray films every month during the first few months and then approximately every 4 months for at least the first 2 years.

Proximal dissections are much more dangerous, and the mortality rate with hypotensive therapy alone is high. Therefore, most authorities agree that surgical intervention is appropriate after a period of medical therapy and immediately if there is severe aortic regurgitation or perforation of the aorta. Surgery is difficult and often involves an aortic graft and replacement of the aortic valve as well as obliteration of the false lumen. In one large series, the mortality rate was 34 per cent when surgery was performed within 14 days of the acute event and 14 per cent when it was deferred beyond 14 days.[15]

ACKNOWLEDGEMENT

The author wishes to thank Dr. Mohandas Shenoy, Chief of Non-Invasive Cardiology Laboratory at Coney Island Hospital, for providing echocardiographic data related to dissecting aneurysms.

REFERENCES

1. Bernstein, E. F., Fisher, J. C., and Varco, R. L.: Is excision the optimum treatment for all abdominal aortic aneurysms? Surgery, 61:83, 1967.
2. Carrascal, L., Marshiah, A., and Charlesworth, D.: Aneurysms of the extracranial carotid arteries. Brit. J. Surg., 65:590–592, 1978.
3. Crawford, E. S., Saleh, S. A., and Scheussler, J. S.: Treatment of aneurysm of transverse aortic arch. J. Thorac Cardiovasc. Surg. 78:383–393, 1979.
4. Crichlow, R. W., and Roberts, B.: Treatment of popliteal aneurysms by restoration of continuity: Review of 48 cases. Ann. Surg., 163:417, 1966.
5. DeBakey, M. E., Crawford, E. S., Cooley, D. A. et al.: Aneurysm of abdominal aorta: Analysis of results of graft replacement therapy 1 to 11 years after operation. Ann. Surg., 160:622, 1964.
6. Dillon, M. L., Young, W. G., and Sealy, W. C.: Aneurysms of the descending thoracic aorta. Ann. Thorac. Surg., 3:430, 1967.
7. Dorazio, R. A., and Ezzet, F.: Arterial Complications of the thoracic outlet syndrome. Amer. J. Surg., 138:246–250, 1979.
8. Edmunds, L. H., Jr., Darling, R. C., and Linton, R. R.: Surgical management of popliteal aneurysms. Circulation, 32:517, 1965.
9. Fomon, J. J., Kurzweg, F. T., and Broadway, R. K.: Aneurysms of the aorta: A Review. Ann. Surg., 165:557, 1967.

10. Friedman, S. A., Hufnagel, C. A., Conrad, P. W., et al.: Abdominal aortic aneurysms: Clinical status and results of surgery in 100 consecutive cases. J.A.M.A., 200:1147, 1967.
11. Gifford, R. W., Jr., Hines, E. A., Jr., and Janes, J. M.: An analysis and follow-up study of 100 popliteal aneurysms. Surgery, 33:284, 1953.
12. Hageman, J. H., Smith, R. F., Szilagyi, D. E., et al.: Aneurysms of the renal artery: Problems of prognosis and surgical management. Surgery, 84:563–572, 1978.
13. Joyce, J. W., Fairbairn, J. F., II, Kincaid, O. W., et al.: Aneurysms of the thoracic aorta. Circulation, 29:176, 1964.
14. McFarland, J., Willerson, J. T., Dinsmore, R. F., et al.: The medical treatment of dissecting aortic aneurysms. New Eng. J. Med., 286:115, 1972.
15. Miller, D. C., Stinson, E. B., Oyer, P. E., et al.: Operative treatment of aortic dissections. Experience with 125 patients over a sixteen-year period. J. Thorac. Cardiovasc. Surg., 78:365–382, 1979.
16. Moore, H. D.: Diagnosis of rupture of abdominal aortic aneurysms. Lancet, 2:184, 1967.
17. Moothart, R. W., Spangler, R. D., and Blount, S. G., Jr.: Echocardiography in aortic root dissection and dilatation. Amer. J. Cardiol., 36:11–16, 1975.
18. Neiman, H. L., Yalo, J. S. T., and Silver, T. M.: Gray-scale ultrasound diagnosis of peripheral arterial aneurysms. Radiology, 130:413–416, 1979.
19. Palmer, R. F., and Wheat, M. W., Jr.: Treatment of dissecting aneurysms of the aorta. Ann. Thorac. Surg., 4:38–52, 1967.
20. Pappas, G., Janes, J. M., Bernatz, P. E., et al.: Femoral aneurysms: Review of surgical management. J.A.M.A., 190:489, 1964.
21. Saltani, B., Savrin, R., and Evans, W. E.: Consumption coagulopathy associated with arterial aneurysms. J. Cardiovasc. Surg., 78:273–278, 1979.
22. Sommerville, R. L., Allen, E. V., and Edwards, J. E.: Bland and infected arteriosclerotic abdominal aortic aneurysms. Medicine, 38:207, 1959.
23. Stanley, J. C., Thompson, N. W., and Fry, W. J.: Splanchnic artery aneurysms. Arch. Surg., 101:689, 1970.
24. Wychulis, A. R., Spittell, J. A., and Wallace, R. B.: Popliteal aneurysms. Surgery, 68:942, 1970.

Acute Pituitary Vascular Accident (Pituitary Apoplexy)

Sheldon Markowitz, M.D.,* Lawrence Sherman, M.D.,†
Howard D. Kolodny, M.D.,‡ and Selim Baruh, M.D.§

Apoplexy is a dramatic and frightening term that signifies the sudden striking down of a patient by a critically placed hemorrhage or infarction. "Pituitary apoplexy" thus refers to a neuroendocrine emergency produced by hemorrhage or infarction of the pituitary gland — usually an adenomatous gland. Pituitary apoplexy is now recognized as a well-defined syndrome, one that occurs in perhaps 5 to 10 per cent of patients with pituitary tumors.[4, 29] Common clinical features include sudden headache, visual disturbances, changes in sensorium, nausea and vomiting, nuchal rigidity, and fever.

The syndrome, once considered rare and almost uniformly fatal, is now recognized more frequently and is considered treatable. Proper treatment requires prompt diagnosis in most cases. Both depend on knowledge of the anatomical relationships and complexity of function of the pituitary.

Because the term "apoplexy" implies a catastrophic event with a high likelihood of fatality, while in reality the illness may be mild or severe, and survival is likely with present methods of treatment, we propose the term "acute pituitary vascular accident" as an alternative to "pituitary apoplexy." This new term has the additional benefit of contributing to the understanding of the pathogenesis of this event, which is thought to be due to acute hemorrhage, ischemia, or both. In this chapter we will use both terms interchangeably.

*Fellow in Endocrinology, Queens Hospital Center Affiliation, Long Island Jewish-Hillside Medical Center.

†Associate Director of Medicine, Queens Hospital Center Affiliation, Long Island Jewish-Hillside Medical Center; Professor of Medicine, School of Medicine, State University of New York at Stony Brook.

‡Professor of Clinical Medicine, School of Medicine, State University of New York at Stony Brook; Attending Physician, Long Island Jewish-Hillside Medical Center.

§Physician-in-Charge, Diabetes, Queens Hospital Center Affiliation, Long Island Jewish-Hillside Medical Center; Assistant Professor of Medicine, School of Medicine, State University of New York at Stony Brook.

Supported in part by an internal research grant (#3-347) from the Long Island Jewish-Hillside Medical Center.

Our purpose is to review current ideas concerning pathophysiology, clinical presentation, and surgical and medical treatment of acute pituitary vascular accident. We shall begin by presenting four characteristic cases of acute pituitary vascular accident — three treated medically, one surgically — and commenting on the significant features of each case.

CASE REPORTS AND COMMENTS

The four cases that follow demonstrate a number of frequently occurring clinical features that will be emphasized later in our discussion. These include: the concomitance of headache, nausea, ocular abnormalities, and mental changes in these patients; the difficulty in differential diagnosis, particularly when fever is present; the finding of abnormal cerebrospinal fluid on "routine" lumbar puncture; the discovery of hormonal defects, both at the time of the acute episode and for months or years thereafter; and the survival of most patients without the need for neurosurgical intervention.

Case 1

A 60 year old woman came to the emergency room of Queens Hospital Center in February 1980 complaining of severe headache of 36 hours duration. The headache, which began suddenly, was located in the frontal and occipital areas. She also complained of nausea and had vomited several times. The patient experienced sudden loss of practically all vision at age 13. Menarche occurred at age 12, menses were regular thereafter, and the patient was fertile. On examination, she was initially afebrile and lethargic. There was ptosis of the left eye, and both pupils were reactive to light. The optic discs were atrophic, but not edematous. Extraocular movements of the left eye were impaired, except for abduction. Skull x-ray showed enlargement of the sella. Lumbar puncture demonstrated a normal opening pressure; cell count was 115 red blood cells, 20 polymorphonuclear leukocytes, and 11 lymphocytes per ml. Glucose was 150 mg per dl and protein 214 mg per dl. A bleeding aneurysm was suspected, and the patient was treated with epsilon amino caproic acid (EACA) and high doses of dexamethasone. Because of a chaotic fever to 105°, brain abscess and meningitis were also considered, and therapy with penicillin and chloramphenicol was initiated. An avascular sellar mass was noted on angiography. CT scan showed an intrasellar mass with suprasellar and left lateral extension, which enhanced irregularly following injection of material. Laboratory testing of serum revealed a low T4 and low TSH, low 8 AM and 4 PM serum cortisol levels, low FSH and LH, and normal prolactin. Gradually, over a 7 day period, the patient improved. The fever and headache disappeared and mentation returned to normal. The patient refused any further therapy (radiation or surgery) and was discharged on maintenance prednisone and synthroid.

COMMENT. This patient demonstrated the frequently seen symptoms of headache, nausea, and vomiting. She also manifested a common sign of pituitary apoplexy: extraocular palsies. In her case, the third and fourth cranial nerves were affected. Though the presence of fever obliged the physician to treat for infection, it should be stressed that fever unaccompanied by infection is often associated with acute pituitary vascular accident. A large sella and abnormal cerebrospinal fluid were additional clues. Both angiography and CT scanning demonstrated the pituitary tumor. Hormonal testing demonstrated hypopituitarism. Steroid replacement therapy was instituted, and headache and fever disappeared. In retrospect, the sudden loss of vision at age 13 may also have been an episode of acute pituitary vascular accident; the present occurrence may then represent the second acute pituitary vascular accident in this patient.

Case 2

A 72 year old man presented to the emergency room of Long Island Jewish-Hillside Medical Center in August, 1973 complaining of a severe, diffuse pounding headache of 8 days duration, accompanied by nausea, vomiting, and drooping of the left eyelid. The patient was lethargic and had a left third nerve palsy and bitemporal hemianopsia. Skull x-ray showed an enlarged sella with a fragmented dorsum sella. Lumbar puncture showed several abnormalities, including xanthochromic fluid, a total protein of 88 mg per 100 ml, and a cell count of 25 mononuclear cells. Cerebral angiography showed no evidence of aneurysm. However, there was narrowing of the right internal carotid artery in its supracavernous portion, and posterior displacement of the basilar arteries. Pneumoencephalogram showed extrinsic pressure on the tip of the third ventricle by a pituitary tumor. The patient was treated with high dose corticosteroids, and improved markedly over the next several days. The left third nerve palsy practically disappeared and his visual fields returned to normal. He was discharged without medication. Subsequent testing during the next year demonstrated a low protein-bound iodine, low gonadotropins, and low 17-hydroxysteroids, with no response to metopirone. He was placed on maintenance thyroid, cortisone, and testosterone, and has done very well over the past 7 years.

COMMENT.   This patient also presented with headache, nausea, and vomiting, and exhibited extraocular palsies and lethargy. The enlarged sella and abnormal cerebrospinal fluid suggested the diagnosis, and the pituitary tumor was visible on pneumoencephalography. Corticosteroid therapy was also employed and his signs and symptoms resolved. Hypopituitarism was subsequently demonstrated, although it is not clear if this antedated the episode of acute pituitary vascular accident or occurred as a result of it.

Case 3

A 45 year old man presented to the emergency room in February 1973 complaining of 3 days of severe frontal headache, fever, and blurred vision. On examination a temperature of 102°F was noted, as well as a right sixth nerve palsy; he was otherwise normal. Skull x-ray was normal. Lumbar puncture was remarkable for a cell count of 30 red blood cells, 14 lymphocytes, 8 neutrophils, and 1 eosinophil, and was otherwise normal. The impression was meningitis, and the patient was treated with antibiotics. Cerebrospinal fluid cultures showed no growth. He did well, with resolution of the fever and headaches, although the sixth nerve palsy persisted. Because he was incidentally found to have a low serum T_4 the patient was discharged on thyroid medicine. Over the next several months he began feeling weak and losing weight. Outpatient testing revealed low 24 hour urinary 17-hydroxy-steroids with no response to metopirone. Serum testosterone and gonadotropins were low. He was begun on maintenance cortisone and testosterone, and has done well over the past 7 years.

COMMENT.   Headache and visual disturbances were the presenting complaints. On admission the patient was noted to have fever, a sixth nerve palsy, and abnormal CSF. Because of fever he was treated for possible meningitis. There was a good response to medical treatment although corticosteroids were not given. The subsequent demonstration of hypopituitarism, persistent sixth nerve palsy, and sterile cerebrospinal fluid was consistent with acute pituitary vascular accident rather than infection.

Case 4

A 47 year old man presented to the emergency room in December 1976, complaining of 2 days of severe frontal headache, nausea, vomiting, and blurred vision in the left eye. Impotence had been present for many years, and an evaluation done just before admission revealed a serum prolactin level of 450 ng per ml (normal <25) and skull x-rays suggestive of pituitary tumor. Examination revealed a confused patient, mild nuchal rigidity, bitemporal hemianopsia, and left pupil larger than right, with poor reaction to light. Skull x-ray showed an enlarged sella with erosion of the floor. Lumbar puncture was remarkable for xanthochromia. Cerebral angiography showed an intrasellar mass with suprasellar extension. A transsphenoidal hypophysectomy was performed because of progressive deterioration of vision, with removal of hemorrhagic tumor and decompression of the optic nerves. Pathology showed a chromophobe adenoma. Because of dilation of both pupils in the recovery room, a craniotomy was performed, but only generalized arterial spasm was found. Postoperatively, the patient had severely impaired vision bilaterally, and exhibited inappropriate behavior with emotional outbursts. His condition is essentially unchanged over three years. Laboratory testing has revealed panhypopituitarism, and appropriate replacement medication has been given.

COMMENT.   Although this patient's acute symptoms were similar to those of the others, this case differs in several ways: the presence of long-standing secondary impotence (probably related to the pituitary tumor and hyperprolactinemia), the nuchal rigidity, and anisocoria. A surgical approach was taken and a hemorrhagic chromophobe adenoma removed. Despite hypophysectomy and decompression, there was no improvement in mental status or vision (permanent optic nerve injury

had probably occurred before admission). Panhypopituitarism was subsequently demonstrated.

DISCUSSION

Hemorrhagic necrosis of a pituitary gland was first described in a
young, clinically acromegalic patient by Bleibtreu[2] in 1905. His patient
had weakness, headache, dizziness, and insomnia for several weeks;
these symptoms resolved spontaneously after 9 days of hospitalization.
When the patient died nearly one year later from pulmonary hemorrhage
secondary to tuberculosis, the autopsy revealed old hemorrhage of the
pituitary, but no adenoma was found. The naming and characterization
of pituitary apoplexy awaited Brougham et al.[3] in 1950, who reported 5
cases verified by autopsy. Between these dates a number of case histo-
ries were published of patients whose illnesses clearly fit this syndrome.
An observation made by Harvey Cushing in 1925 is of interest because it
evinces his customary ability to remember unusual cases and grasp
their significance:

> Though extensive operations for the removal of tumors such as the congenital
> lesions arising from the relics of Rathke's pouch are occasionally followed by a
> slow train of symptoms with fatality from inanition, I have never but once known
> a clinical case in which the symptoms resembled the experimental cachexia
> hypophyseopriva which is so quickly fatal in animals. This case was that of a
> middle-aged woman who, while in normal health, had a sudden headache which
> was soon followed by stupor, coma, and death in three days . . . Nothing whatso-
> ever was found which could possibly account for the death but a small and
> unsuspected pituitary adenoma. Into this adenoma a spontaneous hemorrhage
> had occurred with complete intracapsular destruction of the gland.[6]

Since 1950, several hundred cases of pituitary apoplexy have been
reported in the literature. The syndrome has been seen in cases of
chromophobe, eosinophilic, basophilic, and mixed cell adenoma, as well
as in meningiomas, malignant tumors, and craniopharyngiomas.[16, 17] A
greater frequency of pituitary apoplexy has been reported in patients
with acromegaly and Cushing's syndrome,[3, 23] but others have found that
"silent" (supposedly nonsecretory) chromophobe adenomas predominate.

Before discussing pathogenesis and clinical presentation, it is useful
to review the pertinent anatomical relationships of the pituitary gland.
These are shown in Figure 1. The pituitary gland rests in the sella
turcica, a cavity of the sphenoid bone. Important contiguous anatomic
landmarks include the sphenoid sinus inferiorly and the diaphragma
sella superiorly; the latter, an extension of the dura mater, serves as a
roof for the sella and separates the gland from neural structures —
including the optic chiasm that lies above. Lateral to the sella are the
cavernous sinuses, which are traversed by portions of the internal
carotid arteries, by the third, fourth, and sixth cranial nerves, and by the
ophthalmic and maxillary divisions of the fifth nerve.

Tumors of the pituitary may not only expand and erode the walls of
the sella, but they may also expand beyond the sella inferiorly into the

sphenoid sinus, laterally into the cavernous sinuses with their contained vascular and neural elements, and superiorly to affect the optic chiasm, third ventricle, and the hypothalamus. Lateral extension can obviously cause dysfunction of the third, fourth, or sixth cranial nerves as well as vascular compression. Suprasellar extension may cause enlargement of the blind spot, a decrease in color vision, and defective vision in the superior temporal visual quadrants which may eventuate in bitemporal hemianopsia.

Brougham et al. considered pituitary apoplexy a consequence of rapid tumor growth, with the tumor outgrowing its blood supply.[3] A more complex etiology was proposed by Rovit et al.[23] They noted that the circulation of the anterior lobe of the pituitary is supplied exclusively by the hypophysial-portal system, comprised of an extensive capillary network originating from the superior and inferior hypophysial vessels in the infundibular stem. They theorized that as the tumor enlarges, it attempts to expand superiorly by squeezing itself through a narrow channel between the hypophysial stalk centrally and the surrounding diaphragma sella. Impaction of the tumor at the diaphragmatic notch may therefore compress the fine complex of vessels lying within the adjacent to hypophysial stalk — thus rendering the anterior lobe (as well as the tumor) ischemic, necrotic, and hemorrhagic.

A number of events have been suggested as possible precipitating factors in the development of an acute pituitary vascular accident, including pituitary irradiation,[29] trauma,[3] upper respiratory infection with coughing and sneezing,[9] mechanical respirators,[7] atheromatous emboli,[26] and even the administration of chlorpromazine.[25] In many cases, however, there is no clear precipitating factor. A number of cases have been reported in which the acute episode was the first evidence of pituitary neoplasm.[23]

Clinical Presentation

Common signs and symptoms of an acute pituitary vascular accident fall into six major groupings: (1) headache; (2) visual apparatus disturbances, including diplopia, blurred vision, decreased visual acuity, extraocular muscle weakness or paralysis, and pupillary abnormalities; (3) changes in sensorium featuring lethargy, drowsiness, and altered consciousness; (4) nausea and vomiting; (5) nuchal rigidity; (6) hyperpyrexia.

The onset of pituitary apoplexy may be devastating or insidious. In patients who retain consciousness, headache is a universal symptom.[4] The headache is usually severe and may be of lightning-like onset. It is occasionally generalized but more frequently is retro-orbital or periorbital in location, and may be unilateral at onset, becoming generalized in a brief period of time. Subarachnoid hemorrhage need not accompany the headache. Also, headache need not signify extrasellar extension of the tumor. The mechanism of headache may be due to irritation and stretching of the dura mater, distention of the walls of the sella turcica, or irritation of the upper division of the fifth cranial nerve in the cavernous sinus.[30]

Visual blurring, visual field defects, and varieties of blindness signify involvement of the optic nerves, chiasm, or tracts.[10] Optic atrophy may also be noted. The visual apparatus may suffer the effects of compression or irritation without direct tumor involvement.[4] In nearly all patients who remain conscious, complaints of diplopia accompany those of headache. The nerves to the extraocular muscles (III, IV, VI) occupy a vulnerable position in the cavernous sinus, whose medial walls form the lateral boundary of the pituitary fossa (Fig. 1), and are impaired as this boundary shifts laterally owing to sudden increases in tumor size that accompany acute hemorrhage or necrosis. As with involvement of vision, the presence of extraocular muscle paralysis in pituitary apoplexy is not necessarily evidence of extrasellar tumor extension. If the third cranial nerves are impaired in the process, pupillary enlargement and ptosis will occur. Findings of facial sensory impairment may arise on the same basis.

An altered level of consciousness has been reported to be the most frequent neurologic abnormality.[3] The mechanism is not entirely clear but may be related to subarachnoid hemorrhage, compression of hypothalamic structures, raised intracranial pressure from obstructive hydrocephalus, or an attack of acute adrenal insufficiency accompanied by hypotension and hypoglycemia.

Nausea and vomiting may be related to meningeal irritation, hypothalamic dysfunction, or increased intracranial pressure.[3] Nuchal rigidity may be seen in pituitary apoplexy, possibly secondary to subarachnoid hemorrhage.[14] Hemiplegia and aphasia have also been documented.[3] These are usually attributed to involvement of the internal carotid artery. Hyperpyrexia resulting from hypothalamic involvement may be seen.

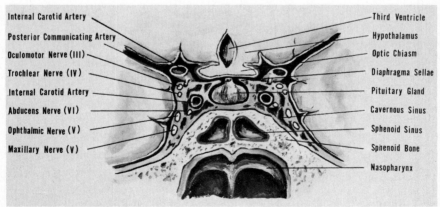

Figure 1.   Pituitary gland anatomical relationships shown in frontal section through the cavernous sinuses. Lateral extension of pituitary contents produced by an acute pituitary vascular accident may compress the internal carotid arteries and cranial nerves 3 through 6; suprasellar extension may compress the optic chiasm, third ventricle, and hypothalamus; and inferior extension may erode into the sphenoid sinus. These patterns of extrasellar extension produce some of the common symptoms and signs associated with an acute pituitary vascular accident.

Cases have also been reported of inappropriate antidiuretic hormone secretion[4] and diabetes insipidus[11] with an acute pituitary vascular accident. These are uncommon complications.

Cerebrospinal Fluid

The cerebrospinal fluid is usually abnormal. If the acute pituitary vascular accident is caused by hemorrhage, the cerebrospinal fluid may be frankly blood-stained or xanthochromic. An excess of white and red blood cells may be seen. Both the protein content and the pressure may be raised.[10] Cerebrospinal fluid pressure is frequently elevated even in the absence of hemorrhage, cerebrospinal fluid pleocytosis, or extrasellar tumor extension. The pathogenesis of this change is unknown, but it may contribute to aspects of the clinical picture such as stupor, confusion, headache, nausea, and vomiting.

Differential Diagnosis

The clinical presentation of a ruptured cerebral aneurysm may be similar to that of an acute pituitary vascular accident. A useful differentiating point: ruptured aneurysms usually produce unilateral oculomotor deficits, while bilateral deficits are associated more commonly with an acute pituitary vascular accident.[18]

Other conditions that may mimic an acute pituitary vascular accident include brain abscess, bacterial meningitis, viral meningoencephalitis, primary intracerebral hemorrhage, cerebrovascular accidents, transtentorial herniation, mesencephalic infarction, and degenerative encephalopathies involving the diencephalon and midbrain.

Skull x-rays will usually show enlargement or erosion of the sella. There are, however, reports of pituitary apoplexy with normal sellae on plain films.[23] Cerebral angiography, pneumoencephalography, and computed tomography may be very helpful in differential diagnosis and evaluation.

Pituitary Function After an Acute Pituitary Vascular Accident

The effect of an acute pituitary vascular accident on pituitary function varies with its location and extent. As can be surmised from Figure 2, which shows normal hypothalamic pituitary relationships, the acute pituitary vascular accident can prevent secretion of hypothalamic releasing hormones, obstruct portal vascular flow, destroy secretory pituitary cells, or do all of these things simultaneously. One detailed study by Pelkonen et al.[19] considered the effects of acute pituitary vascular accident in 9 patients who recovered spontaneously. Four patients had acromegaly, 2 had Cushing's disease, and 3 had "silent" pituitary adenomas. In the 4 patients with acromegaly all had transient or persistent hypogonadotropic hypogonadism. All had poor TSH responses to TRH infusion, although only one was clinically hypothyroid. Two patients developed adrenal insufficiency (hypocortisolism). Also, 3 of the 4 patients were clinically and biochemically "cured" of their acromegaly.

Of the two patients with Cushing's disease, one was "cured" (but developed hypocortisolism) while the other developed excessive ACTH secretion and hyperpigmentation. The other anterior pituitary functions were not substantially altered.

Of the three patients with "silent" pituitary adenomas all had low serum gonadotropin levels initially. Two patients had a low free T_4 index, but were clinically euthyroid. Low serum cortisol was found in one patient, and growth hormone deficiency in two.

An important recent review by Veldhuis and Hammond[28] summarized the literature on endocrine function after pituitary apoplexy. These authors found multiple deficits in anterior pituitary function occurring in neurosurgically proven pituitary apoplexy associated with pituitary tumors. They found that 88 per cent of the patients who were tested had hGH deficiency. Diminished cortisol, ACTH, or compound S secretion occurred in 66 per cent of patients after appropriate stimuli. Diminished thyroid function was present in 42 per cent of cases. Diminished sex steroids occurred in 85 per cent of patients, and diminished LH and FSH secretion in 76 and 58 per cent, respectively (although the data were limited). Of the 4 patients in whom prolactin was investigated, 2 had hyperprolactinemia, and 2 diminished prolactin reserve. Impaired water homeostasis was found to be uncommon: transient diabetes

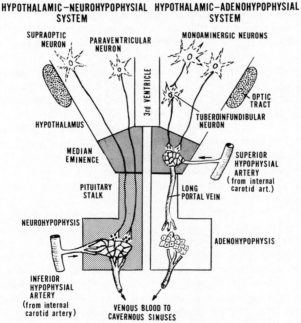

Figure 2. Pituitary gland physiological relationships, schematically showing hypothalamic-neurohypophysial and hypothalamic-adenohypophysial systems. Depending upon its location, an acute pituitary vascular accident may prevent secretion of hypothalamic releasing hormones, obstruct portal vascular flow, prevent attachment of releasing hormones to pituitary receptor sites, or destroy secretory pituitary cells. Transitory or permanent deficiency of one or more pituitary hormones (particularly of the anterior pituitary) may result.

insipidus occurred in 4 per cent, diabetes insipidus in 2 per cent, and the syndrome of inappropriate ADH secretion even more rarely.[33] In addition, Veldhuis and Hammond noted a surprisingly high frequency of apparent hypothalamic dysfunction (inferred from basal deficiency of several adenohypophyseal hormones coupled with preserved responsivity of hormone secretion to hypothalamic releasing factors). Vascular injury of hypothalamic control centers — or possible disruption of normal portal delivery of endogenous hypothalamic hormones to surviving pituitary cells — may have produced this picture of apparent post-apoplexy hypothalamic dysfunction.

It should be noted that the above statistics describing endocrine dysfunction after an acute pituitary vascular accident do not necessarily imply cause and effect. Some of the hormonal deficiencies may have antedated the acute pituitary vascular accident, as they may have been due to effects of the tumor itself.

Autocure of acromegaly after pituitary apoplexy has been noted in a number of cases.[23, 22, 15] In addition, an acute pituitary vascular accident has been followed by complete anterior pituitary insufficiency in some cases,[24, 27] partial pituitary insufficiency in other cases,[13] and only growth hormone deficiency in others.[22]

Treatment

The acute management of pituitary apoplexy — particularly the question of surgical intervention — has been a matter of controversy. Epstein et al.[10] advocated an aggressive neurosurgical approach, particularly if visual loss or neurologic sequelae were present. Their series of 5 patients underwent craniotomies. More recently, transsphenoidal puncture and aspiration under x-ray guidance[1, 33] have been advocated. Aspiration of hemorrhagic fluid has led to dramatic reversal of signs and symptoms in some cases. Also, decompressive surgery via a transsphenoidal approach has been used successfully. However, there have been a number of reports of good neurologic and endocrinologic recovery without surgical treatment in patients with clinically severe disease.[16, 19, 32] One recent set of guidelines proposes deterioration in level of consciousness, visual fields, or visual acuity as indications for surgery, while noting that other focal signs, e.g., ophthalmoplegia, often recover spontaneously.[16] Whether neurosurgery is contemplated or not, it is mandatory that all patients with an acute pituitary vascular accident be treated with corticosteroids, both to protect against secondary adrenal insufficiency and to decrease cerebral edema. The dose should be approximately 100 mg hydrocortisone given intravenously every 6 hours for the first 48 hours, followed by tapering to an oral maintenance dose as the patient's condition warrants. The frequent use of corticosteroids for all types of neurosurgical emergencies is probably one of the reasons mortality from pituitary apoplexy has decreased. Another probable reason for improved survival statistics is the inclusion of milder cases, based on greater awareness of diagnostic signs and symptoms.

After the acute episode it is important to keep in mind the long-term consequences of an acute pituitary vascular accident. Pituitary hormonal deficiencies are common, as discussed above. Therefore, appropriate testing for anterior pituitary hormones should be done, and replacement given for documented deficiencies.

Radiation therapy has little role after an acute pituitary vascular accident episode: pituitary tumors that have undergone acute necrosis respond poorly to radiotherapy.[20] Furthermore, since radiation therapy has been implicated in the etiology of some cases of pituitary apoplexy, it is regarded by some as absolutely contraindicated in such cases.

SUMMARY

1. An acute pituitary vascular accident, or pituitary apoplexy, refers to the neuroendocrine emergency produced by sudden infarction or hemorrhage of the pituitary gland — usually one that is adenomatous.

2. Once considered rare and universally fatal it is now recognized more frequently (in part because milder cases which were previously missed are now being diagnosed), and is considered treatable in most instances.

3. Common signs and symptoms of acute pituitary vascular accident include headache, visual disturbances, changes in sensorium, nausea and vomiting, nuchal rigidity, and hyperpyrexia.

4. An enlarged or eroded sella turcica on skull x-ray or an abnormal cerebrospinal fluid may be clues to the diagnosis.

5. Deficiencies of anterior pituitary hormone secretion after an acute pituitary vascular accident are common. In decreasing frequency they include: growth hormone, gonadotropins, ACTH, and TSH. Posterior pituitary function is nearly always preserved.

6. Management may require neurosurgery (either craniotomy or transsphenoidal approach) or transsphenoidal aspiration, but many patients do well without surgery. All patients should receive corticosteroid therapy.

REFERENCES

1. Berte, G., Heisy, W. G., and Dohn, D. F.: Pituitary apoplexy treated by stereotactic transsphenoidal aspiration. Cleve. Clinic Quart., 41:163–175, 1974.
2. Bleibtreu, L.: Ein Fall von Akromegalie. Munch. Med. Wschr., 52:2079–2080, 1905.
3. Brougham, M., Heusner, A. P., and Adams, R. D.: Acute degenerative changes in adenomas of the pituitary body with special reference to pituitary apoplexy. J. Neurosurg., 7:421–439, 1950.
4. Conomy, J. P., Ferguson, J. H., Brodkey, J. H., et al.: Spontaneous infarction in pituitary tumors: Neurologic and therapeutic aspects. Neurology, 25:580–587, 1975.
5. Cooperman, D., and Malarkey, W. B.: Pituitary apoplexy. Heart and Lung, 7:450–454, 1978.
6. Cushing, H.: The pituitary gland as now known. Lancet, 2:899–906, 1925.
7. Daniel, P. M., Spicer, E. J., and Treip, C. S.: Pituitary necrosis in patients maintained on mechanical respirators. J. Path., 3:135–138, 1973.
8. David, M.: Les formes hemorragiques des adenomes hypophysaires: Aspects cliniques et etiologiques. Presse Med., 77:1887–1891, 1969.
9. Dawson, B. H., and Kothandaram, P.: Acute massive infarction of pituitary adenomas. J. Neurosurgery, 37:275–278, 1972.

10. Epstein, S., Pimstone, B. L., de Villiers, J. C., et al.: Pituitary apoplexy in five patients with pituitary tumors. Brit. Med. J., *1*:267–270, 1971.
11. Gebel, P.: Pituitary apoplexy: Review of the literature with a report of an unusual case associated with diabetes insipidus. Milit. Med., *127*:753–760, 1962.
12. Gurling, K. J.: Diabetic coma and pituitary necrosis in an acromegalic patient. Diabetes, *4*:138–140, 1955.
13. Jacobi, J. D., Lawrence, M. F., and Daroff, R. B.: Pituitary apoplexy in acromegaly followed by partial pituitary insufficiency. Arch. Intern. Med., *134*:559–561, 1974.
14. Jefferson, M., and Rosenthal, F. D.: Spontaneous necrosis in pituitary tumors. Lancet, *1*:342–344, 1959.
15. Lawrence, A. M., Gordon, D. L., Hagen, T. C., et al.: Hypothalamic hypopituitarism after pituitary apoplexy in acromegaly. Arch. Intern. Med., *137*:1134–1137, 1977.
16. Lloyd, M. H., Belchetz, P. E.: The clinical features and management of pituitary apoplexy. Postgrad. Med. J., *53*:82–85, 1977.
17. Lopez, I. A.: Pituitary apoplexy. J. Oslo City Hosp., *20*:17–27, 1970.
18. Nourizadeh, A. R., and Pitts, F. W.: Hemorrhage into pituitary adenoma during anticoagulant therapy. J.A.M.A., *193*:623–25, 1965.
19. Pelkonen, R., Kuusisto, A., Salmi, J., et al.: Pituitary function after pituitary apoplexy. Amer. J. Med., *65*:773–778, 1978.
20. Pennybacker, J.: The treatment of pituitary tumors. Proc. Roy. Soc. Med., *54*:619–621, 1961.
21. Perpetrio, F.: Apoplexia hypofisaria apos pneumencefalograma. Arq. Neuropsiquiatr., *34*:298–300, 1976.
22. Rigolosi, R. S., Schwartz, E., and Glick, S. M.: Occurrence of growth hormone deficiency in acromegaly as a result of pituitary apoplexy. New Engl. J. Med., *279*:362–364, 1968.
23. Rovit, R. L., and Fein, J. M.: Pituitary apoplexy: A review and reappraisal. J. Neurosurgery, *37*:280–286, 1972.
24. Ruiz, A. E., Mazzaferri, E. L., and Skillman, T. F.: Silent reversal of acromegaly: Pituitary apoplexy resulting in panhypopituitarism. Ohio State Med. J., *65*:1017–1020, 1969.
25. Silverman, V. E., Boyd, A. E., McGrary, J. A., et al.: Pituitary apoplexy following chlorpromazine stimulation. Arch. Intern. Med., *138*:1783–1784, 1978.
26. Sussman, E. B., and Porro, R. S.: Pituitary apoplexy: The role of atheromatous emboli. Stroke, *5*:318–323, 1974.
27. Taylor, A. L., Finster, J. L., Raskin, P., et al.: Pituitary apoplexy in acromegaly. J. Clin. Endocrinol. Metabol., *28*:1784–1792, 1968.
28. Veldhuis, J. D., and Hammond, J. M.: Endocrine function after spontaneous infarction of the human pituitary: Report, review, and reappraisal. Endo. Reviews, *1*:100–107, 1980.
29. Weisberg, L. A.: Pituitary apoplexy: association of degenerative change in pituitary adenoma with radiotherapy and detection by cerebral computed tomography. Amer. J. Med., *63*:109–115, 1977.
30. Werth, F. P., VanBuren, J. M.: Referral of pain from dural stimulation in man. J. Neurosurg., *34*:630–642, 1971.
31. Williams, F. W.: Pituitary necrosis in a diabetic during pregnancy. Diabetes, *1*:37–40, 1962.
32. Wright, R. L., and Ojemann, R. G., and Dreq, J. H.: Hemorrhage into pituitary adenomata. Arch. Neurol., *12*:326–331, 1971.
33. Zervas, N. T., and Mendelson, G.: Treatment of acute hemorrhage of pituitary tumors. Lancet, *1*:604–605, 1975.

Queens Hospital Center Affiliation
Long Island Jewish-Hillside Medical Center
82-68 164th Street
Jamaica, New York 11432

Diabetic Ketoacidosis and Coma

Selim Baruh, M.D.,* Lawrence Sherman, M.D.,†
and Sheldon Markowitz, M.D.‡

Diabetic ketoacidosis can present with a wide range of altered sensorium, from quasi-normal consciousness to deep coma. It has been the custom of the Joslin Clinic[4] and others[7] to classify any case of diabetic ketoacidosis as one of "diabetic coma" when the plasma bicarbonate (HCO_3^-) concentration is 9 mEq per liter or less, regardless of the degree of sensorium alteration. A HCO_3^- below 9 mEq per liter, and perhaps more specifically a pH less than 7.1, is only one of the clinical and laboratory findings that imply poor prognosis. Others are extreme hyperglycemia and hyperosmolality, extreme total body water and electrolyte depletion, and cardiovascular collapse.

Ketoacidosis was the main cause of death in diabetes before the discovery and use of insulin in the early 1920's. The decrease in overall mortality from diabetic coma among all Joslin Clinic patients, during the pre-insulin and insulin periods, is eloquently illustrated in Figure 1.[4] However, among patients treated for diabetic ketoacidosis and coma in the insulin period, the mortality rate still varies roughly from 5 to 15 per cent according to the series.[4] The persistence of such a substantial mortality rate stresses the continuing importance of diabetic coma and the vigilance required during therapy not only towards the ketoacidosis per se and its complications, but also toward the causes that precipitate it, such as infections, sepsis, myocardial infarction, thyroid storm, and immunologic insulin resistance. Noteworthy and encouraging are two recent small series (69 cases) with zero mortality.[6, 14]

*Physician-in-Charge, Diabetes, Queens Hospital Center Affiliation, Long Island Jewish-Hillside Medical Center; Assistant Professor of Medicine, School of Medicine, State University of New York at Stony Brook

†Associate Director of Medicine, Queens Hospital Center Affiliation, Long Island Jewish-Hillside Medical Center; Professor of Medicine, School of Medicine, State University of New York at Stony Brook.

‡Fellow in Endocrinology, Queens Hospital Center Affiliation, Long Island Jewish-Hillside Medical Center

Supported in part by an internal research grant (#3-347) from the Long Island Jewish-Hillside Medical Center.

118   SELIM BARUH, LAWRENCE SHERMAN AND SHELDON MARKOWITZ

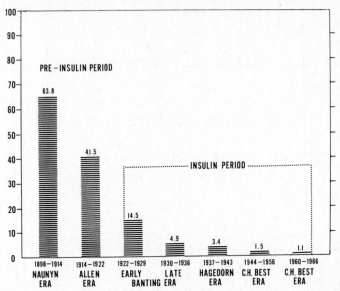

Figure 1.   Percentage of deaths due to diabetic coma among Joslin Clinic patients. (*From*
Bradley, R. F.: Diabetic Ketoacidosis and Coma. In Marble, A., White, P., Bradley, R. F., and
Krall, L. P., eds.: Joslin's Diabetes Mellitus. Philadelphia, Lea & Febiger, 1971, pp. 361–416.
Reproduced by permission).

PATHOGENESIS

Diabetic ketoacidosis, defined as a plasma concentration of total
ketoacids in excess of 3 mM per liter (Nl: 0.15 mM per liter),[20] results
mainly from a relative or absolute shortage of insulin. It is much more
common in insulin-dependent diabetes mellitus, characterized by an
almost total lack of insulin secretion, than in non–insulin dependent
diabetes mellitus, which is usually characterized by a delayed release of
insulin in response to glucose stimulation

It has been suggested that a second prerequisite for the development
of the ketotic state is the concomitant excess secretion of insulin-
counter-regulatory hormones (such as glucagon, catecholamines, cortisol and growth hormone) in response to stress.[23] In other words, diabetic
ketoacidosis would be induced by a marked decrease in the physiologic
ratio of insulin to counterregulatory hormones, whatever the cause. A
large body of literature emphasizing the presumptive role of each hormone in the production of diabetic ketoacidosis has been reviewed and
summarized by Schade and Eaton.[23]

Among the counterregulatory hormones, glucagon shows an excessive increase in plasma levels and has been the object of thorough
investigation. McGarry and Foster[16] have postulated that while the lack
of insulin results primarily in lipolysis at the periphery, thus supplying
the liver with an excess of free fatty acids, glucagon exerts its main
action on the liver by increasing the capacity for fatty acid oxidation
(ketogenic liver) which facilitates ketone body formation. Clinical studies[9] have shown that somatostatin — a potent inhibitor of glucagon

release — can prevent or delay diabetic ketoacidosis in man; this observation supports the role of glucagon in regulating ketogenic potentials.

It would be a mistake, however, to minimize the role of insulin deficiency in the development of ketoacidosis. The "preponderant role of insulin lack" is corroborated by studies in pancreatectomized patients, in whom, despite the absence of glucagon, hyperglycemia and ketosis can develop, though at a slow rate.[2] Furthermore, ketoacidosis has not been reported in cases of glucagonoma presenting with the highest plasma levels of glucagon (above 1,000 pg per ml), unless there is a concomitant deficiency of insulin. It is indeed not difficult to explain the whole picture of diabetic ketoacidosis through the pathophysiologic dynamics of lack of insulin, i.e., stimulation of lipolysis, proteolysis, and gluconeogenesis, coupled with inhibition of glycolysis and of fatty acid and glycogen synthesis. What then is the specific additional role of increased glucagon?

Hepatic ketogenesis has been extensively studied and revised during the last decade by McGarry and Foster.[17] They have tried to elucidate the exact site of action of glucagon in relation to insulin, and to clarify how and where the hormonal signals were translated into biochemical events. The sequence of events can be summarized as follows (Figs. 2 and 3):

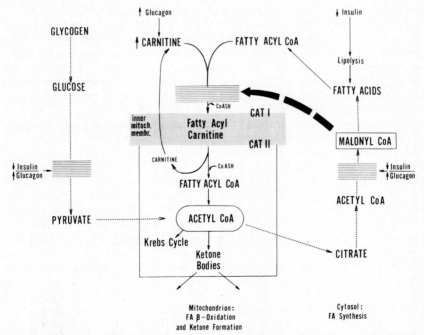

Figure 2. Ketogenesis. Interrelations between the pathways of fatty acid synthesis and oxidation in liver, and their dependence on the presence or absence of glycogen stores and glycolysis. The dotted-line-arrows and the thick broken-line arrow indicate the pathways inhibiting ketogenesis and favoring fatty acid synthesis. The full-line-arrows indicate the pathways stimulating ketogenesis, after depletion of glycogen stores. CAT I and CAT II, Carnitine acyltransferase enzymes I and II. (Modified from McGarry, J. D.: New perspectives in the regulation of ketogenesis. (Lilly Lecture, 1978), Diabetes, 28:517–523, 1979, by permission of the American Diabetes Association, Inc.).

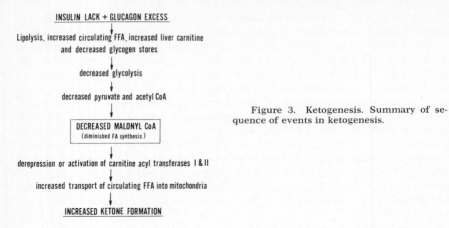

Figure 3.   Ketogenesis. Summary of sequence of events in ketogenesis.

1. Glucagon increases ketogenic activity in isolated liver preparations by increasing the level of cytoplasmic carnitine concentration. Carnitine (L-3-OH-4 trimethyl ammonium butyrate), like fatty acyl CoA, is a substrate for the enzymes carnitine acyltransferase I and II which transport FFA from the cytosol into the mitochondria where they are oxidized. Its increase raises the potential activity of these enzymes.

2. However, the ketogenic liver so produced cannot form ketones as long as glycogen stores are present to provide the means for glycolysis and fatty acid synthesis to continue, even if circulating fatty acids have been increased artificially. On the other hand, there will be ketone formation in conditions leading to glycogen depletion and lipolysis, such as starvation and clinical or experimental diabetic ketoacidosis, both accompanied by a low insulin/glucagon ratio.

3. It became obvious that the two opposing metabolic pathways, fatty acid synthesis and fatty acid degradation cannot be simultaneously active. A step by step search for the "carbohydrate key" to the control of fatty acid oxidation and ketogenesis revealed that *malonyl CoA,* first committed intermediate in the conversion of glucose into fat via acetyl CoA, is the magic metabolic switch: increased malonyl CoA (from increased glycolysis) has been shown to be the most potent inhibitor of the enzyme carnitine acyltransferase at the mitochondrial membrane. Conversely a decreased level of malonyl CoA (decreased glycolysis) activates the enzyme and leads to fatty acid transport and oxidation. Once in the mitochondrion, the rate of ketogenesis is determined in first order fashion by the rate of delivery of free fatty acids to the liver. Like insulin lack, glucagon might also suppress glycolysis and fatty acid synthesis at the pyruvate kinase and acetyl CoA carboxylase steps.

It is, therefore, very likely that in diabetic ketoacidosis "insulin-lack" and "increased glucagon" — and possibly increase of the other counter-regulatory hormones — team up to generate an *overproduction of ketones.* An additional factor which accentuates the already excessive ketonemia is also the peripheral *underutilization of ketones* attributed to insulin deficiency.[26]

With respect to hyperglycemia, the following question still has no satisfactory answer: Why is hyperglycemia in ketoacidosis usually lower than in hyperglycemic hyperosmolar nonketotic coma? While glucagon levels are known to be similarly high in both conditions, we might expect the highest concentrations of glucose to occur in ketoacidosis, when insulin is most deficient.

First, we must recognize that in ketoacidosis in the elderly it is not uncommon to see very high blood sugar levels, sometimes reaching the levels encountered in hyperosmolar hyperglycemic nonketotic coma. In contrast to the rapid occurrence of ketoacidosis in type I insulin-dependent diabetics, the protracted clinical course of these two syndromes in the elderly results in very marked dehydration — more so in hyperosmolar hyperglycemic nonketotic coma—and this in itself may account for the extreme hyperglycemia.[10] Two more possibilities may play an important role in this apparent discrepancy:

1. In diabetic ketoacidosis, unlike hyperosmolar hyperglycemic nonketotic coma, lipolysis and the overwhelming oxidative breakdown of fatty acids in the liver markedly decrease the NAD/NADH* ratio (oxidative redox potential); this, in turn, as in alcohol-induced hypoglycemia,[3] would inhibit the various NAD-dependent paths of gluconeogenesis and decrease hepatic glucose output.

Nevertheless, alanine, the most important substrate for glyconeogenesis is not fully NAD-dependent, and may in part be converted to pyruvate by a transaminase; pyruvate is then easily converted to glucose through the NADH-dependent enzyme glyceraldehyde-3-P-dehydrogenase.

2. Sherwin et al.,[25, 26] have observed a marked decline in plasma concentrations of alanine and glucose following infusion of β-hydroxybutyrate in normal as well as diabetic subjects. In other words, ketones can limit substrate availability for gluconeogenesis and reduce hepatic glucose output. A similar role has been suggested for ketones in prolonged starvation.[25]

It seems reasonable, therefore, to assume that a decrease in NAD/NADH ratio and a decrease in alanine availability to the liver may act together to limit gluconeogenesis and hepatic glucose output in diabetic ketoacidosis. This may explain why hyperglycemia in diabetic ketoacidosis is relatively of lower magnitude than in hyperosmolar hyperglycemic nonketotic coma, in spite of the greater deficiency of insulin in the former.

CLINICAL EVALUATION

IMPORTANT PRECIPITATING FACTORS.   Omission of the daily injection of insulin is a major factor in precipitating diabetic ketoacidosis in patients with insulin dependent diabetes mellitus. A second broad factor in patients with insulin-dependent and non-insulin dependent diabetes

---

*NAD (or DPN) = nicotinamide adenine dinucleotide (hydrogen acceptor); NADH is its reduced form (hydrogen donor).

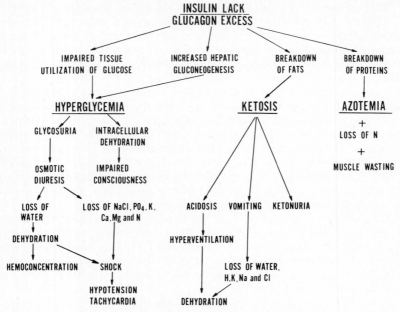

Figure 4.   Metabolic consequences of insulin lack, accelerated by glucagon excess.

mellitus is stress, whatever its nature, including infections, cerebrovascular and cardiovascular events, pancreatitis, pregnancy, trauma, and hyperthyroidism. The most common stressfull trigger is infection, viral or bacterial. The site of infection may be skin, pulmonary tract, urinary tract, abdominal, meningeal, etc. In a good number of cases, however, etiology remains obscure; in Genuth's[8] experience these cases may constitute 35 per cent of all patients with diabetic ketoacidosis.

PROMINENT SYMPTOMS AND SIGNS. Polyuria, polydipsia, fatigue, weight loss, vomiting, and abdominal pain (which can mimic an acute surgical abdomen), Kussmaul breathing (a compensatory rapid and deep breathing when blood pH is below 7.2; it ceases and becomes shallow when a very low pH depresses the respiratory center), water and electrolyte depletion, dehydration (dry skin, sunken soft eyeballs), lethargy, circulatory collapse, and coma (Fig. 4).

LABORATORY FINDINGS. Hyperglycemia (usually 200 to 800 mg per dl), ketonemia (increased beta-hydroxybutyric acid, acetoacetic acid and acetone), decreased pH, HCO_3^-, and $PaCO_2$, more than 2 per cent glycosuria and large ketonuria (may be less in cases with seriously jeopardized glomerular filtration secondary to circulatory collapse or advanced glomerulosclerosis), azotemia caused by increased protein breakdown and diminished renal clearance, hyperuricemia because of diminished competitive urate clearance, increased serum free fatty acids and triglycerides because of accelerated lipolysis in adipose tissue and increased production of triglycerides and very low density lipoproteins in the liver.

SERUM AMYLASE. Acute pancreatitis has often been mentioned as one of the causes of diabetic ketoacidosis, and there is recent autopsy documentation of such cases.[18] Nevertheless, serum amylase can reach very high levels in uncomplicated diabetic ketoacidosis, and is usually accompanied, as in acute pancreatitis, by an unusually high amylase/creatinine clearance ratio.[15] The reason for hyperamylasemia in diabetic ketoacidosis is not clear. Even in patients presenting with abdominal pain and vomiting the clinical impression of acute pancreatitis has been invalidated by autopsy findings.[5] Besides, most of the time, the prompt improvement of abdominal symptoms following a few hours of adequate treatment militates against the initial impression. Neither has the type of amylase shown a consistent isoenzyme pattern. It can be of "pancreatic," "salivary," or "mixed pancreatic and salivary" type.[27] Serum lipase determination could eventually be more helpful than amylase.

The origin of the abdominal pain is obscure; it has been attributed to various processes, such as gastric atony, gastritis, distention of the hepatic capsule, peritoneal dehydration, or rarely, an acute primary intra-abdominal problem which could have precipitated diabetic ketoacidosis. It is, therefore, of vital importance to allow about 4 to 6 hours for energetic correction of the metabolic imbalance before venturing into any surgical intervention in an otherwise very poor risk patient. By then the abdominal symptoms would subside, unless they are due to a primary acute abdomen.

DIFFERENTIAL DIAGNOSIS. The metabolic emergency states that may present some clinical similarities to diabetic ketoacidosis are listed in Table 1 with emphasis on their most relevant laboratory and clinical features.

OUTLINE OF THERAPY

1. FLOW SHEET. Perhaps the most important way to avoid confusion during treatment and make therapeutic adjustments is to record on a comprehensive flow sheet the date and time, clinical state, hourly plasma and urine glucose and ketones, pH, HCO_3 and electrolytes, intake-output, therapy, and so forth.

2. INSULIN. Needless to say, only short-acting insulin should be used.

A. *High-Dose Insulin.* This has been the conventional way of treating diabetic ketoacidosis for more than five decades. First dose: half subcutaneous, half intravenous bolus. Average total dose used: first 3 hours more than 200 units, first 24 hours 300 to 500 units or more. The amount of plasma ketone bodies was empirically used to determine the dosage of insulin.

B. *Low-Dose Insulin.* Reported first from England,[1, 20] Scotland,[24] and Australia,[13] the treatment of diabetic ketoacidosis with low-dose insulin (5 to 10 units per hour) has been tested and investigated since 1973, and its efficacy, compared to that of high-dose insulin treatment, has been confirmed by Kitabchi et al.[14] (Fig. 5).

Table 1. *Diabetic Ketoacidosis and Coma: Differential Diagnosis*

	ACUTE, INSULIN HYPOGLYCEMIA	DIABETIC KETOACIDOSIS	HYPEROSMOLAR HYPERGLYCEMIC NONKETOTIC	ALCOHOLIC KETOACIDOSIS	LACTIC ACIDOSIS
LABORATORY FINDINGS					
Plasma glucose	< 40–50 mg/dl	200–800 mg/dl	800–2500 mg/dl	Low, normal or high	Normal*
Urine glucose	Negative, may be +	4 +	4 +	Negative, may be pos.	Negative*
Plasma acetone	Negative	Large	Negative**	Positive, may be neg.#	Usually negative #
Plasma HCO_3	Normal	Low	Normal***	Low	Low
Blood Pco_2	Normal	Low	Normal***	Low	Low
Blood pH	Normal	Low	Normal***	Low or High ##	Low
Anion gap	Normal	Increased: Ketones (+ L.Ac.)	Normal	Increased: B-OHB + L.Ac.	Increased: L.Ac. (+ B-OHB)
SYMPTOMS AND SIGNS	Anxiety; Palpitations; Inner tremor; Dilated pupils; Bizarre behavior; Blurred vision; Hunger	Blurred vision; Anorexia; Polyuria; Polydipsia; Abdominal pain; Vomiting; Kussmaul Resp.	Blurred vision; Anorexia; Polyuria; Polydipsia	May have symptoms of hypoglycemia; Abdominal pain; Vomiting; Kussmaul Resp. may be present (often primary hyperventilation)	Vary according to primary disease; Kussmaul Resp.

Sweating	Dehydration	Dehydration (most severe)	Dehydration ±	Dehydration ±
Moist skin	Dry skin	Dry skin	Dry skin ±	Dry skin ±
DTR's brisk	Sunken soft eyeballs	Sunken soft eyeballs		
Neuro. focal signs, paresis, paralysis, tonic spasms, etc.	DTR's depressed	DTR's may vary with symptoms		
Convulsions		Neuro. focal signs, paresis, paralysis, tonic spasms, etc.		
		Convulsions	Convulsions may occur Shakes or DT's may be present or follow	
Stupor	Stupor	Stupor	Stupor	Stupor
Coma	Coma	Coma	Coma	Coma
HISTORY OF				
Previous episodes of Hypoglycemia, Insulin & Alcohol abuse	Previous episodes of DKA	In elderly NIDDM, or previously unknown diabetics	Chronic alcoholism, recurrent pancreatitis, previous episodes of alcoholic ketoacidosis	May be combined with DKA (Fatty Acid Oxidation), may be idiopathic (?), or secondary to: Hypoxia, shock, sepsis, tissue hypoperfusion, liver disease, glycogenosis, leukemia, lymphomas, alcohol, Phenformin, isoniazide, streptozotocin.

*May be elevated when lactic acidosis occurs in a diabetic patient.
**May be present in cases of HHNKC mixed with KA.
***May be moderately decreased in cases of HHNKC mixed with KA.
#Because of a markedly decreased NAD/NADH ratio most of the Aceto Acetate is reduced to b-Hydroxybutyrate which does not react with the reagent Na Nitroprusside.
##High pH with low Pco_2 and low HCO_3 is due to primary hyperventilation.
L.Ac. = Lactic Acid, B-OHB = B-Hydroxybutyrate, NIDDM = NonInsulin-Dependent Diabetes Mellitus

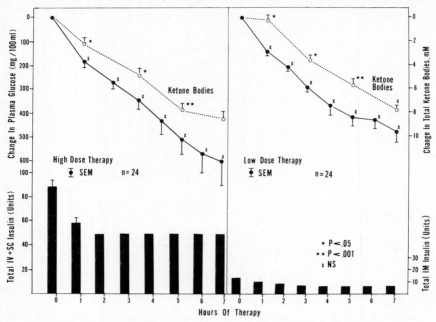

Figure 5.   Effect of insulin and fall in glucose and ketone bodies in ketoacidotic patients treated with high- and low-dose insulin. (*From* Kitabchi, A. E., Ayyagari, V., Guerra, S. M. O., and the Medical House Staff: The efficacy of low-dose versus conventional therapy of insulin for treatment of diabetic ketoacidosis. Ann. Intern. Med., 84:633–638, 1976. Reproduced by permission.)

A study comparing the effectiveness of three various routes of administration of low-dose insulin — continuous intravenous infusion, hourly intramuscular, hourly subcutaneous — showed similarly satisfactory results in lowering blood sugar and ketone bodies to reasonable levels within 6 to 8 hours[6] (Fig. 6). An objection may be raised against the intramuscular and subcutaneous routes in severely dehydrated, hypotensive patients with poor perfusion and poor absorption of the injected insulin. Also, in these patients insulin can accumulate in the tissue and cause late hypoglycemia, especially if it is administered in high doses.

The ideal way appears to be the *continuous intravenous infusion* of a small dose of insulin through an infusion pump or through a pediatric drip set. An objection to insulin administration through a continuous intravenous infusion was that insulin adheres to glassware and plastic tubing, and that this would unpredictably decrease the amount of insulin reaching the circulation. The magnitude of insulin loss, from 20 to 75 per cent, varies with many factors including the concentration of insulin and the duration of the intravenous infusion drip.[21, 28] To decrease insulin loss, human serum albumin can be added into the infusion bottle to form a 1 per cent solution (5 gm in 500 ml); this carries a risk, though very small, of hepatitis. In studies carried out with and without addition of albumin, the results of low-dose insulin infusion proved to be similarly successful despite the loss of some insulin, suggesting that addition of albumin to the infusion is not necessary.[20] For example, if we mix 50 units of insulin within 500 ml of normal saline to run in for 5 hours (and we assume a loss of 50 per cent of the insulin), we end up administering an effective total amount of insulin of 25 units, i.e., 5 units per hour, which is still in the recommended therapeutic dose range.

Those who prefer the intramuscular or subcutaneous route for insulin administration now recommend starting with a supplementary intravenous bolus of 10 units of insulin.

The conventional high-dose insulin treatment may produce a slightly faster decline of the plasma glucose and ketone curves, but this is not always an advantage; on the contrary, slower correction of the metabolic and fluid balance would prevent undesirable sharp osmolar fluctuations.

The recommended dose of 10 U per hour of insulin achieves serum levels of 80 to 200 μU per ml; these are within the range that stimulates maximal rates of glucose transport and utilization in muscle and adipose tissues. It is, however, imperative to monitor the patient very closely in order to prevent the serious consequences that would arise from an otherwise unpredictable high resistance to insulin.[12] If plasma sugar remains unchanged 2 hours after starting treatment, insulin dosage should be substantially increased and it would even be advisable to switch to the purest Pork insulin preparation available.

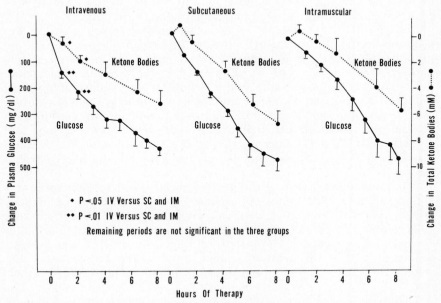

Figure 6.   Change in plasma glucose and total ketone bodies (Beta-hydroxybutyrate plus acetoacetate) after intravenous, subcutaneous or intramuscular low-dose insulin (15 patients in each group). (*From* Fisher, J. N., Shahshahari, M. N., and Kitabchi, A. E.: Diabetic Ketoacidosis: low-dose insulin therapy by various routes. N. Engl. J. Med., 297:238–241, 1977. Reproduced by permission.)

The advantage of this new low-dose insulin method of treating diabetic ketoacidosis is that it significantly lowers the risk of hypoglycemia, hypokalemia,[14] and, possibly, cerebral edema. The theoretical contribution of this new approach to treatment is that it refutes the 50 year old concept of tremendous insulin resistance in ketoacidosis. There is certainly insulin resistance in ketoacidosis, more so when diabetic ketoacidosis is associated with infection, but it is of much smaller degree than assumed in the past.

3. WATER AND SALT.   The degree of water deficit varies according to the type of diabetes, the length of time of the prodromal phase, and the amount of fluid intake and urine output. An estimated water deficit of 10 per cent of body weight can occur and should be replaced in 24 hours. Sodium and chloride deficit reaches approximately 7 and 5 mEq per kg of body weight respectively. The first 2 to 3 liters of fluid should be given as intravenous normal saline solution in 3 to 4 hours. Five per cent Dextrose in water solution should be started when plasma glucose level falls to about 250 mg per dl.

4. POTASSIUM.   Potassium deficit can reach 5 to 10 mEq per kg of body weight. The initial serum K^+ can appear, however, to be normal or elevated due to acidosis (shift of K^+ from intracellular to extracellular space), dehydration, and insulin deficiency. If serum K^+ is normal or low on admission, it is imperative to add potassium chloride into initial intravenous fluids at the rate of 20 to 40 mEq of K^+ per liter. If the initial K^+ level is above normal, administration of potassium chloride should be delayed for 1 or 2 hours. It is imperative to monitor serum K^+ level with repeated electrocardiograms and chemical determinations.

5. SODIUM BICARBONATE.   It is usually not necessary to administer sodium bicarbonate unless pH is below 7.1. When needed, one or two ampules (44 mEq per ampule) of bicarbonate may be given. Rapid correction of acidosis with bicarbonate may be harmful; bicarbonate diffusion through blood-brain barrier is slow; rapid increase in blood pH depresses the respiratory center causing hypoventilation and accumulation of soluble carbon dioxide which diffuses rapidly into the cerebrospinal fluid and lowers its pH; a sharp disequilibrium between blood and cerebrospinal fluid pH may aggravate the state of coma.[19, 22] Sodium bicarbonate increases also the risk of hypokalemia and hypophosphatemia.

6. PHOSPHATE.   During the development of ketoacidosis there is a significant loss of inorganic phosphate (about 1 mM per kg of body weight). As with potassium, there is a marked egress of phosphate from cells so that its plasma concentrations may appear spuriously normal or elevated before treatment is started. An impressive fall, even to below 1 mg per dl, may occur during treatment, as phosphate returns into cells; several days are necessary for serum phosphate level to return to normal.

There is a good correlation between low concentrations of plasma phosphate and red cell 2,3-diphosphoglycerate (2,3-DPG). Red cell 2,3-DPG falls when plasma phosphate falls, with consequent shift of the oxyhemoglobin dissociation curve to the left and decreased tissue oxygenation;* this can be restored to normal with intravenous administration of phosphate (eventually given as potassium phosphate slow drip: 30 to 60 mM of phosphate) with consequent shift to the right and improved tissue oxygenation.** Caution is advised in administering phosphate intravenously: a rapid drip may increase the risk of hypocalcemia.

Metabolic acidosis lowers red cell 2,3-DPG because low pH inhibits glycolysis at the phosphofructokinase step; this, of itself, would cause a marked shift to the left. However, acidosis per se causes a shift to the right (the Bohr effect). Therefore, in diabetic ketoacidosis the oxyhemoglobin dissociation curve remains normal. But, treatment creates an imbalance between 2,3-DPG and pH. It may take 3 to 4 days for 2,3-DPG to return to normal while pH is generally normal within 24 hours. This early restoration of blood pH leads to a shift to the left because of the still low 2,3-DPG unless phosphate is administered. This left shift is accentuated if a large dose of alkali is given early in treatment. Defective oxygen release may account for some findings relating to depth of coma, as well as to high lactate/pyruvate ratio despite an increase in pH. This is another reason for avoidng the hasty use of intravenous bicarbonate.[11]

7. SOME GENERAL MEASURES

A. *Treat circulatory collapse*, if any, *energetically*: plasma dextran in saline; vasopressors only if needed.

B. *Gastric Lavage:* only in case of vomiting, gastric atony and abdominal distention. Use warm saline.

C. *Vitamins:* The use of vitamins such as B complex and ascorbic acid is advisable because of their important role in oxidation and reduction and their increased turnover owing to treatment-induced rapid build-up in carbohydrate, fat, and protein metabolism.

8. FIND AND TREAT PREDISPOSING CAUSE. Infection (genitourinary, respiratory, skin, etc.), diarrhea, myocardial infarction, emotional cause, hyperthyroidism, etc.

9. ORAL FEEDING. About 12 hours after initiation of treatment or as indicated. Start with fluids such as tea with sugar, ginger ale, milk, broth.

10. ROUTINE INSULIN TREATMENT. Can be restored to the precoma pattern about 24 to 48 hours after starting treatment, provided there is no serious and prolonged stressful situation such as infection. The latter would rather require multiple daily injections of regular insulin until stress subsides.

PLASMA KETONES

Plasma ketones derive from the accelerated beta-oxidation of fatty acids to acetyl CoA and formation of *aceto-acetate* (AcAc) via condensation of two melecules of acetyl CoA. Aceto-Acetate is reduced to *beta-*

---

*shift to left: increased affinity of oxygen to hemoglobin, i.e., decreased release of oxygen from hemoglobin to tissues.

**shift to right: decreased affinity of oxygen to hemoglobin, i.e., increased release of oxygen from hemoglobin to tissues.

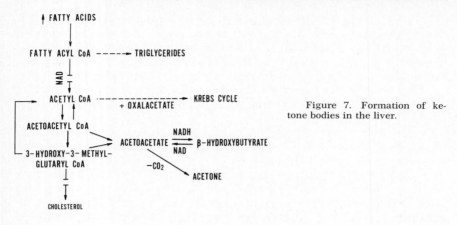

Figure 7. Formation of ketone bodies in the liver.

hydroxybutyrate (β-OHB) by a dehydrogenase and the hydrogen donor NADH. Decarboxylation of AcAc generates *acetone* which is metabolically inert. AcAc and β-OHB cannot be metabolized in the liver and leak out into the circulation, and serve as fuels for those tissues such as heart, kidney, and muscle which possess the appropriate metabolic enzymes. Normal plasma β-OHB/AcAc ratio is 2:1 but in diabetic ketoacidosis this ratio may rise to 6:1 or even more because of the excess of NADH generated during the oxidation of fatty acids (Fig. 7). Therefore, β-OHB is always the most abundant acid in diabetic ketoacidosis.

However, the usual qualitative testing of ketones gives only an approximate and sometimes a false low estimate of the ketosis because the nitroprusside reagent used in the test ("acetone test" — Denco powder, Acetest tablet, or Ketostix strip) reacts only with AcAc and acetone, and not at all with β-OHB. Hence, frequent discrepancies may occur, such as a β-OHB-induced very low pH, coupled with a ketone test result of moderate degree.

During treatment with insulin, the decrease in lipolysis and fatty acid oxidation regenerates NAD and raises the oxidative capacity NAD/NADH; the reaction then shifts toward acetoacetate, and the acetest reagent might then

$$\text{Acetoacetate} + \text{NADH} + \text{H} \underset{}{\overset{\beta\text{-OHBDH}}{\rightleftharpoons}} \beta\text{-hydroxybutyrate} + \text{NAD}$$

show a ketone reaction stronger than that recorded before treatment. The physician should be familiar with this phenomenon in order to avoid overtreating with insulin.

One more cause for a discrepancy between a very low pH and a rather moderately elevated ketone reaction could eventually be a marked increase of plasma lactic acid prior to treatment. The lactic acidosis accompanying diabetic ketoacidosis is also attributed to the alterations of the redox potential NAD/NADH: decreased NAD and increased NADH tend to block the oxidation of lactate to pyruvate, and accelerate the reduction of pyruvate to lactate. Insulin will reverse and normalize the situation

$$\text{Pyruvate} + \text{NADH} + \text{H} \;\overset{\text{LDH}}{\rightleftharpoons}\; \text{lactate} + \text{NAD}$$

Acetone is metabolically inert. Because it is a volatile substance and is soluble in fat tissue it may persist in expired air and in urine after the other blood ketone bodies have returned to normal levels.

CEREBRAL EDEMA (DISEQUILIBRIUM SYNDROME)

Following energetic treatment and improvement of diabetic coma, some patients (about 1 per cent) may develop seizures and lapse into an intractable fatal coma. Autopsy reveals cerebral edema. This has been attributed to a rapid correction of body fluids, of hyperglycemia and/or hypernatremia, which may produce a state of intracellular hypertonicity relative to the extracellular dilution; serum water moves into the intracellular space and results in cellular swelling.[30] Another explanation suggests that accumulation of sorbitol and fructose (polyol pathway) in the brain cells may be responsible for the intracellular hypertonicity and cerebral edema.[29] This fatal complication calls for caution against too rapid hydration of patients with severe ketoacidosis and hyperosmolality, and against the use of hypotonic solutions during the first hours of treatment.

ACKNOWLEDGEMENT

The authors are grateful to librarians Mrs. H. Pilikian and Mrs. V. Frankel for their assistance, and to Miss B. Poskrop for her secretarial help.

REFERENCES

1. Alberti, K. G. M. M., Hockaday, T. D. R., and Turner, R. C.: Small doses of intramuscular insulin in the treatment of diabetic "coma." The Lancet, 2:515–522, 1973.
2. Barnes, A. J., Bloom, S. R., Alberti, K. G. M. M., et al.: Ketoacidosis in pancreatectomized man. New Engl. J. Med., 296:1250–1253, 1977.
3. Baruh, S., Sherman, L., Kolodny, H. D., et al.: Fasting hypoglycemia. Med. Clin. N. Amer., 57:1441–1462, 1973.
4. Bradley, R. F.: Diabetic ketoacidosis and coma. In Marble, A., White, P., Bradley, R. F., et al.: Joslin's Diabetes Mellitus. Philadelphia, Lea & Febiger, 1971, pp. 361–416.
5. Finn, R., and Cope, S.: The plasma amylase in diabetic coma. Diabetes, 12:141–143, 1963.
6. Fisher, J. N., Shahshahani, M. N., and Kitabchi, A. E.: Diabetic Ketoacidosis: low-dose insulin therapy by various routes. New Engl. J. Med., 297:238–241, 1977.
7. Frank, E.: Pathologie des Kohlehydratstoffwechsels. Basel, Benno Schwabe & Co., Verlag, 1949.
8. Genuth, S.: Diabetic ketoacidosis. In Podolsky, S., ed.: Clinical Diabetes: Modern Management. New York, Appleton-Century-Crofts, 1980, pp. 173–207.
9. Gerich, J. E., Lorenzi, M., Bier, D. M., et al.: Prevention of human diabetic ketoacidosis by somatostatin. New Engl. J. Med., 292:985–989, 1975.
10. Gerich, J., Penhos, J. C., Gutman, R. A., et al.: Effect of dehydration and hyperosmolarity on glucose, free fatty acid, and ketone body metabolism in the rat. Diabetes, 22:264–271, 1973.

11. Hockaday, T. D. R., and Alberti, K. G. M. M.: Diabetic coma. Clinics in Endocrinol. Metabol., 1:751–788, 1972.
12. Holt, S.: Insulin resistance during continuous insulin infusion. Lancet, 1:44, 1976.
13. Kidson, W., Casey, J., Kraegen, E., et al.: Treatment of severe diabetes mellitus by insulin infusion. Brit. Med. J., 2:691–694, 1974.
14. Kitabchi, A. E., Ayyagari, V., Guerra, S. M. O., et al.: The efficacy of low-dose versus conventional therapy of insulin for treatment of diabetic ketoacidosis. Ann. Intern. Med., 84:633–638, 1976.
15. Levine, R. L., Glauser, F. L., and Berk, J. E.: Enhancement of the amylase/creatinine clearance ratio in disorders other than acute pancreatitis. New Engl. J. Med., 292:329–332, 1975.
16. McGarry, J. D., and Foster, D. W.: Hormonal control of ketogenesis. Biochemical considerations. Arch. Intern. Med., 137:495–501, 1977.
17. McGarry, J. D.: New perspectives in the regulation of ketogenesis. (Lilly Lecture, 1978). Diabetes, 28:517–523, 1979.
18. Menzel, R., Zander, E., and Jutzi, E.: Treatment of diabetic coma with low-dose injections of insulin. Endokrinologie, 67:230–239, 1976.
19. Ohman, J. L., Jr., Marliss, E. B., Aoki, T. T., et al.: The cerebrospinal fluid in diabetic ketoacidosis. New Engl. J. Med., 284:283–290, 1971.
20. Page, M. McB., Alberti, K. G. M. M., Greenwood, R., et al.: Treatment of diabetic coma with continuous low-dose infusion of insulin. Brit. Med. J., 2:687–690, 1974.
21. Petty, C., and Cunningham, N. L.: Insulin adsorption by glass infusion bottles, polyvinyl-chloride infusion containers, and intravenous tubing. Anesthesiology, 40:400–404, 1974.
22. Posner, J. B., and Plum, F.: Spinal fluid pH and neurologic symptoms in systemic acidosis. New Engl. J. Med., 277:605–613, 1967.
23. Schade, D. S., and Eaton, R. P.: The controversy concerning counterregulatory hormone secretion. A hypothesis for the prevention of diabetic ketoacidosis? Diabetes, 26:596–599, 1977.
24. Semple, P. F., White, C., and Manderson, W. C.: Continuous intravenous infusion of small doses of insulin in treatment of diabetic ketoacidosis. Brit. Med. J., 2:694–698, 1974.
25. Sherwin, R. S., Hendler, R. G., and Felig, P.: Effect of ketone infusions on aminoacid and nitrogen metabolism in man. J. Clin. Invest., 55:1382–1390, 1975.
26. Sherwin, R. S., Hendler, R. G., and Felig, P.: Effect of diabetes mellitus and insulin on the turnover and metabolic response to ketones in man. Diabetes, 25:776–784, 1976.
27. Vinicor, F., Lehrner, L. M., Karn, R. C., et al.: Hyperamylasemia in diabetic ketoacidosis: Sources and significance. Ann. Intern. Med., 91:200–204, 1979.
28. Weisenfeld, S., Podolsky, S., Goldsmith, L., et al.: Adsorption of insulin to infusion bottles and tubing. Diabetes, 17:766–771, 1968.
29. Winegrad, A. I., and Clements, R. S., Jr.: Diabetic ketoacidosis. Med. Clin. N. Amer., 55:899–911, 1971.
30. Young, E., and Bradley, R. F.: Cerebral edema with irreversible coma in severe diabetic ketoacidosis. New Engl. J. Med., 276:665–669, 1967.

Queens Hospital Center
82-68 164th Street
Jamaica, New York 11432

Evaluation and Management of the Bleeding Patient

Kandhasamy Jagathambal, M.D.,*
Hans W. Grünwald, M.D.,†
and Fred Rosner, M.D.‡

Successful management of patients with defective hemostasis and bleeding depends on an accurate diagnosis. An understanding of the normal mechanisms that are required to keep the hemostatic systems in balance is essential to reach the correct diagnosis. In this article, we shall review normal hemostasis, the clinical manifestations of various bleeding disorders, and the diagnostic approach to and management of these disorders.

NORMAL HEMOSTASIS

Normal hemostasis depends on the integrity of blood vessels, normal function of platelets, interaction of circulating procoagulants and platelets, and activation of fibrinolysis.[13] Even though these mechanisms are all interrelated, for the sake of clarity, each will be considered separately.

ROLE OF BLOOD VESSELS. Trauma to blood vessels elicits an immediate vasoconstrictive response. This vasoconstriction is mediated via the autonomic nervous system as well as by direct stimulation of the smooth muscle within the vessel wall. Vasoactive amines such as

From the Division of Hematology, Department of Medicine, Queens Hospital Center Affiliation of the Long Island Jewish-Hillside Medical Center; and the Department of Medicine, Health Sciences Center, State University of New York at Stony Brook

*Assistant Attending, Division of Hematology, Department of Medicine and Physician-in-Charge of Coagulation, Queens Hospital Center Affiliation of the Long Island Jewish-Hillside Medical Center
†Chief, Division of Hematology, Queens Hospital Center Affiliation of the Long Island Jewish-Hillside Medical Center; Associate Professor of Medicine, Health Sciences Center, State University of New York at Stony Brook
‡Director of Medicine, Queens Hospital Center Affiliation of the Long Island Jewish-Hillside Medical Center; Professor of Medicine, Health Sciences Center, State University of New York at Stony Brook

Table 1. *Nomenclature for Procoagulant Factors*

COAGULATION FACTOR	SYNONYMS
I	Fibrinogen
II	Prothrombin
III	Tissue factor, thromboplastin
IV	Calcium ions
V	Proaccelerin; labile factor
VII	Proconvertin; stable factor
VIII	Antihemophilic factor (AHF), antihemophilic globulin (AHG), antihemophilic factor A
IX	Plasma thromboplastin component (PTC), antihemophilic factor B, Christmas factor
X	Stuart factor, Prower factor
XI	Plasma thromboplastin antecedent (PTA)
XII	Hageman factor
XIII	Fibrin stabilizing factor
Prekallikrein	Fletcher factor
High molecular weight kininogen	Fitzgerald factor, Williams factor, Flaujeac factor

epinephrine, serotonin, and thromboxane A_2, released from platelets, promote vasoconstriction. Vasoconstriction in the control of bleeding is dependent on the type of blood vessel involved. Although vasoconstriction is not required for effective hemostasis in the capillaries and venules, it is critical for arterioles.

ROLE OF PLATELETS.   Tissue injury results in the adhesion of platelets to exposed subendothelial structures such as collagen, noncollagenous microfibrils, and amorphous material. In addition to certain plasma proteins, calcium, fibrinogen, and von Willebrand factor are required for normal platelet adhesion. Platelet adhesion is followed by the extrusion of some platelet contents such as ATP, ADP, and serotonin (release reaction). The released ADP causes additional platelets to aggregate, resulting in the formation of the primary hemostatic plug.[19] At first the aggregates can be disaggregated, but with the release of more ADP, the formation of thrombin resulting from the activation of the coagulation cascade, the synthesis and release of prostaglandin endoperoxides and thromboxane A_2, the aggregation process becomes irreversible. During platelet aggregation, a membrane phospholipoprotein (Pf_3) becomes available on the surface of the aggregated platelets. The latter accelerates several steps of the blood coagulation sequence (factor X activation and conversion of prothrombin to thrombin).[11, 14]

ROLE OF PROCOAGULANT PROTEINS.   (See Table 1 for nomenclature of the various procoagulant factors.) Both extrinsic and intrinsic coagulation pathways participate in the activation of factor X to Xa, a step that is essential for the conversion of prothrombin to thrombin. Exposure of the subendothelial structures with contact of blood thereto activates factor XII which, in the presence of prekallikrein and high molecular weight kininogens, activates factor XI. The activated factor XI (XIa), in the presence of calcium, cleaves a peptide from factor IX, producing activated factor IX (IXa). Activated factor IX, in the presence of platelet phospholipid (Pf_3), factor VIII, and calcium, proteolytically converts factor X to Xa.

In the extrinsic pathway, a tissue factor (tissue thromboplastin), released from damaged cells, activates factor X, in the presence of factor VII, and calcium.

The activated factor X (Xa), in the presence of Ca^{++}, factor V, and Pf_3, converts prothrombin to thrombin. Thrombin cleaves fibrinopeptides A and B from fibrinogen to produce fibrin monomer which, in turn, undergoes spontaneous polymerization. Fibrin polymer is cross-linked by activated factor XIII, in the presence of calcium, producing a highly insoluble, hemostatically effective, firm, fibrin clot.

BLEEDING DISORDERS RELATED TO PLATELETS

Platelets may be qualitatively abnormal or decreased in number or both. The most common disorder involving platelets is thrombocytopenia. Clinical manifestations of thrombocytopenia include petechiae, purpura, and mucosal bleeding such as epistaxis, gum bleeding, and menorrhagia. There is a linear relation between the bleeding time and the platelet count.[5] Younger platelets are hemostatically more effective than older platelets. Thrombocytopenic disorders can be classified according to the physiological disturbances relating to platelet production, destruction, and distribution (Table 2).

Decreased platelet production may result from (a) generalized

Table 2. *Causes of Thrombocytopenia*

DECREASED PLATELET PRODUCTION

    Aplastic or hypoplastic marrow
    Infiltrative disease of marrow: carcinoma, leukemia, disseminated infection
    Specific megakaryocytic hypoplasia

INEFFECTIVE PLATELET PRODUCTION

    Folate deficiency
    Vitamin B_{12} deficiency

PLATELET SEQUESTRATION

    Pooling of platelets in enlarged spleen

INCREASED PLATELET DESTRUCTION

    Immune thrombocytopenia
      Autoimmune
      Isoimmune
      Drug-associated
    Consumption coagulopathy
    Mechanical injury of platelets

COMBINATION OF SEVERAL MECHANISMS

hypoplasia of the bone marrow; (b) infiltration of the bone marrow with foreign cells (leukemia, myeloma, metastatic cancer); (c) inhibition of cellular proliferation caused by drugs such as cytotoxic agents, gold, sulfonamides and ethanol; (d) defective production and maturation of cells as in megaloblastic anemias.

Disordered distribution of platelets can occur with massive splenomegaly when up to 80 per cent of all circulating platelets can be trapped in the spleen, resulting in thrombocytopenia due to hypersplenism. Normally, only 30 per cent of circulating platelets are present in the spleen.

Accelerated destruction is a frequent cause of thrombocytopenia. Such platelet destruction may be secondary to immunologic or nonimmunologic mechanisms. The latter includes excessive platelet utilization secondary to consumption coagulopathy, vasculitis, thrombotic thrombocytopenic purpura, and prosthetic valve replacement. Immunologic thrombocytopenia, which is antibody mediated, may be due to (a) autoantibodies, as in idiopathic thrombocytopenia, systemic lupus erythematosus, chronic lymphocytic leukemia, and in association with autoimmune hemolytic anemia; (b) alloantibodies associated with pregnancy and transfusion; (c) antibodies associated with certain drugs such as quinidine and sulfonamides.

Qualitative platelet disorders can be classified into dysfunction related to adhesion, aggregation, or release.[4, 22]

The most common cause of a platelet *adhesion defect* is *von Willebrand's disease* which is most frequently an autosomal dominant disorder. The defective adhesion is due to deficiency of the "von Willebrand factor." Patients with this disorder also have decreased factor VIII procoagulant activity. Platelet aggregation with ADP, collagen, and epinephrine is normal, as is the platelet ADP release reaction. Patients have a life-long history of mucosal bleeding, and easy bruising. They have a prolonged bleeding time, decreased plasma factor VIII level, decreased platelet retention in glass bead columns, and decreased platelet aggregation in response to ristocetin. Normal hemostasis can be restored by infusion of plasma rich in factor VIII.

The *Bernard-Soulier syndrome* is a rare inherited platelet disorder in which platelet adhesion is decreased and platelets do not respond to ristocetin despite normal plasma factor VIII levels. These patients have large platelets and may also have mild thrombocytopenia. Treatment consists of platelet transfusions when necessary.

Primary platelet *aggregation defects* include *Glanzmann's thrombasthenia* which is a rare, autosomal recessive condition, associated with serious bleeding. The platelets do not aggregate with ADP, epinephrine, or collagen. They also fail to support clot retraction. Recent data suggest that the defect is due to an abnormal platelet membrane glycoprotein.[15]

Secondary aggregation defects include a heterogeneous group of congenital and acquired platelet aberrations with a variety of laboratory abnormalities. The common abnormalities include prolonged bleeding time with absence of the secondary wave of platelet aggregation with ADP and epinephrine, and a slow response to collagen; such platelets respond normally to ristocetin. Two major groups of patients with this type of syndrome are those with deficiency of platelet storage pool nucleotides and those with an abnormality in the release mechanism.

Platelet *release defects* are those disorders in which the release of platelet ADP is defective; hence, the second wave of platelet aggregation secondary to endogenous release of ADP is absent. The most common cause of this defect is the ingestion of medications such as aspirin. Aspirin acetylates the platelet cyclo-oxygenase system and thus decreases production of the prostaglandin endoperoxide intermediates that stimulate release of ADP and platelet aggregation. Although aspirin is the commonest offender, other drugs which produce a similar effect are indomethacin, phenylbutazone, tricyclic antidepressants, antihistamines, certain anesthetics, ethyl alcohol, dextran, clofibrate, carbenicillin, and phenothiazines, all of which inhibit the second wave of aggregation of platelets by preventing the release of platelet ADP. An inherited defect in this enzyme system with a similar platelet function abnormality has also been described.

In platelet *storage pool disease,* the release mechanism is normal but there is a lack of releasable stores of ADP and other granules; hence, the name storage-pool disease. This defect may occur as an isolated autosomal dominant disorder or in association with a wide variety of diseases (e.g., leukemia, alcoholic intoxication). These patients have a prolonged bleeding time and defective secondary platelet aggregation.

Acquired platelet defects occur in certain systemic diseases such as uremia. These abnormalities are (a) defective Pf_3 availability; (b) abnormal ADP-induced aggregation; and (c) decreased platelet adhesiveness. These abnormalities improve after dialysis.[20] Liver disease is known to cause thrombocytopenia and abnormal platelet function (decreased aggregation and glass-bead retention) secondary to the increase in circulating fibrin split products. Other disorders known to be associated with platelet functional abnormalities are multiple myeloma, systemic lupus erythematosus, and myeloproliferative disorders.[6, 8]

VASCULAR DISORDERS

Inherited or acquired abnormalities of blood vessel walls comprise a group of disorders which may be associated with clinical bleeding. Bleeding occurs mainly from mucous membranes or into the skin and is generally related to injury or trauma. The platelet count and bleeding time are usually normal. The diagnosis of a vascular defect is often by exclusion. The following conditions may be associated with vascular defects and a bleeding tendency: (a) amyloidosis, (b) vascular purpura (Henoch-Schönlein purpura); (c) hereditary hemorrhagic telangiectasia; (d) pseudoxanthoma elasticum; (e) Ehlers-Danlos syndrome; (f) vasculitis.

DISORDERS OF COAGULATION FACTORS

Bleeding due to impaired coagulation is related to defective production of coagulation factors, their excessive destruction or consumption, pathological inhibition of their activity or a combination of these. Vascular injury always precedes such bleeding; when platelet plug formation is intact, there may be initial hemostasis followed by secondary bleeding within hours because of inadequate fibrin formation. The plasma level of coagulation factor necessary to achieve hemostasis is somewhat variable, depending upon the amount of vascular damage and the competence of the remaining hemostatic mechanisms. Usually, fibrin formation is sufficient when clotting factor activity is maintained at 30 to 40 per cent of normal. Levels of 1 to 5 per cent of normal are necessary to prevent bleeding associated with normal vascular injury of everyday living.

Defective Production of Coagulation Factors

Defective production of coagulation factors can be either hereditary or acquired. *Hereditary defects* involve deficiency of a single coagulation factor which persists at a constant level throughout life. Factor VIII and IX deficiencies are sex-linked recessive disorders. Other hereditary coagulation disorders are inherited in an autosomal manner.

Factor VIII deficiency (hemophilia A) is an "X-linked" abnormality, the average incidence being 1 in 10,000 births. There is defective synthesis of the factor VIII molecule. The severity of the disease closely parallels the plasma level of factor VIII procoagulant activity. In patients with severe hemophilia, factor VIII levels are less than 1 per cent of normal, and such patients develop severe, spontaneous bleeding beginning in infancy with recurrent hemarthrosis as the major clinical event. Moderately severe disease, with factor VIII levels 1 to 5 per cent of normal, is characterized by only occasional hemarthrosis. Mild hemophiliacs (levels 5 to 25 per cent) manifest abnormal bleeding only with extensive hemostatic challenge such as major surgery or trauma.

Factor IX deficiency (hemophilia B) resembles factor VIII deficiency in its mode of inheritance and clinical manifestations. The incidence is five times less than that of hemophilia A.

Factor XI deficiency is less common than factor IX deficiency and occurs most often in Jews. The disease resembles a mild to moderate form of hemophilia and is readily treated with infusions of fresh frozen plasma.

Factor XIII deficiency may be inherited by two different mechanisms: (a) autosomal recessive; (b) x-linked. Fibrin clots formed in this disorder are not cross-linked and are susceptible to dissolution by plasmin and mechanical stress. Excessive bleeding from the umbilical stump, spontaneous abortion, and delayed wound healing occur in patients with this disorder.

Fibrinogen deficiency and dysfibrinogenemia represent a heterogenous group of disorders. Congenital afibrinogenemia is a rare autosomal recessive abnormality manifested by an almost total absence of fibrinogen synthesis, with circulating fibrinogen levels less than 5 mg per 100 ml and a life-long history of repeated bleeding. In congenital hypofibrinogenemia, the fibrinogen levels are 50 to 100 mg per 100 ml and hemorrhagic events are uncommon. Dysfibrinogenemia, characterized by a defective fibrinogen molecule, is associated with a very mild bleeding tendency. There is a disparity between the level of functionally active and immunologically active fibrinogen.

Acquired disorders of coagulation factor production usually involve multiple factor deficiencies because of either *vitamin K deficiency* or *liver disease*. The factor levels may show considerable variability because of differences in their individual rates of synthesis and metabolism. Vitamin K is synthesized in the body by the intestinal flora, and green leafy vegetables also contain vitamin K. Vitamin K is not stored to any great extent in the body. The deficiency occurs in the following settings: malabsorption, the postoperative patient with limited oral intake, and patients receiving broad spectrum antibiotics. Defective production of vitamin K–dependent factors may also develop secondary to the use of oral anticoagulants. Lack of this vitamin results in reduced gamma-carboxylation of specific glutamyl residues located on factors II, VII, IX and X.[21] These factors decrease in the blood in the following order: factor VII first, then factors IX and X, and prothrombin last.

The liver is the main site of synthesis of most of the procoagulant factors. It is also responsible for the clearance of various activated forms of coagulation factors and related enzymes. For example, fibrinolytic enzymes are normally degraded in the liver, and impairment of liver function may result in abnormally accelerated fibrinolysis. However, chronic liver failure also induces a number of non-hematologic abnormalities that may contribute to bleeding (e.g., portal hypertension with esophageal varices, change in the gastric mucus and increased acidity causing peptic ulcer). In patients with splenomegaly, there may be concomitant thrombocytopenia that exacerbates mechanical or anatomical causes of bleeding. In severe liver disease, levels of all coagulation factors may be decreased except factor VIII, but factor V and the prothrombin group (II, VII, IX and X) are the most vulnerable.[2] There is a rough correlation between most clotting factors and the level of serum albumin. In contrast to liver disease, factor V level is normal in vitamin K deficiency. In jaundiced patients with prolonged prothrombin times, correction of this abnormality following vitamin K administration can help to distinguish an obstructive process in which there is poor vitamin K absorption due to absence in the intestine of bile salts, from hepatocellular disease, in which there is little or no response to vitamin K.

Disorders Related to Increased Consumption or Destruction of Coagulation Factors

Under normal conditions, various factors influence the activity of the hemostatic mechanism. These include (a) normal blood flow; (b) hepatic clearance of the activated clotting factors; (c) circulating inhibitors such as antithrombin. Patients with a number of serious illnesses often have excessive activation of coagulation and inadequate protective mechanisms. These disorders can be grouped into: (a) conditions that introduce tissue factor or other activators into the circulation; (b) damage to endothelial surfaces; (c) stagnation of blood flow; and (d) combinations of the above. Such conditions may become manifest as uncompensated or compensated forms of consumption coagulopathy.[18] Patients usually present with an identifiable serious illness that may be accompanied by hypotension, acidosis, and infection. There may be diffuse ecchymoses and mucous membrane bleeding. Laboratory findings are variable depending upon the stage — e.g., in the compensated form of consumption coagulopathy, the coagulation factors that are consumed in the formation of the clot (II, V, VIII, fibrinogen and platelets) may even be increased, reflecting the compensatory activity ("overshoot"); however, in the decompensated stage the above factors are decreased and the screening tests (PT, APTT, and TT) are prolonged and the platelet count is decreased. Fibrin degradation products (FDP) are greatly increased, as the clotting is almost always accompanied by fibrinolysis.

Accelerated destruction of clotting factors occurs in association with varying clinical manifestations, ranging from asymptomatic status to severe bleeding. The hallmark of an acquired inhibitor is an abnormal PTT (sometimes an abnormal PT) that cannot be corrected by the addition of an equal volume of normal plasma. The inhibitors are of two types: antibody inhibitors and non-antibody inhibitors. In the former, the antibody is directed specifically against a particular coagulant component, most commonly against factor VIII. Antibodies against factor V, factor XIII and even factor IX have also been demonstrated. Antibody against factor VIII develops in 5 to 10 per cent of patients with hemophilia A. Factor VIII antibodies have also been described in (a) postpartum women; (b) in disorders of an immunologic nature such as sytemic lupus erythematosus, rheumatoid arthritis, ulcerative colitis, regional enteritis, penicillin reaction; and (c) in old age.[3, 10, 17]

The chemical nature of non-antibody inhibitors is not clear. The activity is directed against the phospholipid component of the prothrombin activator. These inhibitors may not create a clinical problem, in spite of abnormal in vitro test results. This type of inhibitor has been described mostly in association with systemic lupus erythematosus.

DIAGNOSTIC APPROACH TO THE BLEEDING PATIENT

Having summarized the various disorders related to vascular, platelet and procoagulant factor abnormalities, let us now focus on dealing with a patient who presents with clinical bleeding. By far, the most important consideration in evaluating the bleeding patient is the *history.*[16] One should obtain the following data:

Type of Bleeding	Petechiae, purpura, ecchymoses, deep-tissue bleeding (muscles and joints)
Course of Bleeding	Spontaneous or related to trauma; frequency and severity

Relation to surgical procedures	Circumcision, tooth extraction
Associated systemic illness	Systemic lupus erythematosus, liver disease, uremia
Drug history	1. Drugs affecting platelets, e.g., aspirin, phenylbutazone dipyridamole, antihistamines
	2. Drugs affecting coagulation factors such as heparin and coumadin
Family history	Vertical or horizontal transmission

The type of bleeding is an important help in the diagnosis. Spontaneous skin and mucosal bleeding is mostly associated with platelet disorders and is manifest as petechiae and ecchymoses. Bleeding into the deeper tissues, such as muscles and joints, is usually associated with procoagulant factor deficiency. Bleeding, if secondary to the former, generally occurs immediately after the trauma and lasts for a short period, whereas with coagulation factor deficiencies, the bleeding is delayed and lasts longer. Clinical examples of platelet and vascular bleeding are epistaxis, menorrhagia, gastrointestinal bleeding, and purpura. Examples of clotting factor deficiency bleeding are hemarthrosis, deep hematoma, and occasionally epistaxis.

On *physical examination,* the patient should be examined for the following: (1) evidence of petechiae, ecchymoses, and telangiectasia; (2) joint deformities; hemarthrosis and ankylosis due to repeated bleeding; (3) abnormal elasticity of skin and/or hyperextensibility of joints (e.g., Ehlers-Danlos syndrome); (4) evidence of systemic illness e.g., spider angioma, hepatosplenomegaly.

Laboratory Investigation

Despite the leads derived from the history and physical examination, the definitive diagnosis depends on laboratory testing. A systematic approach is necessary for efficient delineation of the hemostatic abnormality in each patient. Initially a battery of rapid tests is used as a screen, following which the defects may be classified on the basis of a physiologic abnormality.

Platelets are first evaluated by examination of peripheral blood smear for number and morphology.

If there is no thrombocytopenia and the patient's history is suggestive of platelet dysfunction, a bleeding time determination is required. If thrombocytopenia is diagnosed, the most common cause, i.e., drug ingestion, should be sought, and examination of the bone marrow aspirate is indicated to rule out a primary bone marrow disease.

If the platelet count is normal and the bleeding time is prolonged, one should consider qualitative platelet disorders secondary to drugs or the presence of systemic illnesses such as uremia and liver disease. Von Willebrand's disease is also associated with a prolonged bleeding time and a slightly prolonged PTT. To confirm this diagnosis, a von Willebrand factor assay (ristocetin induced platelet aggregation) should be done and factor VIII antigen levels measured. Platelet function studies other than the bleeding time do not correlate well with the clinical severity of bleeding.

Procoagulant factors are evaluated by the performance of (a) prothrombin time; (b) activated partial thromboplastin time; (c) thrombin time; and (d) factor XIII screening test. These tests are available in most hospitals and with these four tests it is possible to identify the general locus of the abnormality in the coagulation pathway. Further tests can be done to pinpoint the diagnosis.

The prothrombin time test (PT) is prolonged by significant reduction in the plasma levels of factors VII, X, V, prothrombin, or fibrinogen as occurs in liver disease, or by inhibitors of these factors. The partial thromboplastin time (PTT) is almost always abnormal when any of the plasma procoagulant factor activities involved are reduced to levels which result in abnormal hemostasis. The PTT is thus prolonged by low levels of factors XII, XI, IX, VIII, X, V, prothrombin, and fibrinogen, or by inhibitors of these factors. To differentiate between deficiency and inhibitor, the patient's plasma is mixed with an equal volume of normal plasma; in case of deficiency the prolonged PT, PTT, or TT becomes normal, whereas with an inhibitor, only partial or no normalization occurs (although occasionally the mixture must be incubated for up to 2 hours to demonstrate such inhibition).

Deficiencies of clotting factors are commoner than inhibitors or inactivators. The thrombin time (TT) measures the ability of thrombin to catalyze the transformation of fibrinogen to fibrin; this reaction is prolonged by decreased or abnormal fibrinogen, circulating heparin or fibrin degradation products (resulting from fibrinolysis). A factor XIII screening test is included as one of the initial screening tests since the PT, PTT, and thrombin time measure all clotting factors except factor XIII, and the latter is necessary for the formation of a stable clot.

The four screening procedures described above permit the disorders related to procoagulant factors to be classified into different groups:

1. PT—abnormal   (a) VII deficiency, exceedingly rare (1/500,000)
   PTT, TT, XIII—normal   (b) at the onset of coumadin treatment (factor VII half life 3-5 hours, hence first factor to go down)

2. PTT—abnormal   (a) with no bleeding (XII, prekallikrein, kininogen)
   PT, TT, XIII—normal   (b) with significant bleeding (VIII, IX, XI and von Willebrand factor)

3. PT, PTT—abnormal   (a) deficiency of proteins of the common pathway (II, V, X or multiple factors)
   TT, XIII—normal   (b) mostly acquired disorders, liver disease and vitamin K deficiency

4. PT, PTT, TT—abnormal   (a) hypofibrinogenemia or dysfibrinogenemia
   XIII—normal   (b) interfering substances—heparin, FDP

5. XIII—abnormal   (a) factor XIII deficiency
   PT, PTT, TT—normal

6. Mixed disorders (platelet   (a) von Willebrand's disease
   and coagulation factor   Consumption coagulopathy
   abnormalities)

MANAGEMENT OF THE BLEEDING PATIENT

Management of the bleeding patient is clearly dependent upon the identification of the underlying cause. If thrombocytopenia is present and is due to decreased platelet production (diagnosis made by the examination of the bone marrow aspirate), the treatment of choice would be replacement of the platelets by platelet transfusion. Spontaneous bleeding is unlikely if the platelet count is more than 20,000 per microliter. However, if there is an "open wound," a platelet count of 50,000 per microliter is required for effective hemostasis. In an average individual who has had no previous exposure to blood or blood components, a single unit of platelet concentrate containing approximately 7×10^{10} platelets can be expected to increase the platelet count by 9000-12,000 per microliter. Therefore, transfusion of 8 to 10 units of platelets should be sufficient to raise the platelet count over 100,000 per microliter in the average-sized adult. This transfusion may have to be repeated every 24 to 48 hours, depending upon the underlying disorder.[12]

In immune-mediated thrombocytopenia (both idiopathic and drug-related), transfused platelets are subjected to the same destructive immune interactions as the patient's own platelets, and survive no longer than a few hours. Hence, platelet transfusion is not recommended for such patients, unless there is life-threatening bleeding (e.g., central nervous system hemorrhage). In drug-related thrombocytopenia, withdrawal of the offending drug is followed by a rise in platelet count within 7 to 10 days, though it takes a longer period with drugs that are metabolized and eliminated slowly such as gold thiomalate or diphenylhydantoin. Steroid administration is the initial mode of treatment in autoimmune ("idiopathic") thrombocytopenia.[7]

Platelet transfusion is indicated for excessive bleeding in qualitative platelet disorders. However, correction of the causative factors should be considered. For example, in drug-related qualitative platelet dysfunction, the offending drug should be discontinued, and in cases of uremia, dialysis should be considered to remove the "toxic" metabolites. Plasmapheresis can also be performed to remove the "M" protein in paraproteinemias.

Multiple factor deficiencies which occur in patients with liver disease, vitamin K deficiency, or the "wash-out" syndrome associated with massive blood transfusion, are managed by the administration of fresh frozen plasma. The aim to achieve 20 to 30 per cent of normal clotting factor activity can be accomplished by the initial administration of 15 to 20 ml per kg of fresh frozen plasma, followed by one third the initial dose at 8 to 12 hour intervals. In the "wash-out" syndrome secondary to massive transfusion, dilutional thrombocytopenia often accompanies the clotting factor deficiency and is corrected by platelet transfusion.

In vitamin K deficiency, correction occurs following administration

Table 3. *Replacement Therapy in Hereditary Coagulation Disorders*

DISORDER	PLASMA CONCENTRATION REQUIRED FOR HEMOSTASIS (PER CENT OF NORMAL)	HALF-LIFE OF TRANSFUSED FACTOR UNDER OPTIMAL CONDITIONS	RECOVERY IN BLOOD (AS PER CENT OF DOSE TRANSFUSED UNDER OPTIMAL CONDITIONS)	THERAPEUTIC MATERIAL	LOADING DOSE	MAINTENANCE DOSE
Fibrinogen deficiency	10–25	4 days	50	cryoprecipitate	4 bags/10 kg	1 bag/10 kg daily
Prothrombin deficiency	40	3 days	40–80	stored plasma; purified "prothrombin complex"	20 u/kg	10 u/kg daily
Factor V deficiency	10–15	12–15 hours	? 80	fresh or fresh frozen plasma	20 ml/kg	10 ml/kg every 12 hours
Factor VII deficiency	5–10	4–6 hours	70–80	stored plasma; "prothrombin complex"	10 ml or 10 u/kg	5 ml/kg Q6–24 hrs. 10 u/kg Q6–24 hrs.
Hemophilia A (VIII def.)	10–40	12–15	50–80	cryoprecipitate (80–100 units/bag) purified factor VIII	Minor bleed. Not req. Major bleed. 30 u/kg	10–15 u/kg Q 12 hrs for 2–4 days 15–20 u/kg Q8X1–2d + Q 12 thereafter
Hemophilia B (IX def.)	10–40	20 hours	50	purified prothrombin complex	Minor bleed. 30 u/kg Major bleed. 60 u/kg	10 u/kg Q12HX2–4 days 10 u/kg Q 12 hrs.
Factor X deficiency	10–15	2 days	50	stored plasma; purified "prothrombin complex"	15 u/kg	10 u/kg daily
Factor XI deficiency	?30	3 days	90–100	stored plasma	10 ml/kg	5 ml/kg daily
Factor XIII deficiency	1–5	6 days	?75–100	stored plasma	5 ml/kg weekly	not required

of vitamin K (10 mg vitamin K intravenously every 12 hours for 3 doses). If the PT and PTT have not normalized in 48 hours, another cause for the abnormal clotting tests should be sought. Treatment of consumption coagulopathy should be directed at correcting the underlying disease or triggering event. Patients with diffuse hemorrhage need intensive support with fresh frozen plasma, cryoprecipitate, platelet, and red-cell transfusions. There is some controversy about the efficacy of heparin in treating this syndrome.[9] While heparin usually suppresses the hemostatic system's activity in this disorder, regulation of the dose and prevention of heparin-induced hemorrhage is difficult. Unless the underlying cause of the consumption coagulopathy is treated, the use of heparin or the infusion of various blood components offers only temporary help.

In patients with hereditary procoagulant factor deficiency, blood is tested to determine the level of the deficient factor and, in certain cases, whether or not an inhibitor is present. Therapy of bleeding episodes consists of replacement of the deficient factor in sufficient amounts.[1, 23] The dose of coagulation factor is usually calculated in units. One unit is the activity of the coagulation factor present in one milliliter of normal plasma. A relatively high dosage is required to control extensive hemorrhage or hemorrhage in a potentially dangerous area, such as the head, throat, or abdomen. Calculation of the required dose is based on several variables relating to the biodynamics of the clotting factor which is deficient (i.e., the recovery rate, the in vivo half-life, and the concentration for effective hemostasis). Table 3 summarizes these variables, and cites the therapeutic materials that contain various coagulation factors.

Von Willebrand's disorder is omitted from the table only because the response to cryoprecipitate (the preferred modality of treatment) varies with different patients. One starts with one bag of cryoprecipitate per 10 kg per day and increases or decreases the dose, depending on the response.

REFERENCES

1. Biggs, R.: Human Blood Coagulation, Hemostasis and Thrombosis. 11th Edition. Oxford, Blackwell Scientific Publ., pp. 365–394, 1976.
2. Dymock, I. W., Tucker, J. S., Woolf, I. L., et al.: Coagulation studies as a prognostic index in acute liver failure. Brit. J. Haematol., 29:385–395, 1975.
3. Feinstein, D. I., and Rapaport, S. I.: Acquired inhibitors of blood coagulation. Prog. Hemostasis Thromb., 1:75–95, 1972.
4. Hardisty, R. M.: Disorders of platelet function. Brit. Med. Bull., 33:207–212, 1977.
5. Harker, L. A., Slitcher, S., Jr.: The bleeding time as a screening test for evaluation of platelet function. New Engl. J. Med., 287:155–159, 1972.
6. Inceman, S., and Tangum, Y.: Platelet defects in the myeloproliferative disorders. Ann. N.Y. Acad. Sci., 201:251–261, 1972.
7. Lacey, J. V., and Penner, J. A.: Management of idiopathic thrombocytopenic purpura in the adult. Semin. Thromb. Hemostasis, 3:160–174, 1977.
8. Lackner, H.: Hemostatic abnormalities associated with dysproteinaemias. Semin. Hematol., 10:125–133, 1973.
9. Mant, M. J., and King, E. G.: Severe acute disseminated intravascular coagulation. A reappraisal of its pathophysiology, clinical significance and therapy based on 47 patients. Amer. J. Med., 67:557–563, 1979.
10. Margolius, A. Jr., Jackson, D. P., and Ratnoff, O. D.: Circulating anticoagulants. A study of 40 cases and a review of the literature. Medicine, 40:145–202, 1961.

11. Moncada, S., and Vane, J. R.: Arachidonic acid metabolites and the interactions between platelets and blood vessel walls. New Engl. J. Med., 300:1142–1145, 1979.
12. Murphy, S.: Platelet transfusions. Prog. Hemostasis Thromb., 3:289–310, 1977.
13. Mustard, J. F., and Packham, M. A.: Normal and abnormal hemostasis. Brit. Med. Bull., 33:187–191, 1977.
14. Mustard, J. F., and Packham, M. A.: Clinical pharmacology of platelets. Blood, 50:555–573, 1977.
15. Nurden, A. T., and Caen, J. P.: An abnormal platelet glycoprotein pattern in three cases of Glanzmann's thrombasthaenia. Brit. J. Haematol., 28:253–260, 1974.
16. Owen, A. O., Bowie, E. J. W., and Thompson, J. H.: The diagnosis of bleeding disorders. Boston, Little Brown and Co., pp. 368–384, 1975.
17. Shapiro, S. S., and Hultin, M.: Acquired inhibitors of blood coagulation factors. Semin. Thromb. Hemostasis, 1:336–385, 1975.
18. Sharp, A. A.: Diagnosis and management of disseminated intravascular coagulation. Brit. Med. Bull., 33:265–272, 1977.
19. Sixma, J. J., and Wester, J.: The hemostatic plug. Semin. Hematol., 14:265–300, 1977.
20. Stewart, J. M., and Castaldi, P. A.: Uraemic bleeding: A reversible platelet defect corrected by dialysis. Quart. J. Med., 36:409–423, 1967.
21. Suttie, J. W., and Jackson, C. M.: Prothrombin structure, activation and biosynthesis. Physiol. Rev., 57:1–70, 1977.
22. Weiss, H. J.: Platelet physiology and abnormalities of platelet function. (Parts 1 and 2) New Engl. J. Med., 292:531–541, 580–588, 1975.
23. Wintrobe, M. M.: Therapy of the hereditary coagulation disorders. In Clinical Hematology. Philadelphia, Lea and Febiger, 7th ed., 1974, pp. 1183–1200.

Queens Hospital Center
82-68 164th Street
Jamaica, New York 11432

Acute Tubular Necrosis

Pathophysiology and Management

Leonard A. Arbeit, M.D., *

and Stephen W. Weinstein, M.D. **

Many diseases are associated with acute loss of glomerular and tubular function resulting in abnormalities of fluid and electrolyte balance. Acute tubular necrosis is only one of many causes of such acute renal failure (Table 1) and, in fact, even this entity is heterogenous in etiology and pathophysiology. In any evaluation of the patient with acute respiratory failure one must, of course, delineate the underlying etiologic pathophysiologic causes. This has been extensively reviewed by others.[22, 27] The focus of this review is the subcategory acute tubular necrosis. We will not attempt to review the diagnostic parameters used to differentiate acute tubular necrosis from other types of acute renal failure. For reference, those characteristic abnormalities in urine and plasma used to establish the diagnosis of acute tubular necrosis are given in Table 2.

The goal of this review is to integrate current knowledge of the pathophysiology based upon what is known about human and experimental acute tubular necrosis with the clinical manifestations of the disease. In particular, we will emphasize the rationale for prevention and treatment of these groups of diseases.

PATHOPHYSIOLOGY

The syndrome of acute tubular necrosis occurs in a wide variety of clinical situations. Commonly, the disease follows a period of hypotension and sepsis and appears to result from ischemia. Another type of

*Instructor in Medicine, State University of New York at Stony Brook, Stony Brook, New York

**Associate Professor of Medicine, State University of New York at Stony Brook, Stony Brook, New York

Supported in part by Biomedical Research Grants SO7RR05736-07.

Table 1. *Causes of Acute Renal Failure*

I. Prerenal Azotemia
   Volume depletion
   Congestive heart failure
   Hypoalbuminemia (nephrotic syndrome and cirrhosis)
   Renal ischemia (renal artery stenosis, embolic disease)
II. Postrenal Azotemia
   Obstructive uropathy (stone, papillary necrosis, prostate, extrinsic tumor
   compression or retroperitoneal fibrosis)
III. Parenchymal renal disease
   Nephritis (glomerular and interstitial)
   Vasculitis
   Pyelonephritis
   Hypercalcemia
   Hepatorenal syndrome
   Myeloma kidney
   Uric acid nephropathy
   Acute tubular necrosis
      Ischemia (shock, sepsis)
      Nephrotoxins (aminoglycosides, anesthetics, iodinated contrast media)
      Pigments (hemoglobin and myoglobin)

acute tubular necrosis follows the ingestion of certain drugs (aminogly-
cosides, methoxyflurane anesthetics, and diatrizoate dyes) and appears
to result from a direct toxic effect of these drugs. In other instances the
acute tubular necrosis may follow the exposure of the kidney to various
pigments (myoglobin and hemoglobin). These varied causes of acute
tubular necrosis seen by the physician usually present in the same
manner, with oliguria, diminished glomerular filtration rate, and tubular dysfunction. Most of what is known about the pathophysiology of
these renal abnormalities is based on experimental animal models of
acute tubular necrosis.

In animals, acute tubular necrosis has been created by the administration of a variety of nephrotoxins, such as dichromate, uranyl nitrate,
and mercury, and by renal ischemia induced by renal artery clamping
and by norepinephrine. These models in many respects are similar to
human acute tubular necrosis in that there is diminished glomerular
filtration and tubular dysfunction. Furthermore, like human acute tubu-

Table 2. *Criteria for the Diagnosis of Acute Tubular Necrosis*

Urine sediment	pigmented cast, renal tubular cells
Urine sodium concentration	> 20 mEq/liter
Urine/plasma osmolality	< 1.1
Urine/plasma creatinine	< 10/1
Urine flow rate	Oliguric (<400 ml/day)
	Nonoliguric (~2000 ml/day)
IVP	rapid persistant nephrogram

lar necrosis which is a heterogenous entity, different pathophysiologic events are associated with different experimental models. Another important similarity is that certain pathophysiologic events appear to initiate and others to maintain the renal failure. Unlike human acute tubular necrosis, where the pathological lesion is spotty in nature, characterized by interstitial edema and cellular infiltrate, rare necrosis, and occasional intratubular casts, the pathologic lesions in the experimental models of acute tubular necrosis are usually more uniform in nature and more severe. Such similarities and differences must be kept in mind when applying data from experimental models to the human condition.

Certain authors using micropuncture techniques to study the functions of single nephrons have found dilatation of the tubules and increased intratubular pressure following ischemic acute tubular necrosis.[5] Additional data show that when ATN tubules are perfused at normal tubular flow rates there is a rapid increase followed by a sudden fall in intratubular pressure.[28] These investigators have concluded that during acute tubular necrosis tubules are obstructed by casts which can be washed away by the increased intratubular pressures generated during perfusion of the obstructed nephron. In both human and experimental acute tubular necrosis these casts have indeed been identified in pathological sections. Furthermore, ischemia is known to cause sloughing of the microvillus membrane of the proximal tubule.

More recent data demonstrate that these sloughed microvilli form part of the obstructing casts.[12] Other workers studying the effects of tubular obstruction on renal blood flow have reported that, following 24 hours of tubular obstruction, there is diminished glomerular blood flow.[4] This observation provides one cogent hypothesis explaining oliguric acute tubular necrosis. As shown in Figure 1, ischemia leads to sloughing of the microvillus membrane of the proximal convoluted tubule. This in turn generates obstructive casts further downstream in the tubule (Fig. 1B). This initially, in conjunction with continued glomerular ultrafiltration, produces dilatation and increased pressure within the tubule. When the intratubular pressure increases to equal the net ultrafiltration pressure, glomerular filtration stops. With continued obstruction glomerular blood flow falls resulting in a fall in ultrafiltration pressure (Fig. 1C). As a result intratubular pressure falls. The initiating event in this hypothesis is tubular obstruction, the maintenance of oliguria is ultimately due to reduced glomerular blood flow. In the maintenance phase, the data are controversial as to whether continued tubular obstruction is necessary since certain investigators report reduced intratubular pressure and glomerular filtration rate without evidence of tubular obstruction.

Other data in the literature suggest that other pathogenetic mechanisms may be involved besides tubular obstruction. In the ischemic and nephrotoxic forms of acute tubular necrosis several investigators have found that the damaged tubular epithelium becomes permeable to water and solutes to which it had been previously impermeable.[5, 7, 12] One way this has been demonstrated is by the microinjection of dyes and marker enzymes into the damaged tubules. These compounds normally do not

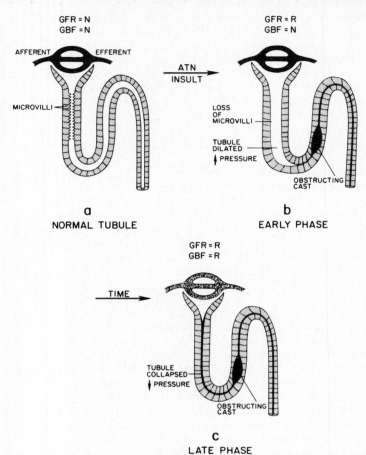

Figure 1.   Role of tubular obstruction in the pathogenesis of acute tubular necrosis. GFR, glomerular filtration rate; GBF, glomerular blood flow; N, normal; R, reduced.

cross the tubular wall, but after ischemia they are consistently found in the interstitial space, suggesting that backleak of tubular fluid occurs. This provides a second reasonable hypothesis explaining oliguric acute tubular necrosis, as shown in Figure 2. The major premise of this hypothesis is that tubular backleak accounts for the entire picture of acute tubular necrosis. Glomerular blood flow and filtration would remain high. All of the tubular contents would leak out into the interstitium and be reabsorbed back into the peritubular blood. Clearly this scenario is inconsistent with all that is known about acute tubular necrosis. The first difficulty is that in all models of acute tubular necrosis studied, cortical blood flow and single nephron glomerular filtration rate are reduced. The second is that the available evidence suggests that only 10 to 15 per cent of ultrafiltrate can backleak,[12] an amount insufficient to account for the oliguria and reduced inulin and creatinine clearance

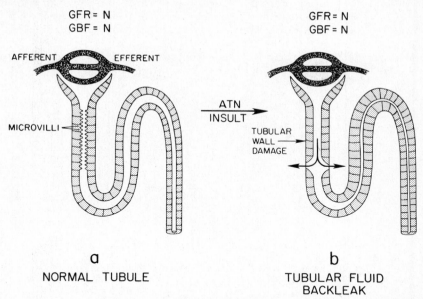

Figure 2. Role of tubular fluid backleak in the pathogenesis of acute tubular necrosis. GFR, glomerular filtration rate; GBF, glomerular blood flow; N, normal.

noted. However, the evidence for backleak is substantial, suggesting that this mechanism does play a significant role in the genesis and maintenance of acute tubular necrosis.

Another factor that may be important in the pathogenesis of acute tubular necrosis is diminished renal blood flow (Fig. 3). This has been observed in experimental acute tubular necrosis caused by nephrotoxins[14] and ischemia.[5] A great deal of effort has been devoted to establishing the mechanism by which renal blood flow is decreased. Several investigators have examined the role of humoral mediators in controlling renal blood flow in acute tubular necrosis.[30] It has been postulated that macula densa, an intratubular sensor, is responsible for the release of humoral mediators resulting in decreased renal blood flow.

The renin-angiotensin system has been suggested as a possible mediator of the diminished renal blood flow in experimental and human acute tubular necrosis. This is based on the finding that plasma renin activity is usually increased under these conditions[11] and angiotensin II infusion can decreased renal blood flow and cause acute tubular necrosis. Against this hypothesis however is the abundant evidence that suppression of the renin-angiotensin system by the administration of anti-renin antibodies and angiotensin II blockers does not prevent the development of acute tubular necrosis in experimental models or in man. Thus, it seems that the renin-angiotensin system is not the only cause of the decrease in renal blood flow observed. Another vasoconstrictor hormone present in the kidney, one whose activity is increased by tubular obstruction, is thromboxane, a member of the

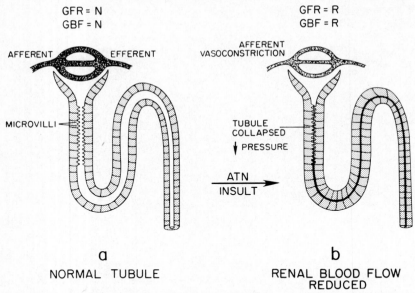

Figure 3.   Role of diminished blood flow in the pathogenesis of acute tubular necrosis. GFR, glomerular filtration rate; GBF, glomerular blood flow; N, normal; R, reduced.

prostaglandin family of compounds.[24] It remains to be determined whether this potent vasoconstrictor is an important mediator of the diminished renal blood flow seen in acute tubular necrosis.

The maintenance of renal blood flow in normal physiologic circumstances is not only a function of the presence or absence of vascular constrictors but may be equally regulated by specific renal vasodilator hormone systems (i.e., prostaglandins and kallikrein-kinin). There has been recent interest in the role played by these systems in maintaining the diminished renal blood flow seen in acute tubular necrosis. In the glycerol model of acute tubular necrosis, prostaglandin inhibition worsens the ATN but intrarenal prostaglandin levels are not diminished in animals treated with glycerol alone. Autotransplantation of medullary renal tissue (prostaglandin-producing tissue) in rabbits diminishes mortality and protects renal function in ischemic acute tubular necrosis. Furthermore, plasma renin activity falls in rabbits with the medullary transplants. Based upon these observations, these investigators have hypothesized that the fall in renal blood flow in acute tubular necrosis is due to an imbalance in vascular constrictors and dilators which in their model was corrected by the autotransplantation.[32]

Only preliminary studies on the kallikrein-kinin system in acute tubular necrosis have been performed. Like prostaglandins, this system is important in regulating renal blood flow. In one study of human acute tubular necrosis the urinary excretion of kallikrein has been shown to be diminished. Whether this is a result of the acute tubular necrosis or part of the pathogenesis of acute tubular necrosis is not known. The finding of a diminished excretion rate suggests that these renal vasodilators may be important in the maintenance of decreased renal blood flow in acute tubular necrosis.

A nonhumoral mechanism that has been proposed to explain the reduction in renal blood flow is based upon the occurrence of endothelial cell swelling. The investigators who support this hypothesis[27-30] have concluded that the initial ischemic insult leads to endothelial swelling, obstructing the microvasculature. Although this remains an attractive hypothesis, at the present time the evidence supporting it is not strong.

The final area of importance in investigation of the pathogenesis of acute tubular necrosis involves direct analysis of glomerular function and pathology. By light microscopy the glomerulus is histologically normal but by electron microscopy there are several abnormalities that have been noted in the epithelial podocytes of the glomerulus. Furthermore, studies using micropuncture techniques have measured the ultrafiltration coefficient (K_f) of the glomerulus during acute tubular necrosis induced by uranyl nitrate[7] and by gentamicin administration. In both studies a decrease in K_f was observed. Since K_f is determined by two factors, total glomerular capillary surface area and permeability per unit of capillary surface area, its reduction could explain the oliguria and decreased glomerular filtration observed in either of two ways. This is illustrated in Figure 4. The first would be a reduction in the number of capillaries perfused in the glomerulus. The second is reduction in glomerular capillary permeability. It certainly is possible that both play a role; however, techniques are not currently available to measure either of these factors separately.

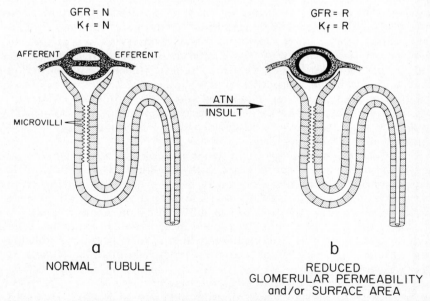

Figure 4.   Role of decreased glomerular function in the pathogenesis of acute tubular necrosis. GFR, glomerular filtration rate; K_f, glomerular ultrafiltration coefficient; N, normal; R, reduced.

The above represents data derived entirely from animal models. What is the relevance of this evidence in patients with acute tubular necrosis? At the bedside a number of important observations can be made. The criteria for establishing the diagnosis, as given in Table 2, provide important clues as to the possible mechanisms involved in human acute tubular necrosis. The oliguria and decreased creatinine clearance are consistent with all of the hypotheses derived from the animal studies. The inappropriately high urine sodium concentration, inability to concentrate the urine, presence of abundant tubular epithelial cell casts and tubular epithelial cells per se provide unequivocal evidence of tubular damage. These observations, in conjunction with experimental evidence that proximal convoluted tubular brush border antigen is present in the urine of patients with acute tubular necrosis,[33] supports the hypothesis of tubular obstruction. However, these same observations can be used to support loss of tubular wall integrity with backleak.

Levinsky[22] has proposed that the backleak hypothesis with preservation of glomerular filtration is strongly suggested by the intravenous pyelogram finding of the rapidly occurring persistent nephrogram commonly seen in acute tubular necrosis. A nephrogram requires filtration of the dye used for intravenous pyelography at a near normal glomerular filtration rate. Thus, in acute tubular necrosis, contrast material might be filtered then leaked into the interstitium and recirculated. Pure tubular obstruction would result in a diminished glomerular filtration rate and the delayed appearance of the neprhogram during the intravenous pyelogram. Thus, tubular venting caused by increased tubular permeability seems important in explaining this finding. These mechanisms of obstruction and backleak may be particularly important in myoglobin-induced and hemoglobin-induced acute tubular necrosis where abundant obstructing tubular casts are observed. In ischemic and nephrotoxin-induced human acute tubular necrosis, obstructing casts have not been uniformly found. This suggests that tubular obstruction may not be an important pathologic mechanism in these forms of acute tubular necrosis. However, it appears more likely that the casts were washed away before the tissue examined was obtained. We are inclined to believe that obstruction and backleak are important in all forms of human acute tubular necrosis.

The factor of diminished renal blood flow has been found as ubiquitously in human as in experimental acute tubular necrosis.[25, 26] As in the experimental models, there currently is no evidence as to the exact causative role of decreased renal perfusion in patients with this disease. However, restoration of blood flow by administration of vasodilators,[21, 26] once the disease is established, does not reestablish excretory renal function. This provides strong evidence that, at least in fully established acute tubular necrosis, factors other than reduced renal blood flow must play a role.

Data concerning the role of glomerular permeability and capillary surface area in human acute tubular necrosis is lacking. However, ultrastructural analysis by electron microscopy shows podocyte abnor-

CAUSES   MECHANISMS   EFFECTS

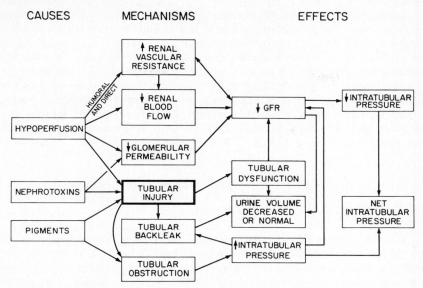

Figure 5.   Summary of the pathogenetic mechanisms operative in acute tubular necrosis.

malities in humans similar to those found in experimental acute tubular necrosis. This is consistent with the glomerular hypothesis presented in Figure 4.

The evidence therefore suggests that all the mechanisms found in the experimental models are important in the human. This being the case, interactions amongst these various mechanisms appear likely in the genesis and maintenance of human acute tubular necrosis. In addition, it is probable that for any given renal insult one or more of these mechanisms may predominate. Our view of this interaction is synthesized in Figure 5. This figure lists the three causative categories of acute tubular necrosis, i.e., hypoperfusion, nephrotoxins, and pigments. Hypoperfusion appears, on the basis of clinical and experimental evidence, to produce renal failure by four mechanisms. It reduces renal blood flow directly and by increasing renal vascular resistance further decreases renal blood flow. It appears to also reduce the glomerular ultrafiltration coefficient and, in addition, produces tubular injury. All four of these factors ultimately result in a reduction of glomerular filtration rate. This in turn leads to a reduction in urine volume. Further reduction in urine volumes may result from tubular backleak, a mechanism enhanced by increased intratubular pressure. In contrast, tubular dysfunction, secondary to tubular injury, tends to increase urine volume. The net effect of these factors may in any given case produce oliguric or nonoliguric renal failure. Also in any given case net intratubular pressure may vary depending upon the relative degree of tubular obstruction versus reduction in glomerular filtration rate.

Nephrotoxins appear to act primarily by producing tubular injury and perhaps by reducing glomerular permeability. Their ultimate effect through these particular mechanisms are similar to those described for hypoperfusion. Pigment-induced acute tubular necrosis, i.e., caused by hemoglobin or myoglobin, appears to act mainly through tubular obstruction with pigment casts and tubular injury. Again the mechanisms of renal failure so induced are similar to those described above and are clearly depicted in Figure 5. The remainder of this review will be devoted to the maneuvers used to prevent the occurrence of or hasten the recovery from acute tubular necrosis. We will also briefly highlight the management of the sequellae of acute renal failure.

PREVENTION AND MANAGEMENT

PREVENTION

In both man and experimental animals, several investigators have attempted to modify the course of acute tubular necrosis. The treatment regimens have been directed against the specific pathogenic mechanisms identified in Figure 5. We will review those regimens designed to prevent the decreased renal blood flow, the tubular injury, and the tubular obstruction.

The decrease in renal blood flow associated with experimental acute tubular necrosis has been prevented by volume expansion, vasodilators, and angiotensin II antagonists. Even though these maneuvers can uniformly increase renal blood flow after acute tubular necrosis has been established, they fail to reverse the diminished glomerular filtration rate and tubular dysfunction which are the hallmarks for the disease. Chronic volume expansion prior to the onset of acute tubular necrosis has a protective effect in some experimental forms of the disorder.[10, 23] The mechanism offered to explain this protective effect is suppression of the renin angiotensin system. Since angiotensin antagonists do not provide a similar protective effect, this explanation appears incorrect.

As previously mentioned, in man renal blood flow has been returned to normal or supernormal levels by the infusion of vasodilators such as acetylcholine and prostaglandins. Despite the increase in renal blood flow, the renal failure does not improve. In fact, the failure of the normalization of renal blood flow to reverse acute tubular necrosis is the most damaging piece of evidence against the hypothesis that diminished renal blood flow is central in pathophysiology.

Though increases in renal blood flow induced as above do not reverse acute tubular necrosis, two compounds, mannitol and furosemide, increase renal blood flow and may ameliorate the severity of acute tubular necrosis. Under normal physiological conditions intravenous mannitol increases renal blood flow as well as urine output in both man and the experimental animal. In the hypoperfused rat kidney, i.e., with systemic arterial pressure reduced to 40 mm Hg, mannitol increases renal blood flow and, by altering glomerular hemodynamics, increases glomerular filtration pressure.[19] As a result glomerular filtration, previously absent, is partially restored. In the norepinephrine-induced model of acute tubular necrosis, pretreatment with mannitol reduces the fall in glomerular filtration rate to less than that which occurs in the animals not pretreated with mannitol.[8] Based on these experiments these investigators conclude that mannitol pretreatment has a dual action in preventing acute tubular necrosis. First the increase in renal blood flow and decrease in afferent arteriolar constriction produced by mannitol results in increased glomerular capillary hydrostatic pressure. This results in an increase in glomerular filtration rate. The increase in filtration rate results in an increase in intratubular pressures, dislodging obstructing casts, and thus allows glomerular filtration rate to increase further. This work in an animal model of acute tubular necrosis provides a strong rationale for the use of this compound in man.

Unfortunately, prospective, well controlled studies using mannitol in man are not yet available. Those that are available suggest that pretreatment with mannitol may be helpful in reducing the severity of human acute tubular necrosis. In patients undergoing vascular surgery or open heart surgery, pretreatment with mannitol has been shown to decrease the incidence of postoperative renal failure.[2] In a group of patients with nonsurgical disease caused by ischemia or pigments (myoglobin), mannitol has been reported to reverse acute tubular necrosis.[13] A recent report concludes that in patients with diabetes mellitus, mannitol can decrease the incidence of acute tubular necrosis following the administration of diatrizoate (IVP) dyes.[3] So at least in a select group of patients, mannitol has been demonstrated to be effective in reducing the incidence of acute tubular necrosis. In most clinical circumstances, mannitol can be administered without significant side-effects. However, one should keep in mind that mannitol will cause intravascular expansion, especially in the patient with oliguria and intractable renal failure. This could precipitate congestive heart failure, especially in a patient with limited cardiac reserve. If this should occur, the volume expansion produced by mannitol must be corrected by acute dialysis.

As is the case with mannitol, the mechanism and efficacy of the loop diuretics (furosemide and ethacrynic acid) in reversing acute tubular necrosis remains unresolved. Unlike mannitol, furosemide does not increase renal blood flow or increase glomerular filtration rate in the hypoperfused kidney. Similar to mannitol, however, furosemide pretreatment has been shown to protect against the development of acute tubular necrosis in certain experimental models. In the norepinephrine model, it has been suggested that the protective effect is a result of the solute diuresis with the resultant increase in urine flow rate raising intratubular pressure and washing away obstructing casts.[9] In other experimental models of acute tubular necrosis, furosemide has not been effective in preventing renal failure.

In man, except for several uncontrolled studies, furosemide has not proved effective in preventing acute tubular necrosis.[20] However, there is evidence that oliguric acute tubular necrosis can be converted to nonoliguric acute tubular necrosis with diuretics. Whether the diuretics act on a small population of functionally intact nephrons or change intratubular or intraglomerular dynamics is not known. Whatever the case, one clear benefit of the diuresis produced is that sodium and water balance can be achieved with greater ease and overall prognosis may be improved. Caution must be exerted in the use of these diuretics since ototoxicity can occur. This is especially troublesome in acute renal failure where potentially high blood levels can occur owing to the decreased renal excretion. Furthermore, the use of these diuretics in a patient with prerenal azotemia, already volume contracted, may lead to further reduction in extracellular volume resulting in acute tubular necrosis rather than preventing it. We, therefore, recommend that until the efficacy of diuretics is more firmly established, they should be reserved for the patient with acute tubular necrosis who is clearly volume overloaded and should be given with the goal of controlling volume rather than reversing acute tubular necrosis.

Other investigators have examined modalities which would hasten the repair of damaged tubules after acute tubular necrosis has been established. Most promising in this respect has been the infusion of essential amino acids. In the experimental animal with nephrotoxin-induced ATN the tubular epithelium repairs faster in the animal pretreated with essential amino acids.[31] Furthermore, the severity of the renal failure is less. Though no definite site of action of the amino acids is known, it has been postulated that they stimulate epithelial cell membrane synthesis which results in more rapid tubule repair. Essential amino acids and glucose have been administered to surgical patients in whom acute tubular necrosis developed.[1] In a prospective double blind study, the survival rate was significantly higher in those patients who received essential amino acids and glucose than in those who received glucose alone. In this study, patients who received essential amino acids also had a significantly better survival rate if extrarenal complications such as pneumonia, generalized sepsis, or gastrointestinal bleeding occurred. Thus, it appears that the essential amino acids not only accelerate the renal repair but also enhance the ability of the patient to fight systemic complications.

Management

The management of patients with established acute tubular necrosis has been reviewed in two previous articles in this series.[17, 29] We will update these reviews and summarize our approach to acute tubular necrosis. The goal of all such regimens is to maintain water and mineral balance while preventing development of the uremic state. All treatment is supportive and is based on the premise that the patient will eventually recover renal function.

Hyperkalemia

Hyperkalemia is reviewed elsewhere in this issue. This potentially life threatening complication is very common in acute tubular necrosis. Hyperkalemia is of special concern in trauma, postoperative renal failure, rhabdomyolysis-induced acute tubular necrosis, following the administration of blood, and after development of severe acidosis. The presence of hyperkalemia is a medical emergency and requires rapid treatment.

Fluid and Electrolytes

The primary goal is to maintain water and electrolyte balance, neither exceeding requirements nor allowing deficits to occur. An accurate record of the fluid and electrolyte output of the patient (including urine volume, gastrointestinal losses, and tube drainage) must be maintained. The volume lost should be replaced such that output and insensible losses are balanced. Specific electrolyte and mineral concentrations may become deranged. Hyponatremia and hypernatremia most often reflect over or underhydration since the damaged tubules are no longer able to regulate water balance by excreting concentrated or diluted urine. Thus, volume expansion should always be accomplished with isotonic solutions to prevent these complications. As an example, a patient whose fluid output is 400 ml of urine per day and 1000 ml of gastric juice per day containing 75 mEq per liter of sodium will need replacement with 2000 ml of fluid to balance urinary, gastrointestinal, and net insensible losses. Replacement fluid should be approximately half normal saline since the patient is losing 75 mEq per liter of sodium chloride in the output. Hyponatremia would occur if the patient received only dextrose in water. Essential to the fluid management of a patient is the measurement of daily weight to insure that estimates of balance are correct. In the patient receiving adequate nutrition, body weight should remain constant if balance is to be achieved. In the fasted patient, balance will be achieved if the patient's weight decreases 0.5 kg per day. The scrupulous management of fluid and electrolyte balance will avoid complications in the already difficult course of acute renal failure.

Nutrition

As previously reviewed, proper nutrition may not only hasten kidney repair but appears to promote wound healing, decrease catabolism of muscle, and decrease mortality from sepsis. Essential amino acids for infusion are available from several different manufacturers. Glucose or lipid must be given simultaneously to meet the caloric needs of the patient. Specific recommendations as to the caloric and protein content have been reviewed previously. The administration of hyperalimentation solutions to patients with oliguric acute tubular necrosis frequently requires the initiation of dialysis since azotemia may progress more rapidly. If dailysis is readily available, the nutritional benefits of these solutions far outweigh any problems associated with dialysis. Unlike previous recommendations where a patient was thought to be in balance if he lost 0.5 to 1 kg per day, in the patient receiving hyperalimentation optimum treatment enables the patient to maintain his body weight.

The complications of hyperalimentation in renal failure do exist and include the trauma related to placing a subclavian vein catheter, the potential metabolic acidosis form amino acid solutions containing arginine hydrochloride, the increased potential for excess volume expansion, and increased incidence of infection from the indwelling central venous catheter. The most ominous complication secondary to hyperalimentation in acute tubular necrosis is sepsis.

Infection

In general, the incidence of infection in acute tubular necrosis is high. This results in serious morbidity and a high mortality. Based upon this observation, all potential sources of infection should be assessed daily and removed at the earliest possible time. These include indwelling bladder catheters which are usually not needed in the management of acute tubular necrosis, intravenous access sites, arterial lines, and pressure monitoring devices. Frequently these potential sources of infection are left in place too long because the information generated is helpful in the management of acutely ill patients.

Prophylactic antibiotics are not recommended because of superinfection with resistant organisms. However, patients with febrile episodes must be thoroughly evaluated and properly treated as quickly as possible. When antibiotics are needed, dosages should be regulated to the level of renal function and dialysis clearance.[6]

Dialysis

In the past dialysis treatment was only considered when uremic complications (e.g., nausea, vomiting, or pericarditis) developed or when fluid and electrolyte balance could no longer be managed by conservative measures. Today we are more aggressive in our dialytic approach to the oliguric patient with acute renal failure. We no longer wait for uremic symptoms to appear but dialyze early so as to prevent the onset of uremia. This policy allows the patient to be given adequate nutrition, and prevents complications such as bleeding due to coagulopathy, sepsis, acidosis, and life-threatening electrolyte abnormalities. Dialysis, therefore, should be started early in the catabolic patient, especially if receiving hyperalimentation, in all oliguric patients with a creatinine of 10.0, and certainly at the first symptom suggestive of uremia. Most cases of nonoliguric renal failure do not require dialysis. For most patients peritoneal dialysis, the slower form of dialysis, is the treatment of choice since the uremic state can be reversed without a large shift in intracerebral fluid and electrolytes (dysequilibrium). Hemodialysis should be reserved for those patients who have had recent abdominal surgery, intra-abdominal adhesions, or are highly catabolic. Peritoneal dialysis causes considerable protein loss across the peritoneum and cannot be used in the patient who has had abdominal surgery, while hemodialysis requires an indwelling vascular access (Scribner shunt), requires anticoagulation during dialysis and may cause aberrent shifts in fluid and electrolyte balance (dysequilibrium). Despite these complications, we feel that early dialysis is preferable in the treatment of acute tubular necrosis.

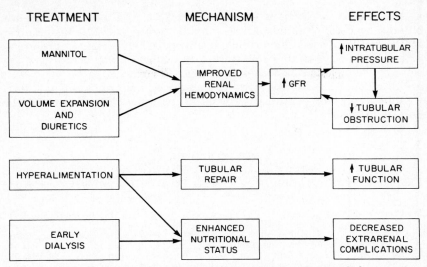

Figure 6.   Therapeutic modalities involved in the prevention of acute tubular necrosis.

PROGNOSIS

Despite the advances in dialysis and fluid and electrolyte management, the mortality of acute tubular necrosis remains between 40 and 60
per cent. This bleak prognosis reflects more the type of patient being
treated than the managerial acumen of the physician. Acute tubular
necrosis now appears to be primarily a disease of the elderly, septic, and
postoperative patient. Rarely do patients die of uremic symptoms but
rather from complications such as sepsis and shock attributable to their
underlying disease. Thus, the underlying disease appears to be the best
prognosticator of ultimate outcome. Patients with burns or postoperative
renal failure have the worst prognosis while those with nephrotoxic
renal failure have the best survival. Subgroups among these categories
suggest that patients past the fourth decade have a worse prognosis than
younger patients with the same cause for their acute tubular necrosis.
Also, oliguric patients have a worse prognosis and higher morbidity than
nonoliguric patients. Despite the managerial expertise acquired over the
past 10 years, the reversal of the high morbidity and mortality associated
with acute tubular necrosis remains a major challange as yet un-
solved.

New effective treatment regimens are clearly necessary in order to
improve the poor prognosis of this disease entity. Our current recommendations for management of these patients in order to improve prognosis
are summarized in Figure 6. The preventative and managerial regimens
which seem appropriate based on the pathophysiology of acute tubular
necrosis are outlined. In any one patient all or one of these treatments

may be used based on the particular needs of the patient. Mannitol, volume expansion, and diuretics act by improving renal hemodynamics resulting in increased glomerular filtration rate. Hyperalimentation and early dialysis have a dual function in that they enhance recovery and they decrease extrarenal complications. It remains to be seen with careful prospective stuides whether these treatment regimens will have an impact on the overall prognosis of patients with acute tubular necrosis in the 1980's.

REFERENCES

1. Abel, R. M., Beck, C., Abbott, W. M., et al.: Improved survival from acute renal failure after treatment with intravenous L-amino acids and glucose. New Eng. J. Med., 288:695–699, 1973.
2. Abbott, W. M., and Austen, W. G.: The reversal of renal cortical ischemia during aortic occlusion by mannitol. J. Surg. Res., 16:482–489, 1974.
3. Anto, H. R., Chou, S. Y., Porush, J. G., et al.: Mannitol prevention of acute renal failure associated with infusion pyelography. Clin. Res. 407A, 1979.
4. Arendshorst, W. J., Finn, W. F., and Gottschalk, C. W.: Nephron stop-flow pressure response to obstruction for 24 hours in the rat kidney. J. Clin. Invest., 53:1497–1500, 1974.
5. Arendshorst, W. J., Finn, W. F., and Gottschalk, C. W.: Pathogenesis of acute renal failure following temporary renal ischemia in the rat. Circ. Res., 37:558–568, 1975.
6. Bennett, W., Mather, R. S., Parker, R. A.: Drug therapy in renal failure. Dosing guidelines for adults. Ann. Intern. Med., 93:62–89, 1980.
7. Blantz, R. C.: Mechanism of acute renal failure after uranyl nitrate. J. Clin. Invest., 55:621–635, 1975.
8. Burke, T. J., Cronin, R. E., Duchin, K. L., et al.: Ischemia and tubular obstruction during acute renal failure in dogs: Mannitol and protection. Amer. J. Physiol., 238:F305–F314, 1980.
9. DeTorrente, A., Miller, P. D., Cronin, R. E., et al.: Effect of furosemide and acetylcholine in norepinephrine-induced acute renal failure. Amer. J. Physiol., 235:F131–F136, 1978.
10. DiBona, G. F., McDonald, D., Flamenbaum, W., et al.: Maintenance of renal function in salt-loaded rats despite severe tubular necrosis induced by $HgCl_2$. Nephron, 8:205–220, 1970.
11. DiBona, G. F., and Sawin, L. L.: The renin angiotensin system in acute renal failure in the rat. Lab. Invest., 25:528–532, 1971.
12. Donohoe, J. F., Venkatachalam, M. A., Bernard, D. B., et al.: Tubular leakage and obstruction in acute ischemic renal failure. Kid. Internat., 10:567, 1976.
13. Eneas, J. F., Schoenfeld, P. Y., and Humphreys, M.: The effect of infusion of mannitol sodium bicarbonate on the clinical course of myoglobinuria. Arch. Intern. Med., 139:801–805, 1979.
14. Flamenbaum, W., Huddleston, M. L., McNeal, J. S., et al.: Uranyl nitrate-induced acute renal failure in the rat: Micropuncture and renal hemodynamic studies. Kid. Internat., 6:408–418, 1974.
15. Flores, J., DiBona, D. R., Beck, C. H., et al.: The role of cell swelling in ischemic renal damage and the protective effect of hypertonic solute. J. Clin. Invest., 51:118–126, 1972.
16. Frega, N. S., DiBona, D. R., Guertte, B., et al.: Ischemic renal injury. Kid. Internat. 4(Suppl. 6):S17–S25, 1976.
17. Hedger, R. W.: The conservative management of acute oliguric renal failure. Med. Clin. N. Amer., 58:121–135, 1971.
18. Hollenberg, D., Epstein, M., Rosen, S., et al.: Acute oliguric renal failure in man: Evidence for preferential renal cortical ischemia. Medicine, 47:455–474, 1968.
19. Johnston, P., Bernard, D. B., and Levinsky, N. G.: Effect of volume expansion on hemodynamics of the hypoperfused rat kidney. J. Clin. Invest., 64:550–558, 1979.
20. Kleinknecht, D., Guneval, D., Gonzales-Dique, L. A., et al.: Furosemide in oliguric acute renal failure. A controlled trial. Nephron, 17:51–58, 1976.

21. Ladefoged, T., et al.: Effect of dihydralazine and acetylcholine on renal blood flow, mean circulation time for plasma and renal resistance in acute renal failure. Pathogenesis and clinical findings with renal failure. Edited by U. Gessler, K., Schroder, H., Weidinger. Stuttgart Georg Thieme Verlag, 1971, p. 7–15.
22. Levinsky, N. G.: Pathophysiology of acute renal failure. New Eng. J. Med., 296:1453–1458, 1977.
23. McDonald, F. D., Thiel, G., Wilson, D. R., et al.: The prevention of acute renal failure in the rat by long term saline loading. A possible role for the renin angiotensin axis. Proc. Soc. Exper. Biol. Med., 131:610–614, 1969.
24. Morrison, A. R., Nishikowa, K., and Needleman, P.: Unmasking of thromboxane A_2 synthesis by ureteral obstruction in the rat kidney. Nature, 267:259, 1977.
25. Reubi, F. C. and Vorburger, C.: Renal hemodynamics in acute renal failure after shock in man. Kid. Internat., 10:S137–S143, 1976.
26. Reubi, F. D.: The pathogenesis of anuria following shock. Kid. Internat., 3:106–110, 1974.
27. Stein, J., Myer, H., Lifschitz, D., et al.: Current concepts on the pathophysiology of acute renal failure. Amer. J. Physiol., 3:F171–F181, 1978.
28. Tanner, G. A., and M. Steinhausen: Tubular obstruction and ischemia-induced acute renal failure in the rat. Kid. Internat., 10:565–573, 1976.
29. Thomson, G. L.: Acute Renal Failure. MED. CLIN. N. AMER., 57:1579–1589, 1973.
30. Thurau, K., and Baylon, J. W.: Acute renal success: The unexpected logic of oliguria in acute renal failure. Amer. J. Med., 61:308–315, 1976.
31. Toback, F. G.: Amino acid enhancement of renal regeneration after acute tubular necrosis. Kid. Internat., 12:193–198, 1977.
32. Torres, V. E., Storng, C. G., Romero, J. C., et al.: Indomethacin enhancement of glycerol-induced acute renal failure in rabbits. Kid. Internat., 7:170–178, 1975.
33. Zager, R., and Carpenter, C. B.: Radioimmunoassay of urinary renal tubular antigen: A potential marker of tubular injury. Kid. Internat., 13:505–512, 1978.

Division of Nephrology and Hypertension
Department of Medicine
State University of New York
Stony Brook, New York 11794

The Emergency Treatment of Hyperkalemia

Cheryl L. Kunis, M.D.,*
Jerome Lowenstein, M.D.†

Potassium is the major intracellular cation. Unlike other cations such as calcium, which exist largely in bound and complexed forms, potassium is thought to exist as a free ion. Ninety eight per cent of total body potassium is located intracellularly at a concentration of 150 mEq per liter; the extracellular concentration normally ranges from 3.5 to 5.0 mEq per liter. The steady state transcellular potassium gradient is important for the transmission of electrical impulses and may also be necessary for optimal synthesis of nucleic acid, protein, and glycogen.[20]

Hyperkalemia is defined as a serum potassium concentration greater than 5.0 mEq per liter. Although extracellular potassium represents only 2 per cent of total body stores, changes in the extracellular concentration are associated with significant changes in the transcellular potassium gradient which result in alterations in cellular function. An understanding of the factors which determine the distribution of potassium between cells and the extracellular space, and of the mechanisms responsible for homeostasis, provides a framework for the rational treatment of life-threatening hyperkalemia.

THE TRANSCELLULAR POTASSIUM GRADIENT

The resting membrane potential is the voltage difference a cell maintains across its membrane in the steady state. The resting potential is determined largely by the concentration gradient for potassium.[11, 17, 19] Alterations in the transcellular potassium gradient influence the mem-

*Instructor in Medicine, New York University Medical Center, New York, New York
†Professor of Medicine, New York University School of Medicine, New York, New York

Supported in part by the Jane Hilder Harris Fund.

brane potential and exert diverse effects on electrical activity in excitable tissues such as nerve and muscle.

There is a constant passive efflux of potassium from the cell along a concentration gradient. Maintenance of the high intracellular potassium concentration is dependent upon the presence of Na^+-K^+-dependent ATPase in the cell membrane. Energy derived from the conversion of ATP to ADP is used to pump potassium into the cell from the extracellular space and to extrude sodium from the cell.

Changes in extracellular pH can alter the potassium gradient. In acute acidosis, hydrogen ions move into cells to be buffered by cellular proteins and potassium shifts to the extracellular compartment to maintain electroneutrality. In alkalosis the converse is true and potassium moves into cells.

In addition to the Na^+-K^+-dependent ATPase pump and extracellular pH, circulating levels of insulin, aldosterone, and catecholamines affect the transcellular potassium gradient. Following potassium loading, secretion of insulin and aldosterone is enhanced, promoting cellular uptake of potassium. The mechanism whereby insulin moves potassium into cells appears to be separate from its effect on uptake of glucose; glucose and potassium do not enter cells in a coupled fashion.[4, 29, 30] Whether aldosterone plays a significant role in affecting the potassium gradient under acute conditions, as insulin does, is not well established. Catecholamines have been shown to produce an initial release of potassium by hepatocytes, followed by the uptake of potassium in liver and skeletal muscle.[28] This latter effect is mediated by beta-adrenergic receptors. Although beta-adrenergic agonists can promote release of insulin, insulin does not seem to play a role in catecholamine-induced movement of potassium into cells.[28]

RENAL EXCRETION OF POTASSIUM

Potassium is added to the extracellular fluid by intestinal absorption of dietary potassium and by endogenous cellular breakdown. The normal diet contains 50 to 100 mEq of potassium per day, almost all of which is absorbed, and 90 per cent of which must be eliminated by the kidney. Only 5 to 10 mEq are normally lost through the gastrointestinal tract; potassium loss through the skin is insignificant. Following ingestion and absorption, potassium is rapidly transferred into cells and thus, changes in the serum concentration are minimal. Renal excretion of the ingested potassium is completed in 6 to 8 hours.

Potassium is freely filtered by the glomerulus, and 90 per cent of the filtered load is reabsorbed in the proximal tubule and loop of Henle. Whereas renal sodium excretion is determined by glomerular filtration and reabsorption, potassium excretion is dependent almost entirely on secretion by the distal tubule and collecting duct. The potassium concentration in the distal tubular cell is of primary importance in determining the amount of potassium secreted into the lumen. In general, the greater

Table 1. *Determinants of Renal Potassium Secretion*

Distal cellular potassium concentration
    Dietary intake
    pH
    Aldosterone (also increases luminal membrane permeability to K^+)
Distal tubular flow rate
    Distal luminal potassium concentration
Distal luminal sodium concentration

the potassium load, the higher the concentration in the distal tubular cell. Since the intracellular potassium is greater than the luminal concentration, potassium moves into the distal tubular fluid passively along a concentration gradient. Thus, low luminal potassium concentrations facilitate secretion. Since acute acid-base abnormalities produce transcellular shifts in potassium, the gradient is altered between the distal tubular cell and the lumen which, in turn, affects renal excretion. For example, in acute acidosis, a decreased potassium concentration in distal tubular cells reduces the cell-to-lumen concentration gradient and leads to decreased potassium secretion. Acute alkalosis, conversely, promotes kaliuresis. The effects of chronic acid-base disturbances on the renal handling of potassium are less well defined.

Distal sodium delivery, distal tubular flow rate, and the circulating aldosterone concentration also influence renal secretion of potassium (Table 1). Aldosterone is thought to enhance secretion by increasing the permeability of the luminal membrane to potassium, as well as by stimulating active transfer of potassium into cells at the peritubular membrane.[16] The reabsorption of sodium in the distal tubule creates a potential difference across the epithelial cell with the lumen becoming more electronegative. Secretion of potassium is facilitated by the greater electrical gradient.

Recent evidence suggests that flow rate in the distal tubule may be much more significant than sodium concentration in modulating potassium secretion.[14] The distal luminal potassium concentration is usually less than 1 mEq per liter. Since potassium diffusion into the distal tubule and collecting duct appears to reach equilibrium rapidly, an increase in distal tubular flow rate is associated with more potassium secretion. In vivo microperfusion studies in the rat distal tubule have demonstrated that increasing flow without changing the sodium concentration augments excretion of potassium; conversely, increasing the sodium concentration without changes in flow rate has no effect on secretion of potassium.[14] When luminal potassium concentrations were increased to levels greater than the cellular concentration in these microperfusion studies, passive reabsorption of potassium could be demonstrated.[14]

Potassium secretion by the distal tubule thus appears to be dependent upon distal cellular potassium concentration, distal tubular flow, luminal sodium and potassium concentrations, and aldosterone.

MANIFESTATIONS OF HYPERKALEMIA

Hyperkalemia produces changes in the electrical properties of cell membranes which may result in neuromuscular and cardiac manifestations. Neuromuscular symptoms are the most common complaints. Paresthesias and weakness may progress to an ascending paralysis which classically begins in the hands and feet. Cardiac conduction disturbances are commonly seen and may result in cardiac standstill.

The magnitude of the transmembrane resting potential, determined largely by the potassium gradient, affects the rate of rise of the cellular action potential; this, in turn, determines the speed of impulse conduction in nervous tissue.[8] Hyperkalemia, by diminishing the ratio of intracellular to extracellular potassium, reduces the resting membrane potential; i.e., the membrane potential becomes less negative. This diminishes the rate of rise of the action potential and slows conduction.[8] This effect may contribute to the severe muscle weakness which characterizes hyperkalemia.

When a stimulus transiently reduces the resting membrane potential to the threshold potential, an action potential results. The action potential is produced by the opening of sodium channels which permits a rapid entry of sodium into the cell.[17] Hyperkalemia has two effects on this process. The first effect is a reduction in the resting membrane potential, as discussed above. This reduction in the resting potential toward threshold allows stimuli of lesser intensity to evoke action potentials. The second effect of hyperkalemia on the development of the action potential is to inactivate sodium channels.[17] This prevents the development of an action potential independent of the magnitude of the stimulus. When the rise in the serum potassium is small, the first effect predominates. The cell becomes hyperexcitable, giving rise to muscle twitching and paresthesias. When hyperkalemia is profound, the second effect predominates. When all the sodium channels are inactivated, a stimulus is unable to produce an electrical response.[17] This may account for the paralysis seen in hyperkalemia.

The abnormalities in electrophysiologic activity are frequently reflected in the electrocardiogram, as cardiac tissue is especially susceptible to the changes in membrane potential induced by hyperkalemia. Early repolarization, manifested by peaked T waves and shortening of the QT interval, is usually the first electrocardiographic finding. The decreased rate of rise of the cellular action potential is manifested on the electrocardiogram by prolongation of the QRS complex, atrioventricular block (reflecting slowed conduction in the His-Purkinje system), and flattening and eventual disappearance of the P wave. The QRS may continue to widen until the "sine wave pattern" emerges. Ventricular fibrillation or asystole may follow. Cardiac standstill, which is most characteristic of hyperkalemia, is produced by the same mechanism as that described for peripheral muscle paralysis.

There is usually a good correlation between the degree of hyperkalemia and the presence of cardiac conduction disturbances. However, some circumstances may exaggerate the effects of mild to moderate hyperkalemia and produce life-threatening cardiac arrhythmias. These include a rapid rise in the serum potassium concentration,[25, 26] acidosis, hyponatremia, and hypocalcemia.

ETIOLOGY OF HYPERKALEMIA

Hyperkalemia may be produced by three mechanisms: (1) an increase in the potassium load, (2) a change in the transcellular gradient for potassium, and (3) a primary decrease in renal excretion (Table 2).

It is very uncommon for exogenous potassium loading to induce hyperkalemia when renal function is normal. As long as distal tubular flow is adequate, potassium secretion and homeostasis are usually maintained; as discussed previously, the rapid cellular uptake of potassium minimizes changes in serum potassium concentration until renal excretion is completed. However, in the patient with reduced renal function, potassium loading can induce hyperkalemia. Exogenous sources of potassium include "salt substitutes," many of which are potassium salts, or medications containing potassium (for example, K^+-penicillin). Hypercatabolism can also produce an increased potassium load. Such increased endogenous potassium loads are observed following surgery, trauma, burns, corticosteroid therapy, cell destruction caused by chemotherapeutic agents, and rhabdomyolysis.

Hyperkalemia may be due to alterations in the transcellular distribution of potassium. This is most frequently seen in acute acidosis. Less commonly, hyperkalemia may be seen with severe digitalis intoxication in which potassium accumulates in the extracellular space due to poisoning of the Na^+-K^+-dependent ATPase pump. Since potassium is released from the muscle cell during depolarization, patients treated with depolarizing muscle relaxants, such as succinylcholine, experience a small, clinically insignificant rise in serum potassium. Patients with renal failure or neuromuscular diseases, or who have suffered trauma, however, may develop life-threatening hyperkalemia following administration of such depolarizing agents.[6]

Another iatrogenic cause of hyperkalemia is the administration of arginine hydrochloride which is used in treating metabolic alkalosis or in testing pituitary function. There appears to be a direct intracellular exchange of arginine for potassium.[14] Hyperkalemic periodic paralysis is an uncommon familial disease in which small increments in the extracellular potassium concentration cause severe symptoms of muscle weakness and paralysis. The etiology of the altered transcellular distribution of potassium in this disease is not well understood. Finally, hyperosmolality and insulin-deficient states have been associated with hyperkalemia. Hyperglycemia can produce hyperkalemia by increasing the serum osmolality which results in the movement of fluid containing potassium out of cells.[7] In nondiabetic patients, this effect is counteracted by the release of insulin. In diabetic patients, however, hyperglycemia can cause life-threatening hyperkalemia. There is some controversy as

Table 2. *Mechanisms of Hyperkalemia*

INCREASED POTASSIUM LOAD

Increased ingestion
    KCl supplementation (and salt substitutes)
    Potassium-containing medications
Blood transfusion
Cell destruction
    Rhabdomyolysis
    Surgery
    Trauma and Burns
    Tumor necrosis
    Corticosteroid therapy

TRANSCELLULAR POTASSIUM SHIFT

Acute acidosis
Digitalis intoxication
Succinylcholine
Arginine hydrochloride
Hyperkalemic periodic paralysis
Hyperosmolality
Insulin deficiency

DECREASED RENAL EXCRETION

Acute renal failure
Chronic renal failure
Hypoaldosteronism
Volume depletion
Potassium-sparing diuretics

PSEUDOHYPERKALEMIA

Thrombocytosis
Leukocytosis
Blood sampling with cell lysis or release of potassium from muscle

---

to whether hypoaldosteronism, in addition to insulin deficiency, is necessary for hyperkalemia to develop under these circumstances.[2, 7, 13]

    Alterations in the mechanisms influencing distal cellular secretion can reduce renal potassium excretion and lead to hyperkalemia. Hyperkalemia is common in acute oliguric renal failure, regardless of etiology, because the diminished distal tubular flow impairs potassium secretion. Hyperkalemia is much less frequent in nonoliguric acute renal failure. When acute renal failure occurs in a setting in which potassium release is enhanced, as with rhabdomyolysis, or in which there is a transcellular shift, as in sepsis with metabolic acidosis, life-threatening hyperkalemia may develop very rapidly.

    In chronic renal failure the excretion of potassium is usually maintained despite a marked decrease in nephron mass. As nephrons are lost, those remaining secrete increasing amounts of potassium per nephron. This adaptation may be mediated by increased Na^+-K^+-ATPase activity in the renal tubular membrane.[24] Increased flow rate per nephron in chronic renal failure also contributes to enhanced potassium secretion per nephron. In addition to these renal responses, an extrarenal adaptive mechanism develops which allows a more rapid transfer of potassium into cells.[1] This cellular adaptation may be mediated by aldosterone; adrenalectomy has been shown to prevent this transcellular shift.[1] Increased potassium loads in patients with chronic renal failure may produce hyperkalemia due to limitation in the adaptive responses when the glomerular filtration rate falls below 5 to 10 ml per minute.

Hyperkalemia is seen in some patients with only moderate reduction in glomerular filtration rate (30 to 80 ml per minute). Typically this is seen in patients with diabetes or chronic tubulointerstitial renal disease and has often been associated with hyporeninemia and selective hypoaldosteronism. Hypoaldosteronism, which appears to be responsible for the hyperkalemia, may be secondary to hyporeninemia or may be due to a separate adrenal defect.[23] The etiology of the diminished renin secretion by the juxtaglomerular apparatus is unknown. In addition to hyperkalemia, approximately 50 per cent of such patients manifest hyperchloremic acidosis. Hyperkalemia, as well as reduction in nephron mass, is associated with decreased renal cortical ammonia production.[27] This, in turn, diminishes the amount of hydrogen ion which can be excreted as ammonium and may contribute to the acidosis seen in this disorder. In addition, experimental studies have demonstrated that hyperkalemia per se reduces proximal tubular bicarbonate reabsorption.[5, 22]

Other states of mineralocorticoid deficiency may also be associated with hyperkalemia. In Addison's disease diminished potassium secretion may be due not only to hypoaldosteronism, but also to volume depletion which diminishes potassium secretion by reducing distal tubular flow. With dehydration, movement of potassium into cells also appears to be impaired by mechanisms which have not been well defined.[3] Mineralocorticoid antagonists, such as spironolactone, or other potassium-sparing diuretics may cause reduced potassium excretion. Diabetic patients are particularly susceptible to the hyperkalemic effects of these agents. This probably results from abnormalities in insulin release and/or effect, associated renal disease, or hypoaldosteronism, all of which are commonly seen in diabetes.

Lastly, under some circumstances an elevated measured serum potassium may result from the in vitro release of potassium during blood clotting (pseudohyperkalemia). Normally this produces a rise in the serum potassium of approximately 0.5 mEq per liter. With thrombocytosis, the amount of potassium released is increased and pseudohyperkalemia develops. This entity can also be seen in myeloproliferative disorders with marked leukocytosis. In addition, difficulty in blood sampling that produces cell lysis can falsely elevate the measured serum potassium concentration. A similar artifact may be produced in vivo by exercising the forearm prior to blood sampling; this releases potassium from muscle cells. These entities should be considered when an etiology cannot be found for an elevated serum potassium concentration or when symptoms or electrocardiographic changes are absent in the face of moderate to severe hyperkalemia.

Table 3. *Acute Treatment of Hyperkalemia*

REVERSAL OF MEMBRANE ABNORMALITIES

Calcium gluconate
Hypertonic sodium solutions

ALTERATION IN THE TRANSCELLULAR GRADIENT

Glucose and insulin
Sodium bicarbonate

REMOVAL OF POTASSIUM FROM THE BODY

Diuretics
Cation exchange resins (Kayexalate)
Dialysis (peritoneal or hemodialysis)

TREATMENT

Treatment of hyperkalemia will depend on the degree to which the potassium is elevated, the etiology, and the presence or absence of symptoms and electrocardiographic findings. In general, a serum potassium concentration between 5.0 and 6.5 mEq per liter is considered mild hyperkalemia, 6.5 to 8.0 mEq per liter is moderate, and a potassium greater than 8.0 mEq per liter is severe hyperkalemia. Moderate and severe hyperkalemia should always be treated. The presence of neuromuscular symptoms requires acute treatment, and evidence of electrocardiographic abnormalities constitutes a true medical emergency. Frequently the diagnosis of hyperkalemia can be suspected from the clinical setting and the electrocardiogram. For example, loss of P waves and a widened QRS complex in an oliguric patient is highly suggestive and justifies emergency treatment for hyperkalemic even before laboratory documentation is available.

The acute treatment of hyperkalemia aims to (1) reverse the membrane abnormalities, (2) restore the transcellular gradient by moving potassium into cells, and (3) remove the excess potassium from the body (Table 3).

Reversal of Membrane Abnormalities

Membrane excitability is defined as the difference between the resting and the threshold potentials. When the resting potential is reduced in the presence of hyperkalemia, increasing the extracellular calcium concentration reduces the membrane threshold potential and restores normal membrane excitability. In the presence of severe neuromuscular symptoms or life-threatening cardiac conduction disturbances, calcium gluconate, 10 to 30 ml of a 10 per cent solution, should be given intravenously over 3 to 4 minutes. Continuous electrocardiographic monitoring is necessary, and the conduction abnormalities usually reverse within several minutes. The effect is transient since the serum potassium concentration is unchanged and the calcium is rapidly excreted or is taken up by bone. Calcium gluconate may be repeated if there is no effect after 5 to 7 minutes or if symptoms recur. The administration of calcium is only a temporizing measure, pending the effects of further therapeutic intervention.

In addition to calcium, hypertonic sodium solutions have been used to reverse the membrane alterations of hyperkalemia. They are useful primarily in hyperkalemic patients with associated hyponatremia, since the decreased serum sodium concentration exaggerates the effects of hyperkalemia on cardiac conduction.[12] Isotonic sodium chloride to which 44 to 88 mEq of sodium bicarbonate have been added may be used effectively.

Restoration of the Transcellular Gradient

In the hyperkalemic patient, movement of potassium into cells restores the transcellular gradient without altering total body potassium. This may be accomplished by the administration of either glucose and insulin, or sodium bicarbonate. Fifty ml of 50 per cent dextrose (25 gm) may be administered intravenously over 2 to 3 minutes together with 10 units of regular insulin subcutaneously (1 unit of insulin per 2 to 3 grams of glucose). The serum potassium should fall 1 to 2 mEq per liter within 30 minutes following administration of glucose and insulin. The effect lasts for several hours and the administration of glucose and insulin may be repeated.

Glucose may also be given alone since it stimulates release of insulin. Five hundred ml of a 10 per cent glucose solution may be given intravenously over 30 to 60 minutes in nondiabetic patients. In diabetic patients glucose should not be given without insulin since hyperglycemia can worsen hyperkalemia if hyperosmolality develops.[2, 7, 13]

Since acidosis promotes transfer of potassium out of cells, the use of sodium bicarbonate to reverse the movement of potassium in an acidotic patient is a logical therapeutic measure. One ampule of sodium bicarbonate (44 mEq) should be given intravenously over several minutes. Administration of sodium bicarbonate can be repeated as long as severe alkalosis does not ensue. Because of its sodium content, bicarbonate therapy can produce both fluid overload and hyperosmolality. It should therefore be used with caution in patients with congestive heart failure or other forms of fluid overload.

Although alkalinization potentiates the shift of potassium into cells, the effect of sodium bicarbonate may be more than just that of changing serum pH. Recent experimental studies have demonstrated that the administration of sodium bicarbonate causes a shift of potassium into cells even when the pH is not changed.[9, 10] Thus, the administration of sodium bicarbonate may be effective in hyperkalemic patients in whom arterial pH is normal as well as in those with metabolic acidosis. In addition to affecting the transcellular gradient, sodium bicarbonate can enhance renal potassium secretion by increasing delivery of bicarbonate to the distal tubule where it acts as a poorly reabsorbable anion.

The electrophysiologic dysfunction produced by hyperkalemia in severe digitalis intoxication may be resistant to conventional therapy. Although the Na^+-K^+-dependent ATPase pump is inhibited, the use of insulin and sodium bicarbonate to move potassium back into cells may be unable to reestablish a normal membrane potential.[21] Digitalis antibody, if available, would appear to be the treatment of choice if life-threatening arrhythmias or markedly elevated serum potassium concentrations are present.

Removal of Potassium from the Body

If there is a total body potassium surfeit, removal of the excess potassium is necessary. The therapeutic modalities described thus far, i.e., reversing the membrane effects with calcium or hypertonic sodium, and driving potassium into cells with glucose, insulin, and bicarbonate, are only temporary measures. Within minutes to hours their effects disappear. With normal or minimally compromised renal function, diuretic therapy can be attempted to remove the excess potassium from the body. Diuretics increase distal tubular flow and delivery of sodium, thereby optimizing the cell-to-lumen concentration and electrical gradients for potassium secretion. Thiazides, furosemide, or ethacrynic acid may be useful in patients who have received an increased oral or intravenous potassium load, potassium-sparing diuretics, or in whom hyperkalemia is secondary to hypercatabolic states. If hyperkalemia is secondary to volume depletion and oliguria, diuretics can be used in conjunction with fluid therapy to replete the volume and enhance the urine flow rate. The doses should be those normally used to promote a diuresis. Diuretics are relatively ineffective in causing kaliuresis in patients with renal failure.

Cation exchange resins promote potassium excretion via the gastrointestinal tract. The most commonly used resin is sodium polystyrene sulfonate (Kayexalate) which acts by exchanging its sodium for potassium in the colon. It cannot be used effectively in patients who have undergone colectomy. Approximately 1 mEq of potassium is excreted for each gram of resin used. Twenty gm of Kayexalate may be given orally with 100 ml of a 20 per cent sorbitol solution. Fifty to 100 gm of resin may be administered with 50 to 100 ml of 70 per cent sorbitol by retention enema. The enema must be retained for at least 30 minutes to allow for adequate potassium exchange. Sorbitol, acting as an osmotic cathartic, prevents constipation and sometimes even produces diarrhea which enhances potassium excretion. The administration of Kayexalate can be repeated every 4 hours. Because the resin releases sodium in exchange for the bound potassium, it can cause significant fluid retention and should be used cautiously in patients with cardiac or renal failure.

In patients in whom the serum potassium concentration cannot be adequately controlled by the above procedures, dialysis may be necessary. Typically this need arises when tissue catabolism results in a large potassium load or when fluid overload makes administration of Kayexalate hazardous. Either peritoneal or hemodialysis may be employed. Peritoneal dialysis against a potassium-free dialysate can remove up to 15 mEq of potassium per hour, but the amount removed is quite variable. The rate of potassium removal depends upon peritoneal blood flow and the time required for the dialysate to be infused and drained. In a hypotensive patient in whom severe mesenteric vasoconstriction may exist, the peritoneal exchange process may be markedly impaired.

Hemodialysis is more efficient than peritoneal dialysis in removing potassium. Up to 50 mEq can be removed hourly. If hemodialysis is available, the decision as to which form of dialysis to institute will depend upon the patient's clinical condition, taking into account the risks of both procedures. Dialysis should be looked upon as a last resort in the hyperkalemic patient, although a very effective mode of therapy. In most cases the serum potassium concentration can be controlled by the administration of calcium, glucose and insulin, sodium bicarbonate, diuretics, and/or the use of potassium exchange resins.

REFERENCES

1. Alexander, E. A., and Levinsky, N. G.: An extrarenal mechanism of potassium adaptation. J. Clin. Invest., 47:740, 1968.
2. Ammon, R. A., May, W. S., and Nightingale, S. D.: Glucose-induced hyperkalemia with normal aldosterone levels. Ann. Intern. Med., 89:349, 1978.
3. Anderson, H. M., and Laragh, J. H.: Renal excretion of potassium in normal and sodium depleted dogs. J. Clin. Invest., 37:323, 1958.
4. Andres, R., Baltzan, M. A., Cader, G., et al.: Effect of insulin on carbohydrate metabolism and on potassium in the forearm of man. J. Clin. Invest., 41:108, 1962.
5. Brandis, M., Keyes, J., and Windhager, E. E.: Potassium-induced inhibition of proximal tubular fluid reabsorption in rats. Amer. J. Physiol., 222:421, 1972.
6. Cooperman, L. H.: Succinylcholine-induced hyperkalemia in neuromuscular disease. J.A.M.A., 213:1867, 1970.
7. Cox, M., Sterns, R. H., and Singer, I.: The defense against hyperkalemia: The roles of insulin and aldosterone. New Engl. J. Med., 299:525, 1978.
8. Fisch, C.: Relation of electrolyte disturbances to cardiac arrhythmias. Circulation, 47:408, 1973.
9. Fraley, D. S., and Adler, S.: Correction of hyperkalemia by bicarbonate despite constant blood pH. Kidney International, 12:354, 1977.
10. Fraley, D. S., and Adler, S.: Isohydric regulation of plasma potassium by bicarbonate in the rat. Kidney International, 9:333, 1976.
11. Gadsby, D. C., and Cranefield, P. F.: Two levels of resting potential in cardiac purkinje fibers. J. Gen. Physiol., 70:725, 1977.
12. García-Palmieri, M. R.: Reversal of hyperkalemic cardiotoxicity with hypertonic saline. Amer. Heart J., 64:483, 1962.
13. Goldfarb, S., Cox, M., Singer, I., et al.: Acute hyperkalemia induced by hyperglycemia: Hormonal mechanisms. Ann. Intern. Med., 84:426, 1976.
14. Good, D. W., and Wright, F. S.: Luminal influences on potassium secretion: sodium concentration and fluid flow rate. Amer. J. Physiol. 236 (2):F192, 1979.
15. Hertz, P., and Richardson, J. A.: Arginine-induced hyperkalemia in renal failure patients. Arch. Intern. Med., 130:778, 1972.
16. Hierholzer, K., and Wiederholt, M.: Some aspects of distal tubular solute and water transport. Kidney International, 9:198, 1976.
17. Hodgkin, A. L., and Horowicz, P.: The influence of potassium and chloride ions on the membrane potential of single muscle fibres. J. Physiol., 148:127, 1959.
18. Hodgkin, A. L., and Huxley, A. F.: The dual effect of membrane potential on sodium conductance in the giant axon of Loligo. J. Physiol., 116:497, 1952.
19. Huxley, A. F., and Stämpfli, R.: Effect of potassium and sodium on resting and action potentials of single myelinated nerve fibers. J. Physiol., 112:496, 1951.
20. Lubin, M.: Intracellular potassium and macromolecular synthesis in mammalian cells. Nature, 213:451, 1967.
21. Reza, M. J., Kovick, R. B., Shine, K. I., et al.: Massive intravenous digoxin overdosage. New Engl. J. Med., 291:777, 1974.
22. Roberts, K. E., Magida, M. G., and Pitts, R. F.: Relationship between potassium and bicarbonate in blood and urine. Amer. J. Physiol., 172:47, 1953.
23. Schambelan, M., Sebastian, A., and Biglieri, E. G.: Prevalence, pathogenesis, and functional significance of aldosterone deficiency in hyperkalemic patients with chronic renal insufficiency. Kidney International, 17:89, 1980.

24. Silva, P., Hayslett, J. P., and Epstein, F. H.: The role of Na^+-K^+-activated adenosine triphosphatase in potassium adaptation. Stimulation of enzymatic activity by potassium loading. J. Clin. Invest., 52:2665, 1973.

25. Surawicz, B., Chlebus, H., and Mazzoleni, A.: Hemodynamic and electrocardiographic effects of hyperpotassemia. Differences in response to slow and rapid increases in concentration of plasma K. Amer. Heart J., 73:647, 1967.

26. Surawicz, B., and Gettes, L. S.: Two mechanisms of cardiac arrest produced by potassium. Circ. Res., 12:415, 1963.

27. Szylman, P., Better, O. S., Chaimowitz, C., et al.: Role of hyperkalemia in the metabolic acidosis of isolated hypoaldosteronism. New Engl. J. Med., 294:361, 1976.

28. Vick, R. L., Todd, E. P., and Leudke, D. W.: Epinephrine-induced hypokalemia: Relation to liver and skeletal muscle. J. Pharmacol. Exper. Therapeut., 181:139, 1972.

29. Zierler, K. L.: Effect of insulin on potassium efflux from rat muscle in the presence and absence of glucose. Amer. J. Physiol., 198:1066, 1960.

30. Zierler, K. L.: Hyperpolarization of muscle by insulin in a glucose-free environment. Amer. J. Physiol., 197:524, 1959.

Renal Section
Department of Medicine
New York University Medical Center
550 First Avenue
New York, New York 10016

Acute Arthritis

Catherine T. Marino, M.D.,[*]
and Robert A. Greenwald, M.D.[†]

The complaint of pain in an extremity is the most frequent manifestation of acute musculoskeletal disease. The physician must first ascertain that the pain is indeed of articular origin and not derived from circulatory compromise, neurologic disease, or other systemic illness. If this appears to be the case, the next step is to determine if the pain has arisen from inflammation within a joint space (arthritis), from a mechanical disorder within the joint, or from a periarticular structure (non-articular rheumatism). The distinction is obviously important, since the nonspecific use of anti-inflammatory agents may ameliorate the symptoms of any of these conditions and mask a destructive inflammatory process such as sepsis or crystal-induced arthritis.

Goldenberg[13] has summarized some of the features which distinguish arthritis from periarthritis. Inflammation and pain in a tendon or a bursa, especially if accompanied by mild swelling and limitation of motion, can simulate acute joint disease. The most reliable sign of joint inflammation is the presence of an effusion which usually distends the joint capsule and is associated with diffuse tenderness. The swelling (if any) associated with periarthritis is usually quite localized and does not distend the joint capsule; similarly, localized (rather than diffuse) tenderness is more often the rule. Arthritis usually results in an equal loss of active and passive range of motion, while acute tendinitis or bursitis may impede the patient's active range of motion more than the passive range of motion. Careful physical examination will usually indicate whether or not acute arthritis is actually present.

The acute or subacute presentation of pain in certain joints, especially the knee, should also alert the physician to the possibility of a mechanical or osseous disorder such as a torn meniscus, torn collateral

[*]Physician-in-charge, Division of Rheumatology, Queens Hospital Center Affiliation/Long Island Jewish-Hillside Medical Center, Jamaica, New York; Assistant Professor of Medicine, State University of New York at Stony Brook

[†]Chief, Division of Rheumatology, Long Island Jewish-Hillside Medical Center, New Hyde Park, New York; Associate Professor of Medicine, State University of New York at Stony Brook

or anterior cruciate ligament, osteonecrosis, and osteochondritis. As summarized by Polley and Hunder,[27] a variety of historical and physical findings can alert the physician to such diagnoses, including a history of joint "locking," a snapping sensation within the joint, a history of abrupt (almost instantaneous) onset of pain, tenderness localized along the joint line, and pain elicited by a variety of abduction or adduction maneuvers. The sudden onset of pain in the region of the medial femoral condyle should suggest osteonecrosis, a diagnosis which may be confirmed by radiographs and bone scan.[29]

In most instances, the diagnosis of acute monoarticular arthritis will be self-evident, since these disorders are generally highly inflammatory and are accompanied by severe pain and tenderness, an obvious effusion, heat emanating from the joint, and erythema. Acute monoarticular arthritis is the situation in which synovial fluid analysis is of greatest value to the physician, and unless the diagnosis is immediately obvious from ancillary information, arthrocentesis should be performed in virtually all such cases for accuracy of diagnosis. Space does not permit a detailed discussion of the principles of joint fluid examination, which are discussed in detail elsewhere.[5, 6] Observation of the gross appearance of the fluid, determination of the cell count and differential, microscopic analysis (wet prep, Gram stain, polarizing microscope), and measurement of synovial fluid glucose are the standard minimum tests which should be done on all fluid samples in such cases.

Once the presence of acute arthritis has been established, the differential diagnosis generally centers about two types of diseases: inflammation induced by crystals or infectious processes. Arthritic disorders of infectious etiology can be due to direct infection (septic joint disease) or can be reactive, i.e., mediated by immune complex phenomena resulting from the response of the host to the infecting agent. Included in the latter category would be the arthritis-dermatitis prodrome of infectious hepatitis and Reiter's disease. This article will deal with acute arthritis produced by crystal deposition and by infectious processes.

CRYSTAL-INDUCED ARTHRITIS

Four types of crystalline material are known to be capable of producing acute arthritis: monosodium urate monohydrate (gout), calcium pyrophosphate dihydrate (pseudogout), hydroxyapatite, and crystals of depot steroid preparations. The mechanism by which crystals induce inflammation is only partially understood (see McCarty[21] for a detailed discussion), but it is clear that phagocytosis of the crystal by a polymorphonuclear leukocyte is a crucial step. Phagocytosis is followed by rupture of phagolysosome membranes, release of enzymes into the surrounding space, generation of superoxide radicals, and production of chemotactic factors, all of which lead to accelerating joint fluid leukocytosis and inflammation. Both motion and heat have been shown to increase joint fluid white counts in animal models of crystal-induced arthritis, suggesting that treatment of acute gouty joints with rest and surface cooling would appear to be rational.

Acute gout is recognized by its occurrence in characteristic settings and by its typical clinical features. The usual patient with acute gout is a middle-aged man; onset before age 30 or in a premenopausal woman is most unusual. Historical factors which should alert the physician to the diagnosis include a family history of gout and/or hyperuricemia, a known background of elevated serum urate levels, or a history of renal stone formation (although patients with hyperparathyroidism also have elevated serum urate levels). Predisposing factors for acute gout include trauma (such as surgery), ingestion of ethanol (leading to increased serum lactate which competes with urate for renal excretory sites), and a large number of drugs which can elevate serum urate (including most diuretics, phenytoin, levodopa, and ethambutol). Other disorders can lead to secondary gout when hyperuricemia is the result of hematologic diseases, especially polycythemia vera, plumbism (Saturnine gout) and occasionally psoriasis or the use of cytotoxic drugs. The latter is more commonly associated with a rapid elevation in uric acid level and acute tubular necrosis, rather than with gouty arthropathy.

Acute gout is characteristically a highly inflammatory, exquisitely painful, monoarticular arthritis of the first metatarsal phalangeal joint (podagra), instep, ankle, heel, knee, wrist, and/or elbow. While most first attacks are monoarticular, subsequent episodes are often oligoarticular or polyarticular and may be associated with constitutional symptoms such as fever, leukocytosis, and so forth, thus mimicking an infectious process. The natural history of an untreated attack is usually that of resolution over a 10 day period, and patients with acute gout will often have a background of prior, milder attacks which did not require medical attention. The physical findings of a highly inflammatory arthritis will be readily evident and may even mimic a cellulitis. Confirmation of the diagnosis requires arthrocentesis and the identification of intracellular, needle-shaped, negatively birefringent crystals typical of monosodium urate monohydrate.

When gout is suspected on clinical features but arthrocentesis fails to reveal the crystals (or the procedure cannot be done), the treatment of choice is the intravenous administration of 2 to 3 mg of colchicine injected over a 2 to 5 minute period with care being taken to avoid extravasation. Although it appears that some attacks of pseudogout, apatite disease, or sarcoid arthritis may respond to colchicine, a dramatic response to this medication, 90 per cent resolution in 48 hours, will reinforce the diagnostic impression of gout. The limiting gastrointestinal side-effects of multiple-dose oral colchicine are eliminated by parenteral administration. If the diagnosis has been established by background or by synovial fluid analysis, any of the nonsteroidal anti-inflammatory agents may be used. A short course of treatment with indomethacin, sulindac, or naproxen is usually successful, and these agents have replaced phenylbutazone as the drug of choice owing to their lesser toxicities. Treatment of the acute attack should be followed by evaluation to characterize the nature of the hyperuricemia (primary or secondary, overproducer or underexcretor), and long-term treatment should be instituted with patient education, prophylactic oral colchicine, uricosuric drugs, or allopurinol as needed.

The second most common form of crystal-induced arthritis is that produced by the deposition of calcium pyrophosphate dihydrate. Calcium pyrophosphate dihydrate crystals appear to have their origin in articular cartilage, where they constitute the asymptomatic condition known as chondrocalcinosis. If the crystals are released into the joint space because of a change in equilibrium conditions between calcium and pyrophosphate ions in the snyovial fluid, or by mechanical or enzymatic disruption of cartilage matrix, an inflammatory arthritis can supervene. Crystals of calcium pyrophosphate dihydrate, like those of monosodium urate, induce inflammation only after phagocytosis by polymorphonuclear leukocytes. Arthrocentesis of affected joints will often reveal intracellular, weakly birefringent crystals with the characteristic morphology of calcium pyrophosphate dihydrate.

Pseudogout, the monoarticular or pauciarticular form of disease characterized by deposition of calcium pyrophosphate dihydrate, is characterized by acute or subacute attacks, often self-limited, lasting one day to several weeks.[22] Trauma, surgery, or medical illness may provoke the attack. More than 50 per cent of acute attacks occur in the knee, with the wrist, elbow, shoulder, and occasionally other joints also being susceptible. In contrast to gout, men outnumber women only slightly in the incidence of pseudogout. The onset may be more gradual, and a prodrome of minor attacks is also more frequent with pseudogout. It is not uncommon for patients with pseudogout to have an elevated serum urate, emphasizing the need for precise diagnosis by arthrocentesis. Joint fluid leukocytosis averages 20,000 cells per cu mm, quite similar to gout.

Pseudogout has been associated with hyperparathyroidism, osteoarthritis, hemochromatosis, and hypothyroidism, and can even coexist with urate gout. Chondrocalcinosis, diagnosed radiogically by the finding of punctate and/or linear calcification of the fibrocartilaginous menisci of the knee, the distal radioulnar joint, and/or articular cartilage in a variety of other locations, is a frequent finding in these cases. Acute or subacute arthritis of the knee associated with radiologically demonstrable chondrocalcinosis is probably the most common, easily recognizable form of pseudogout and should be a straightforward diagnosis. Other presentations of calcium pyrophosphate dihydrate deposition disease include a rheumatoid-like arthropathy, pseudoneurotrophic joints, and progressive degeneration of multiple joints.[22]

Treatment of acute pseudogout arthritis starts with diagnostic confirmation by arthrocentesis, and it has been widely observed that removal of fluid often ameliorates the symptoms of inflammation. Colchicine appears to be moderately effective, and most of the nonsteroidal antiinflammatory drugs will probably work quite well, indomethacin being the personal choice of the authors. Deposition of calcium pyrophosphate dihydrate crystals cannot be halted or reversed, but underlying or associated conditions can be sought and treated if found.

The third form of crystal-induced arthritis is that due to hydroxyapatite, which is the crystalline form of calcium phosphate that is found in bone mineral, in calcific periarthritis (tendinitis and bursitis), in synovial chondromatosis, and in the subcutaneous calcifications of the connective tissue diseases. It has been recognized recently that small (750 to 2500 nm in diameter), needle-shaped crystals of apatite can be identified within vacuoles in phagocytic cells in fluid obtained from inflamed joints,[30] and that injection of such crystals into dog knee joints causes an acute synovitis. In cases of otherwise unexplained monoarticular synovitis, apatite crystal-induced inflammation should be considered, especially if the synovial fluid leukocytosis is less than expected. Unfortunately, the diagnosis is difficult to make with certainty, since the crystals may be too small to be seen with an ordinary light microscope, and definitive diagnosis requires electron microscopy, electron probe analysis, or treatment of synovial fluid preparations with special stains such as alizarin red or van Kossa. Colchicine may be effective but nonsteroidal drugs should relieve the symptoms in most cases.

Finally, it should be mentioned that most depot steroid preparations form crystals upon storage and/or after injection into joints, and postinjection flares of arthritis can readily occur owing to an inflammatory reaction elicited by such material. In view of this phenomenon, plus the adverse effects of intra-articular steroids on the biochemical integrity of cartilage,[1] intrasynovial corticosteroid therapy should be used very sparingly and selectively in the management of arthritic disorders.

INFECTIOUS ARTHRITIS

Infectious agents are associated with both acute and chronic joint symptoms. Intra-articular multiplication of bacteria or fungi generally causes an acute monoarticular, or occasionally oligoarticular, "septic" arthritis. Viral agents, on the other hand, usually produce a polyarticular disease presumed to be mediated by immune complex formation, although virus has been recovered from synovial fluid in patients with rubella[36] and varicella-associated arthritis.[28]

Viral Arthritis

Virus-associated arthritis is generally self-limited and may require no specific treatment. Hepatitis B virus, rubella, adenovirus, arbovirus, and rarely the agents responsible for infectious mononucleosis and varicella-zoster have all been linked to the acute onset of arthralgia or arthritis.[9, 23, 28, 32, 37]

The reported frequency of articular involvement during the prodromal stage of serum hepatitis (hepatitis B) varies between 10 and 50 per cent.[23] It typically begins suddenly with symmetric joint pain and swelling. Synovial effusion is common, while palpable synovitis is infrequent. Morning stiffness is present in many patients and the picture may mimic rheumatoid arthritis. Articular symptoms last from days to months, but the usual duration is 4 weeks.[8] Abatement of joint disease generally occurs with the onset of jaundice, except in anicteric cases where symptoms persist for the duration of the hepatitis.[36]

Abnormal liver enzymes and hepatitis surface antigen (Hbs Ag) are found in 50 to 80 per cent of patients at the initial presentation. Hbs Ag may be demonstrated in the synovial fluid,[23] while serum hepatitis surface antibody (Hbs Ab) occurs later in the course of the illness after the arthritis has subsided. Rheumatoid factor and antinuclear antibody (ANA) are present in 10 to 15 per cent cases; cryoglobulins and decreased C_3, C_4, and CH 50 have also been noted.[8] Synovial fluid examination is non-diagnostic and consists of leukocytosis with a variable predominance of cell type. Immunofluorescent studies of synovial tissue have demonstrated the presence of hepatitis B antigen.[23]

Naturally acquired rubella and attenuated rubella vaccination have been associated with joint symptoms in a significant number of patients, especially young women.[32, 37, 40] In the naturally acquired infection, symmetric arthralgia or arthritis occurs within 1 to 7 days of the rash. Fingers, wrists, and knees are commonly involved; carpal tunnel syndrome and tenosynovitis occur. Duration of symptoms is usually less than 3 weeks and the arthritis is nonrecurrent. Vaccination-induced joint disease occurs 8 to 55 days after injection and knee pain is the most prominent sign. Chronic joint disease has been reported.[32, 37] Rheumatoid factor may be present (10 to 20 per cent cases) and there can be a slight elevation in the erythrocyte sedimentation rate. Treatment of the arthritis is symptomatic and most analgesic or anti-inflammatory agents may be used depending on the severity of joint pain.

Arthralgia or arthritis has occasionally been seen with infectious mononucleosis and varicella. Resolution of joint symptoms is usually complete and analgesic agents are given when needed. Synovial fluid aspiration is nondiagnostic, except in instances in which varicella has been cultured.[28]

Lyme Arthritis

Steere et al. in 1975 described an entity now termed "Lyme" arthritis after its occurrence in the vicinity of Lyme, Connecticut. The syndrome consists of a brief, but often recurrent, large joint arthritis, especially of the knee, that is frequently preceded by a characteristic rash—erythema chronicum migrans.[34] This lesion begins as an erythematous papule that expands, leaving an area of central pallor. It is accompanied by headache, stiff neck, fever, malaise, and fatigue. Cryoglobulin and elevated IgM levels appear in the serum of some patients with erythema chronica migrans and may predict the subsequent development of arthritis.[33] With each episode of arthritis, serum cryoglobulins reappear and the IgM level increases. Arthrocentesis reveals an inflammatory fluid with the white count varying between 4,000 and 100,000 cells per cu mm with a predominance of polymorphonuclear leukocytes. Synovial fluid protein levels are similarly elevated.

The tick, *Ixodes dammini*, is felt to be the vector for an as yet unidentified etiologic agent.[35] Treatment of patients with erythema chronica migrans with penicillin and tetracycline, but not erythromycin, might lessen the severity of the rash and attenuate the arthritis. Neurologic and cardiac complications are not favorably altered by these drugs.[35] Lyme arthritis has been reported in Wisconsin,[7] Rhode Island, Cape Cod, and Long Island.[33]

Reactive Arthritis

Abrupt onset of polyarthritis can occur after infection with salmonella, shigella and *Yersinia enterocolitica*.[19] Large peripheral joints are most frequently involved; manifestations include pain and mild effusion, which are characteristically sterile. An association between the HLA B 27 antigen and the development of arthritis has been noted in 85 to 94 per cent of these cases.[19]

Reiter's syndrome, a pentad of urethritis, conjunctivitis, arthritis, circinate balanitis, and keratoderma blennorrhagica, is also felt to be a reactive arthropathy.[19, 25] It has been reported after a shipboard epidemic of *Shigella flexneri* dysentery[26] and after chlamydial urethritis. In many cases, however, no etiologic agent has been isolated.

The arthritis of Reiter's is commonly pauciarticular and recurrent episodes can lead to chronic joint disease.[3] Sacroiliitis may be prominent and HLA B 27 is similarly noted in a high percentage of patients with this syndrome. Current treatment includes aspirin and the nonsteroidal anti-inflammatory agents, especially indomethacin.

Septic Arthritis

Infection with bacteria or fungi can disseminate hematogenously and cause a septic arthritis. Generally, this is a monoarticular or oligoarticular process and deserves prompt medical attention because of attendant morbidity (loss of joint function) and mortality.[11, 12]

Suspicion of a septic arthritis is the first step in proper management, while confirmation of infection requires arthrocentesis and culture of synovial fluid. As mentioned above, the synovial fluid cell count and differential count, preparation and examination of a Gram stain and observation of the appearance of the fluid are carried out routinely. Joint fluid leukocytosis with a predominance of polymorphonuclear leukocytes is usual, although a low white count should not dissuade one from the diagnosis.[20] A Gram-stained preparation frequently aids the physician in identification of an organism and enhances appropriate antibiotic selection. The demonstration of elevated synovial fluid lactic acid levels has recently been reported[3] but its application to clinical management is not yet established.

Several factors predisposing individuals to septic arthritis are recognized.[12] Chronic debilitating disease, prior antibiotic or immunosuppressive medications, or a previous history of joint damage is found in a large number of patients with nongonococcal septic arthritis.[11, 12] A primary focus of infection, distant from the joint, and positive blood cultures are present in up to 50 per cent of patients.[12] Patients with rheumatoid arthritis and diabetes, as well as increasing age over 40, are likely to have staphylococcal joint infection. Septic arthritis in children ages 6 months to 2 years is frequently caused by *H. influenzae*, while staphylo-

Table 1. *Distribution of Infectious Causes of Arthritis with Age*

AGE	COMMON ORGANISMS
0 to 6 months	*Staphylococcus aureus* *E. coli*
6 months to 2 years	*H. influenzae*
2 years to adolescents	Gram-positive cocci
Adolescents to young adults	*N. gonorrhoeae*
Increasing age over 40	*Staphylococcus aureus*

cocci and *E. coli* predominate in the neonate.[39] The most common causative agent of septic arthritis among adolescents and young adults is the gonococcus.[2, 10] The majority of disseminated gonococcal infections occur in women with asymptomatic anogenital infections and dissemination is usually during pregnancy (1st to 3rd trimeseter) or during menstruation.[2, 18] Cases of disseminated gonococcal infection in men frequently arise from asymptomatic infection of the anogenital area or pharynx and are analogous to the carrier state in women.[18] Less than 3 per cent of all primary gonococcal infections disseminate[23] and the recent finding of deficiencies of the late components of the complement system has been implicated in the pathogenesis of this disease.[16]

Two phases of disseminated gonococcal infection have been reported.[10, 18] An early bacteremic stage has been associated with fever, chills, rash, migratory polyarthralgia, tenosynovitis, peripheral leukocytosis and positive blood cultures; the later "joint" phase is associated with a more prominent arthritis that is frequently polyarticular,[10, 18] positive synovial fluid cultures, and negative blood cultures. Clear-cut differentiation of these two stages is frequently impossible,[2] and in a given patient, the signs and symptoms may be variable.

Recovery of *N. gonorrhoeae* from body fluids is difficult. Joint fluid and blood are best cultured on chocolate agar or TSY broth, while anogenital cultures may be taken on Thayer Martin media. Synovial fluid leukocytosis ranges from several thousand cells to greater than 100,000 per cu mm with a predominance of polymorphonuclear leukocytes. The synovial fluid is generally turbid and a Gram stain of the material occasionally reveals the organism.

The characteristic skin lesion is found in one third of the cases. It begins as a small erythematous macule which may become petechial or vesicular. The vesicles may then become pustular and a dark necrotic center forms. This rash may also be seen with *N. menigitides*, *H. influenzae*, and *S. moniliformis* infections.[3] Culture of the skin lesion is infrequently positive, but gonococcal antigen may be demonstrated with fluorescein-conjugated antibody.[31] In the absence of confirmed blood or synovial fluid cultures, the combination of the characteristic rash, arthritis, and a positive anogenital or pharyngeal culture, as well as a rapid response to appropriate antibiotic therapy are highly suggestive of disseminated gonococcal infection.

Table 2.   *Distribution of Infectious Causes of Arthritis with Underlying Disease*

Rheumatoid arthritis	*Staphylococcus aureus*
Diabetes mellitus	*Staphylococcus aureus,* other gram-positive organisms, gram-negative organisms
Lymphoproliferative disorders	Gram-positive and gram-negative organisms
Intravenous drug users	*Pseudomonas aeruginosa* *Serratia marcescens* *Staphylococcus aureus*
Other chronic illnesses, including liver disease	Gram-positive cocci, especially *S. aureus* Gram-negative organisms

Treatment of disseminated gonococcal infection has recently been modified and one of several regimens is satisfactory.[15] Basically, a loading dose of 3.5 gm of oral ampicillin, followed by 2 gm daily for 10 days or 10 million units of aqueous penicillin intravenously for 3 days followed by oral ampicillin, 2 gm daily for 7 more days, are currently in vogue. Tetracycline is an alternative agent for patients with penicillin allergy.

The Gram-positive cocci account for the majority of cases of nongonococcal septic arthritis in adults. The commonest organisms are *S. aureus* and various streptococci including *S. pneumoniae*. Gram-negative infections were once infrequent, but there has been a steady rise over the years. Twenty-six per cent of isolates from nongonococcal septic joints were due to Gram-negative organisms in the series reported by Goldenberg et al.[11] *E. coli, Pr. mirabilis, P. aeruginosa, S. marcescens* and Salmonella species accounted for 13 of the 50 infections. Nongonococcal septic arthritis is commonly monoarticular or oligoarticular; rarely are more than three joints involved.[12] Peripheral leukocytosis, low-grade fever and joint pain, tenderness and swelling are almost always present. Evaluation should include blood and synovial fluid cultures; sputum, urine, skin and spinal fluid cultures are obtained where appropriate. Examination of synovial fluid demonstrates turbidity, decreased viscosity and a leukocytosis frequently in excess of 50,000 per cu mm. The Gram stain reveals organisms in up to 60 per cent of fluids examined.[12] Morbidity and mortality are related to the severity of the underlying illness, virulence of the infecting organism, and time elapsed from onset of infection to diagnosis and treatment. Outcome is substantially improved when treatment is initiated within the first week of disease.[11, 12] Infection with staphylococcus and Gram-negative organisms is associated with significant joint morbidity and increased mortality.[11]

Treatment consists of an appropriate antibiotic administered parenterally, as dictated by initial Gram stain and later by results of joint fluid culture and sensitivity. Intra-articular usage of antibiotic is generally not suggested. Daily or twice-daily joint aspiration is mandatory. An attempt at "draining the joint dry" should be made. This allows for observation of fluid reaccumulation and changes in the white count; it removes "pus" from the joint space and alleviates pain. Synovial fluid should be sent for culture since ineffectual therapy will not sterilize the joint. Maximal inhibitory concentration of antibiotic within the joint fluid should be tested where available and especially, if the infection is persistent. Failure of optimal medical management will require surgical intervention, i.e., open drainage of the involved joint.

SUMMARY

Acute or subacute onset of monoarticular or pauciarticular arthritis may result from crystal deposition within the joint, infection, or trauma. Arthrocentesis with examination of synovial fluid is performed and often provides a rapid diagnosis when crystals are found with the polarizing microscope or bacteria are identified by gram-stain.

Several types of crystals can induce inflammatory changes and have been clearly associated with the development of arthritis. Monosodium urate monohydrate and calcium pyrophosphate dihydrate are the most common. Calcium hydroxyapatite crystals have been found by electron microscopic examination of some synovial fluids.[30]

Infectious arthritis is associated with bacterial, fungal, and viral agents. The viruses presumably induce an immune complex–mediated synovitis, while bacteria and fungi multiply within the joint space. The commonest cause of septic (bacterial) arthritis is the gonococcus, especially in a younger patient population. Rheumatoid arthritis, diabetes, and increasing age over 40 predispose to infection with *Staphylococcus aureus*. The Gram-negative organisms have recently been shown to be responsible for about 25 per cent of all nongonococcal septic arthritis and have a worse prognosis than Gram-positive infections with the possible exception of *Staphylococcus aureus*.

Treatment of a nongonococcal septic arthritis includes parenteral administration of an antibiotic and daily or twice daily arthrocentesis. Antibiotic selection is aided by the results of the Gram stain. We generally begin intravenous nafcillin in a dose of 1 to 2 gm every 4 hours when a Gram-positive coccus is identified and intravenous or intramuscular gentamicin when the gram-stained slide reveals a Gram-negative agent. A combination of nafcillin and gentamicin is begun when no organisms are initially identified. Antibiotics are appropriately altered when culture and sensitivity reports are available.

REFERENCES

1. Behrens, F., Shepard, N., and Mitchell, N.: Alteration of rabbit articular cartilage by intra-articular injections of glucocorticoids. J. Bone Joint Surg., 57A:70–75, 1975.
2. Brandt, K. D., Cathcart, E. S., and Cohen, A. S.: Gonococcal arthritis. Arthrit. Rheum., 17:503–510, 1974.
3. Brook, I., Rexa, M. J., Bricknell, K. S., et al.: Synovial fluid lactic acid. Arthrit. Rheum., 21:775–779, 1978.

4. Butler, M. J., Russel, A. S., Percy, J. S., et al.: A Follow-up Study of 48 patients with Reiter's syndrome. Amer. J. Med., 67:808–810, 1979.
5. Cohen, A. S., Brandt, K. D., and Krey, P. R.: Synovial fluid. In Cohen, A. S., ed.: Laboratory Diagnostic Procedures in the Rheumatic Diseases. Boston, Massachusetts, Little Brown, 2nd ed., 1975, pp. 1–64.
6. Cohen, A. S., and Skinner, M.: Synovial fluid. In Cohen, A. S., ed.: Rheumatology and Immunology. New York, Grune and Stratton, 1979, pp. 113–116.
7. Dryer, R. F., Goellner, P. G., and Carney, A. S.: Lyme arthritis in Wisconsin. J.A.M.A., 241:498–499, 1977.
8. Duffy, J., Lidsky, M. D., Sharp, J. T., et al.: Polyarthritis, polyarteritis and hepatitis B. Medicine, 55:19–37, 1976.
9. Fernandez, R., and McCarty, D. J.: The arthritis of viral hepatitis. Ann. Intern. Med., 74:207–211, 1971.
10. Gelfand, S. G., Masi, A. T., and Garcia-Kutzbach, A.: Spectrum of gonococcal arthritis: Evidence for sequential stages and clinical subgroups. J. Rheumatol., 2:83–90, 1975.
11. Goldenberg, D. L., Brandt, K. D., Cathcart, M. D., et al.: Acute arthritis caused by gram-negative bacilli: A clinical characterization. Medicine, 53:197–208, 1974.
12. Goldenberg, D. L., and Cohen, A. S.: Acute infectious arthritis. Amer. J. Med., 60:369–377, 1976.
13. Goldenberg, D. L.: Acute monoarticular arthritis. In Cohen, A. S., ed.: Rheumatology and Immunology. New York, Grune & Stratton, 1979, pp. 113–116.
14. Goldin, R. H., Chow, A. W., Edwards, J. E., et al.: Sternoarticular septic arthritis in heroin users. New Eng. J. Med., 289:616–618, 1974.
15. Handsfield, H. H., and Holmes, K. K.: Treatment of the gonococcal arthritis-dermatitis syndrome. Ann. Intern. Med., 82:661–667, 1976.
16. Handsfield, H. H.: Disseminated gonococcal infection. Clin. Obstet. Gynec., 18:131–134, 1975.
17. Handsfield, H. H.: Gonorrhea and non-gonococcal urethritis. Med. Clin. N. Amer., 62:925–943, 1978.
18. Holmes, K. K., Counts, G. W., and Beaty, H. N.: Disseminated gonococcal infection. Ann. Intern. Med., 74:979–993, 1971.
19. Julkunen, H.: Reactive arthritis. Bull. Rheum. Dis., 29:1002–1005, 1978, 1979.
20. Krey, P. R., and Bailen, D. A.: Synovial fluid leukocytosis. Amer. J. Med., 67:436–442, 1979.
21. McCarty, D. J.: Pathogenesis and treatment of crystal-induced inflammation. In McCarty, D. J., ed.: Arthritis and Allied Conditions. Philadelphia, Lea and Febiger, 1979.
22. McCarty, D. J.: Calcium pyrophosphate deposition disease. In Arthritis and Allied Conditions. Philadelphia, Lea and Febiger, 1979.
23. McCarty, D. J.; ed.: Infectious arthritis. In Arthritis and Allied Conditions. Philadelphia, Lea and Febiger, 1979.
24. Medical Letter on Drugs and Therapeutics, 21::53–54 (June 29) 1979.
25. Noer, H. R.: An experimental epidemic of Reiter's syndrome. J.A.M.A., 198:693–698, 1966.
26. Paronen, I.: Reiter's disease. A study of 344 cases observed in Finland. Acta Med. Scand. (Suppl. 212), 131:1–114, 1948.
27. Polley, H. F., and Hunder, G. G.: Physical Examination of the Joints. Philadelphia, Saunders Co., 2nd ed., 1978.
28. Priest, J. R., Urick, J. J., Groth, K. E., et al.: Varicella arthritis documented by isolation of virus from joint fluid. J. Pediatr., 93:990–992, 1978.
29. Rozing, P. M., Insall, J., and Bohne, W.: Spontaneous osteonecrosis of the knee. J. Bone Joint Surg., 62A:2–7, 1980.
30. Schumacher, H. R., Somlyo, A. P., Tse, R. L., et al.: Arthritis associated with apatite crystals. Ann. Intern. Med., 87:411–416, 1977.
31. Sharp, J. J., Lidsky, M. D., Duffy, J., et al.: Infectious arthritis. Arch. Intern. Med., 139:1125–1130, 1979.
32. Spruance, S. L., Metcalf, R., Smith, C. B., et al.: Chronic arthropathy associated with rubella vaccination. Arthrit. Rheum., 20:741–747, 1977.
33. Steere, A. C., Hardin, J. A., Ruddy, S., et al.: Lyme arthritis: Correlation of serum and cryoglobulin IgM with activity, and serum IgG with remission. Arthrit. Rheum., 22:471–483, 1979.
34. Steere, A. C., Malawista, S. E., Hardin, J. A., et al.: Erythema chronicum migrans and lyme arthritis: The enlarging clinical spectrum. Ann. Intern. Med. 86:685–698, 1977.
35. Steere, A. C., Malawista, S. E., Newman, J. H., et al.: Penicillin Therapy in lyme disease. Morbid. Mortal. Weekly Rep., 29:237–238, 1980.

36. Stevens, D. P., Walker, J., Crum, E., et al.: Anicteric hepatitis presenting as polyarthritis. J.A.M.A., 220:687–689, 1972.
37. Tingle, A. J., Ford, D. K., Price, G. E., et al.: Prolonged arthritis in identical twins after rubella immunization. Ann. Intern. Med., 90:203–204, 1979.
38. Ward, J. R., and Atcheson, S. G.: Infectious arthritis. Med. Clin. N. Amer., 61:331–329, 1977.
39. Wolski, K. P.: Staphylococcal and other Gram-positive coccal arthritides. Clinics in Rheumat. Dis., 4:181–196, 1978.

Division of Rheumatology
Queens Hospital Center
82-68 164th Street
Jamaica, New York 11432

Acute Neuromuscular Disorders

*David Grob, M.D.**

A variety of disorders may affect one part or another of the neuro-muscular or motor system (Table 1). Weakness occurs in almost all disorders and is usually the presenting complaint. In some disorders there is also atrophy, and in a few, stiffness, spasm, pain, tenderness, or abnormal movements (Table 2).

In the initial approach to the patient with neuromuscular disease, it is helpful to localize the cause anatomically, and then to consider etiology.[6] Anatomic localization is aided by considering the path taken by the motor stimulus down the motor system: frontal lobes to upper motor neuron (motor cortex and corticospinal tract) to lower motor neuron (anterior horn cells and motor nerve) to neuromuscular junction to muscle (Table 1).

Lesions of the upper motor neuron are recognized by characteristic changes: weakness with spasticity, increased tendon reflexes, clonus, and extensor plantar reflex, but no atrophy unless this occurs from disuse. Lesions of the lower motor neuron and most diseases of muscle produce weakness with atrophy, flaccidity, and decreased tendon reflexes. Other diseases of muscle, and disorders of neuromuscular transmission produce weakness without atrophy. A few disorders of the neuromuscular system are associated with pain or with abnormal tone or movements.

When weakness is of acute onset, it is often more difficult to localize the site of the lesion than when it is of longer duration. Signs indicative of an upper motor neuron lesion may not appear for several hours or days after onset, until spinal "shock" has worn off, but if these signs do not appear in one to two days it is unlikely that such a lesion is present. Muscle atrophy may not be evident until two or three weeks after onset of weakness caused by a lower motor lesion, or months after the onset of muscle disease that produces atrophy, but if atrophy is not present after weakness of this duration, lower motor neuron lesions are unlikely to be the cause of the weakness.

---

*Director, Department of Medicine, Maimonides Medical Center; Professor of Medicine, State University of New York, Downstate Medical Center, Brooklyn, New York

Table 1. *Disorders of the Neuromuscular System*[6]

I. *Central Nervous system*	
Emotional	
Upper motor neuron	Vascular, infection, tumor, trauma, demyelinating disease,
Extrapyramidal	hereditary
Cerebellum	
II. *Lower Motor Neuron*	
Anterior horns cells	Poliomyelitis, progressive muscular atrophy,
	syringomyelia, myelitis, tumor, disc, trauma
Nerves	Peripheral neuritis (*infections* : mononucleosis,
	polyneuritis, herpes zoster; *toxins* : diphtheria, lead,
	arsenic; *deficiency* : thiamine, nicotinic acid,
	vitamin B$_{12}$; *metabolic* : diabetes; porphyria,
	amyloidosis; *vascular* : periarteritis)
	Tumor, disc, trauma
III. *Neuromuscular Junction*	
Chemical agents	Depolarizing: anticholinesterases, decamethonium,
	succinylcholine
	Competitive: d-tubocurarine
	Electrolytes: potassium, calcium, magnesium
Toxins	Botulinus, tetanus, venoms
Disease	Myasthenia gravis
IV. *Muscle*	
Infectious and debilitating	Trichinosis, epidemic myalgia, neuromyasthenia, other
diseases	
"Mesenchymal"	Dermatomyositis, myositis, scleroderma, lupus,
tissue diseases	periarteritis
Endocrine diseases	Hyper or hypofunction of thyroid, adrenal cortex, anterior
	pituitary, parathyroid
Unknown cause	Muscular dystrophy, myotonic dystrophy, myoglobinuria

Limb weakness that develops within minutes is most likely to be due
to a lesion of the upper motor neuron of the cerebrum or the brain stem in
the case of hemiplegia or monoplegia, of the spinal cord in paraplegia, or
of either site in quadriplegia. Limb weakness that develops over hours or
days is attributed to a lesion of the lower motor neuron if atrophy
eventually ensues. A sensory level or bladder paralysis indicates a lesion
in the cord, while distal sensory and motor loss point to a lesion of the

Table 2. *Manifestations of Dysfunction of the Neuromuscular System*[6]

Weakness	In almost all disorders
Wasting	In diseases of the lower motor neuron and of muscle
Stiffness or spasm	In diseases of the upper motor neuron and extrapyramidal system, poliomyelitis, tetany, tetanus, myalgia, scleroderma, muscle trauma, occasionally polymyositis
Pain	In poliomyelitis, spinal tumor, disc or osteoarthritis, some causes of peripheral neuritis, trichinosis, paroxysmal myoglobinuria, epidemic myalgia, occasionally polymyositis
Abnormal movements	In some diseases of the extrapyramidal system, tetany, tetanus; fasciculations in progressive muscular atrophy and anticholinesterase poisoning

peripheral nerves. Disorders of the neuromuscular junction or muscle are uncommon causes of weakness of acute onset, but must be considered if there are no upper motor signs, no atrophy, and no sensory disturbance, and particularly if there is a history of previous episodes of weakness.

WEAKNESS WITH SIGNS OF UPPER MOTOR NEURON LESIONS

Hemiplegia is the most common distribution of severe weakness or paralysis. It almost always results from an upper motor neuron lesion, in over 90 per cent of patients from cerebral vascular disease: 72 per cent arterial thrombosis, 12 per cent intracerebral hemorrhage, 10 per cent subarachnoid hemorrhage, and 6 per cent cerebral embolus. Other causes (Table 3) are less common. The onset of a cerebral vascular "accident" is usually rapid, with maximum weakness attained within minutes to hours after onset. However, at least 15 per cent of patients have premonitory manifestations for hours or days, consisting of headache, drowsiness, mental disturbances, and focal neurologic signs, especially transient hemiparesis, aphasia, or paresthesias over half the body.[10] Aspirin and dipyramidole (Persantine) may have some prophylactic value.

Headache is prominent at the onset of weakness in all patients with subarachnoid hemorrhage, 60 per cent of those with intracerebral hemorrhage, 25 per cent of those with cerebral embolus, and 6 per cent of those with thrombosis. Vomiting at onset occurs in half of patients with hemorrhage and in 10 per cent of those with embolus or thrombosis. Coma at onset occurs in half of those with hemorrhage and one fourth of those with embolus or thrombosis, and convulsions at onset in 15, 9, and 7 per cent, respectively. Hence, the occurrence of headache, vomiting,

Table 3. *Causes of Hemiplegia* [6]

Vascular	Arterial thrombosis (intracranial, extracranial); embolus (from auricle, mural thrombus, bacterial endocarditis); arterial hemorrhage (hypertension, atheroma, aneurysm, thrombocytopenia, hypoprothrombinemia); venous or sinus thrombosis; infarction due to hypotension resulting from heart block, ventricular tachyarrhythmia, or other cause; hypertensive encephalopathy
Infection	Bacterial: meningitis, abscess Tuberculous: meningitis, tuberculoma Viral: encephalitis Fungal: cryptococcosis, moniliasis, aspergillosis, mucormycosis Syphilitic: meningovascular
Neoplasm	Primary, metastatic, tumor meningitis
Hypersensitivity	Polyarteritis, lupus erythematosus
Congenital	Aneurysm: berry, arteriovenous
Trauma	Laceration, subdural hematoma, birth injury
Toxic	Lead encephalopathy
Demyelination	Disseminated sclerosis, Schilder's disease

coma, or convulsions at the onset of a cerebral vascular accident suggests that it is due to hemorrhage, but does not exclude embolus or thrombosis. Stiffness of the neck is usually, though not always, present after hemorrhage, and is only occasionally present after embolus or thrombosis, but cervical osteoarthritis, which is common in the elderly, may simulate this sign. Cheyne-Stokes or labored respiration, pupillary changes, conjugate deviation of the eyes, quadriplegia, and bilateral extensor plantar reflexes are also more common after hemorrhage. The spinal fluid is grossly bloody in all patients with subarachnoid hemorrhage, in 85 per cent of those with intracranial hemorrhage (the remainder having encapsulated bleeding which can be seen on CT scan), and 15 per cent of those with cerebral embolus.

Approximately one fourth of patients with cerebral vascular accidents are said to have extracranial thrombosis of the carotid, vertebral, or subclavian artery, which should be suspected if a bruit is heard and demonstrated by arteriography. This must be performed before the hemiplegia is complete if arterial reconstruction is to have any value.

The mortality of patients with cerebrovascular accident varies with the cause: about 20 per cent after cerebral thrombosis, 30 per cent after cerebral embolus or subarachnoid hemorrhage, and over 80 per cent after cerebral hemorrhage. In about one third the cause of death appears to be cerebral, in about one third cardiac, and one third respiratory infection, or, occasionally, pulmonary embolus. Aspiration of saliva and food results in pneumonia more commonly than is appreciated. Evaluation of the electrocardiogram and serum levels of creatine phosphokinase may disclose unsuspected myocardial damage.[2]

Paraplegia of acute onset is relatively infrequent, and is usually due to a lesion of the corticospinal tracts below the cervical cord. When paralysis occurs suddenly, in a matter of minutes, it is usually the result of traumatic or vascular necrosis of the spinal cord produced by fracture or dislocation of the spine, bleeding from a tumor, or, rarely, from a vascular malformation, bleeding diathesis or hypertension, or occlusion of a spinal artery by a dissecting aneurysm or thrombosis. When paralysis or weakness develops over hours or days, it may be the result of disseminated sclerosis, postinfectious or postvaccinal transverse myelitis, meningovascular syphilis, or spinal cord compression by vertebral metastases, epidural abscess. Pott's disease, tumor, cervical disc, or spondylosis.

When paraplegia begins as a result of spinal cord compression it is vital to localize the lesion by myelography and relieve the compression by laminectomy before thrombosis of spinal vessels occurs and paraplegia becomes complete and irreversible. Paraplegia is often preceded by evidence of compression of posterior nerve roots, resulting in pain, paresthesia, and sensory loss of segmental distribution, and of anterior nerve roots, resulting in lower motor neuron signs of weakness, diminished tendon reflexes, sometimes fasciculations, and eventually atrophy of segmental distribution.

Quadriplegia occurs if the lesion affecting both corticospinal tracts is in or above the cervical cord. If the damage is above the cranial nerve nuclei concerned with swallowing pseudobulbar palsy will ensue. The most common causes of quadriplegia are repeated cerebral vascular accidents or basilar artery insufficiency leading to bilateral hemiplegia. Other causes are the same as those noted for paraplegia, or, less frequently, disease of the lower motor neuron or of muscle.

WEAKNESS WITH ATROPHY

Weakness with atrophy, flaccidity, and decreased tendon reflexes results from lesions of the lower motor neuron (neuropathy) and from most diseases of muscle (myopathy). When weakness develops over hours to days, and atrophy after weeks, poliomyelitis and polyneuritis must be considered, particularly if there is a preceding febrile illness. Poliomyelitis may usually be differentiated by the occurrence of meningeal signs, asymmetric distribution of paralysis, pleocytosis of the spinal fluid, and absence of sensory impairment. Encephalitis may produce similar signs, but is less likely to produce limb weakness and more likely to produce drowsiness. Polyneuritis is usually characterized by symmetric paralysis, paresthesias, sensory diminution, and increased protein in the spinal fluid. When weakness develops more slowly, over weeks, with atrophy and without sensory diminution, disease of muscle must also be considered. In neuropathy, the distribution of weakness and wasting tends to be more distal, and the wasting and decrease in tendon reflexes tend to be more severe. Fascicular twitching and sensory changes do not occur in myopathy; if present, these signs point to neuropathy, but they may be absent, in which case laboratory studies may be needed to localize the lesion (Table 4).

The *electromyogram* in lower motor neuron disease will usually

Table 4. *Differentiation between Weakness Arising from Disease of Lower Motor Neuron (Neuropathy) and of Muscle (Myopathy)*[6]*

DIFFERENCES	NEUROPATHY	MYOPATHY
Site of weakness	Distal	Proximal
Tendon reflexes	Decreased early	Decreased late
Muscle response to direct percussion	Present	Decreased (except in myotonia and hypothyroidism)
Sensory loss	May be present	Absent
Fasciculations	May be present	Absent
Complete paralysis	May occur	Rare (except in periodic paralysis)
Electromyogram: nerve conduction	May be delayed	Normal
Fibrillations and fasciculations	May be present	Rare
Biopsy: atrophy of muscle fibers	Grouped	Diffuse
Serum enzymes: aldolase, creatine phosphokinase, glutamic oxalacetic transaminase, lactic dehydrogenase	Normal	Usually elevated

*Similarities: weakness with wasting, flaccidity, and decreased tendon reflexes.

Table 5. *Causes of Peripheral Neuropathy*[6]

Infectious	Bacterial: leprosy
	Viral: infectious mononucleosis, herpes zoster
Hypersensitivity	Serum sickness, polyarteritis nodosa
Congenital	Peroneal muscular atrophy, hypertrophic interstitial polyneuropathy, hereditary sensory neuropathy
Deficiency	Thiamine deficiency, alcoholism, pellagra, pernicious anemia, sprue, pyridoxine deficiency
Toxic	Bacterial: diphtheria
	Tick: Dermacentor andersoni
	Chemical: heavy metals (As, Hg, Bi, Pb, Th), carbon monoxide, organic phosphates, sulfonamides, vincristine, vinblastine, isoniazid
Metabolic	Diabetes, uremia, porphyria, amyloidosis, Refsum's syndrome
Neoplastic	Pressure (e.g., Pancoast tumor), carcinomatous neuropathy
Vascular	Arterial or venous thrombosis
Trauma	Spondylosis, protruded intervertebral disc, carpal tunnel syndrome, pressure, fracture, dislocation, wound
Unknown cause	Acute "infective" polyneuritis (Guillain-Barré), chronic polyneuritis

show spontaneous electrical discharges from muscle fibers and groups of fibers (fibrillation potentials and positive sharp waves) and from motor units and groups of motor units (fasciculation potentials). The latter are more frequent in diseases of the anterior horn cells than in diseases of the ventral roots, and least common in diseases of the peripheral nerves.

The *serum levels of enzymes derived from muscle,* such as creatine phosphokinase, are normal or only slightly elevated in diseases of the lower motor neuron, and are markedly elevated in some diseases of muscle.

Muscle biopsy is of value in distinguishing between lower motor neuron disease, which results in grouped atrophy, and muscle disease, which causes diffuse atrophy and usually infiltration with round cells.

Peripheral Neuropathy, Predominantly Motor

The most abrupt onset, occurring over minutes or hours and suggesting vascular occlusion, is seen in diabetes mellitus, periarteritis nodosa, or ischemic neuritis. A course with onset over several days, a peak within about 2 weeks, and gradual improvement over several months is seen in the Guillain-Barré syndrome, and much less commonly after exposure to toxins as in acute intermittent porphyria, which can be recognized by porphobilinogen in the urine, diphtheria, or tick-bite, or chemicals such as heavy metals or tricresyl phosphate.[4, 6]

Guillain-Barré syndrome (acute "infective" polyneuritis) is the most common diffuse, predominantly motor neuropathy. In two thirds of the patients there is a prodromal illness. After a latent period of 5 to 18 days rapidly progressive, symmetric weakness begins, usually in the legs, and ascends to the arms and face. There is often low-grade fever, headache, pain in the limbs and back, and occasionally vomiting. The distribution of weakness differs from that seen in most other types of neuropathy, which involve predominently the distal musculature, in that the proximal muscles may be involved to the same degree as the distal, or to even a greater degree, and over three fourths of the patients have facial diplegia. Half have weakness of the muscles of swallowing and speech, and one fourth have respiratory weakness. Extraocular muscles are seldom impaired. Muscular weakness reaches its peak 2 to 21 (average 12) days after onset. Muscle wasting occurs to a moderate degree, and tendon reflexes are diminished. Sensory manifestations usually occur, and are initially of stocking or glove distribution, with paresthesias, dysesthesias, pain, muscle tenderness, and impairment of all forms of sensibility. Occasionally sensory manifestations are minimal or absent. About 15 per cent of patients die of respiratory failure, aspiration pneumonia, pulmonary embolism, or hypotension and arrhythmia attributed to autonomic neuropathy.[8] The remainder gradually improve over a period of 3 to 6 months, with most recovering completely, though some have residual disability or even chronic relapsing polyneuropathy.

Spinal fluid protein is characteristically elevated (50 to 1000 mg per 100 ml), and there is usually no pleocytosis. However, in 25 per cent of patients the initial examination of the spinal fluid is normal, and the protein rises after the first week. In 20 per cent there is an increase in lymphocytes in the spinal fluid (10 to 100 per cu mm).

During the first 2 to 21 (average 12) days of progressive weakness, the vital capacity should be frequently evaluated, endotracheal intubation and assisted ventilation begun if needed, and tracheostomy performed while the tube is in place. The value of corticosteroids is debated, but many physicians administer it when respiratory failure occurs.

Peripheral Neuropathy, Predominantly Sensory

Alcoholism, diabetes, and trauma are the common causes of predominantly sensory neuropathy. Symptoms of *alcoholic* neuropathy include burning, prickling, and jabbing discomfort in the feet and hands, often made worse by exercise. The muscles may be tender, and there may be associated weakness, atrophy, and areflexia. Improvement may occur after the administration of large doses of thiamine.

Diabetes of 10 or more years' duration may result in several types of neuropathy. The most common is sensory neuropathy, manifested by aching or burning pain in the legs, especially the calves, and sometimes by paresthesias. The pain can be differentiated from intermittent claudication caused by peripheral vascular insufficiency by the more striking relation of the latter to exercise. In sensory neuropathy examination will reveal hyperesthesia or hypoesthesia in the distal extremities, decreased vibratory sensation, and sometimes decreased proprioception. Motor neuropathy may or may not be present. Diabetes may also produce motor neuropathy, with or without sensory neuropathy. A single motor nerve may be affected, most commonly the third cranial nerve, resulting in ocular palsy, with or without ptosis and pupillary change. A number of motor nerves may be involved, as in mononeuritis multiplex or diabetic amytrophy, or, less often there may be widespread polyneuropathy resembling the Guillain-Barré syndrome, though of more gradual onset and longer duration. Diabetes may also cause neuropathy affecting the sympathetic nervous system, resulting in decreased sweating in affected areas, nocturnal diarrhea, orthostatic hypotension, and impotence.

Traumatic injury to a peripheral nerve or nerve root may result from bone fracture, joint dislocation (especially at the shoulder), protrusion of a cervical or lumbar intervertebral disc, entrapment in carpal tunnel (median nerve) or thoracic outlet syndrome, pressure palsy of the radial nerve (wrist drop) or external popliteal nerve (foot drop after squatting), or knife or bullet wounds. Disc protrusion occurs most commonly in the fourth, fifth, or, rarely, third lumbar interspace, and less commonly in the fifth, sixth, or, rarely, seventh cervical interspace. The protrusion occurs posteriorly into the spinal canal, resulting in pressure on one or more nerve roots, or occasionally on the cervical cord.

Lumbar disc protrusion produces recurring attacks of low backache, with or without sciatic pain, usually unilateral. The patient usually walks with a limp on the involved side. The erector spinae muscles are likely to be in spasm. Motion of the spinal column is limited and may aggravate the pain, and raising the extended leg on the involved side may reproduce the pain. The Achilles tendon reflex is usually diminished or absent, and there may be hypalgesia in the distribution of the first sacral root. If the protrusion is more marked, there is also weakness and mild atrophy of the lower leg. Severe weakness and wasting of the entire limb is rarely caused by disc lesions; only in the rarely seen massive disc protrusion is there flaccid paraplegia with or without loss of bladder and bowel control and extensive sensory loss, resembling the signs of tumor of the cauda equina.

Cervical disc protrusion is the most common cause of root pain extending from the neck down an upper extremity. It is accompanied by spasm of the neck muscles, loss of normal curvature of the cervical spine, and pain on motion of the neck. The tendon reflexes, particularly of the biceps or triceps, may be diminished, and paresthesias or dermatome hypalgesia may be present.

The spinal fluid protein is usually elevated to between 40 and 100 mg per 100 ml; higher concentrations are more suggestive of neoplasm. Radiologic examination may show narrowing of an intervertebral space; in the cervical region this is suggestive of disc protrusion, but in the lumbar or thoracic region it is of less significance. If bed rest and traction do not result in amelioration of symptoms, or if there are gross signs of nerve deficit, a myelogram should be performed to demonstrate and localize the lesion and to evaluate the desirability of intrathecal corticosteroid or surgical removal of a lumbar disc. Cervical discs are seldom operated on because of the danger of impairing cord blood supply.

Disease of Muscle

The most common primary diseases of muscle are polymyositis and muscular dystrophy; the former is more common in adults, the latter in children. These, like the most common secondary diseases of muscle, hyperthyroidism and steroid myopathy, produce weakness and wasting which usually develop gradually over many weeks and months. Except for muscular dystrophy, onset of these disorders may occasionally occur more rapidly, over several days.[6]

Polymyositis occurs alone in 30 per cent of patients, and is accompanied by dermatitis in 40 per cent, lupus, polyarteritis, or scleroderma in 20 per cent, and malignant disease in 15 per cent (30 per cent if onset is after the age of 40). The initial symptom is weakness, usually of the legs, in half the patients, dermatitis in one fourth, and muscle or joint pain or Raynaud's phenomenon in one fourth. The proximal muscles of the legs become weak in almost all patients, and those of the arms in 80 per cent, while only 35 per cent develop weakness of distal muscles. The neck flexors become weak in 65 per cent, and some dysphagia eventually occurs in 50 per cent. Facial and extraocular muscles are seldom affected. Pain or tenderness of muscles occurs in half the patients. Severe atrophy and weight loss develop in half and contractures in one third. Tendon reflexes and the contractile response of affected muscle to direct percussion are usually diminished.

Approximately 40 per cent of patients have an erythematous eruption which usually begins on the face or upper trunk, with edema, erythema, and a pink "heliotrope" hue. The periorbital areas are particularly involved, and malar erythema may occur, as in lupus erythematosus. The hands are frequently involved, especially the extensor surfaces and nail beds, and sometimes the feet. Pigmentation, hardness, and even calcinosis of the skin and subcutaneous tissues may occur later.

Approximately one third of patients have Raynaud's phenomenon, one third have joint pains, and a few have arthritis which may be indistinguishable from rheumatoid arthritis. About 8 per cent have significant intestinal hypomotility, and 2 per cent recurring pneumonitis. Fever is variable.

The serum enzymes derived from muscle are almost always elevated, sometimes markedly, during active stages of the disease, and usually decline toward normal levels with spontaneous improvement or following treatment. The decline usually precedes by 3 to 4 weeks any improvement in strength, and relapse of the disease is often heralded by a rise in serum enzymes. The enzyme levels may be normal during chronic stages of the disease and, rarely, during active stages. Biopsy of involved muscle shows degeneration and diffuse atrophy of muscle fibers and round cell infiltration, and is helpful in diagnosis. Skin changes are not pathognomonic.

Management relies on corticosteroid, which must be given in doses of about 60 mg of prednisone daily for weeks or months before improvement occurs. If this is unsuccessful, immunosuppressant drugs such as methotrexate, azathioprine, or cyclophosphamide may be tried.[7]

Hyperthyroidism results in weakness and wasting in 70 per cent of patients. This is usually mild or moderate, but is pronounced in a small proportion. The commonest generalized myopathy is the gradual development of pronounced weakness and wasting, to which the term chronic thyrotoxic myopathy has been applied. The commonest localized myopathy is weakness of one or more of the extraocular muscles, usually accompanied by exophthalmos, and in its most severe form manifested as exophthalmic ophthalmoplegia. Much less common is the acute onset in patients with fulminating hyperthyroidism of severe weakness, usually accompanied by evidence of central nervous system dysfunction, and termed acute thyrotoxic myopathy or encephalomyopathy. In 2 per cent of patients hyperthyroidism occurs in association with myasthenia gravis or, more rarely, with hypokalemic periodic paralysis.

Acute thyrotoxic encephalomyopathy is characterized by the acute development of severe weakness, dysphagia, and dysarthria simultaneously with all the nervous disturbances of thyroid "storm" or "crisis". There is rapid progression of weakness of muscles innervated by the cranial nerves, with bulbar paralysis and weakness of the limbs and trunk. There may be marked tremor, agitation or depression, psychosis, delirium, and semicoma or coma. This disorder is more properly termed encephalopathy, since it is probably due mainly to central neural dysfunction, although some patients described with bulbar paralysis may have had undetected fulminating myasthenia gravis appearing as a complication of hyperthyroidism. In the absence of treatment (iodide, propranolol, propylthiouracil, corticosteroids) most patients with encephalomyopathy have died within 1 to 2 weeks after its onset, although a subacute form has been described.

Hyperadrenocorticism (Cushing's syndrome) results in weakness in 80 per cent of patients, whether due to hyperplasia, adenoma, or carcinoma of the adrenal cortex, to basophilic adenoma of the pituitary, to carcinoma of nonendocrine tissue, particularly the lung, or to prolonged administration of corticosteroids. The weakness is gradual in onset, rarely acute, involves the extremities and trunk, and is usually accompanied by wasting of the muscles of the extremities.

WEAKNESS WITHOUT SIGNS OF UPPER MOTOR NEURON LESION OR ATROPHY

When weakness develops over minutes to hours without signs of an upper motor neuron lesion or sensory disturbance, one must consider not only a lower motor neuron lesion, which will result in atrophy in 2 to 3 weeks, but also some of the uncommon toxic and metabolic disorders of the neuromuscular junction or muscle, which do not result in atrophy.[6] Botulism is recognized by the progression of ocular, bulbar, and then trunk and limb weakness and by fixed dilated pupils. The metabolic disorders are characterized by recurring attacks of weakness, which in some instances follow exercise. Attacks of periodic paralysis are painless, while those due to phosphorylase deficiency or paroxysmal myoglobinuria are accompanied by muscle pain and tenderness. When weakness develops over days to weeks without signs of an upper motor neuron lesion, atrophy, or sensory disturbance, one must consider myasthenia gravis or muscle disease that has not yet produced discernible atrophy.

Botulism. The weakness produced by the toxin of *Clostridium botulinum* is due to deficient release of acetylcholine from the motor nerve endings, but is unresponsive to anticholinesterase drugs. Both voluntary and smooth muscle are affected. Symptoms begin 12 to 48 hours after the ingestion of contaminated food. One third of patients have nausea, vomiting, and diarrhea, but over half have constipation, as well as urinary retention. The eye muscles are usually affected early, resulting in diplopia, ptosis, dilated and often fixed pupils, and blurring of near vision due to paralysis of accommodation. The bulbar muscles are affected next, resulting in difficulty in swallowing, speaking, and chewing. Finally the skeletal and respiratory muscles are affected, resulting in generalized weakness and respiratory distress. Patients with mild botulism recover in about 2 weeks. In former years patients severely ill with botulism died in 4 to 14 days of respiratory paralysis, aspiration, or pneumonia. Today, if patients can be kept alive by the use of tracheostomy, assisted ventilation and antibiotic treatment of pneumonia, function begins to return in 7 to 14 days and recovery is complete. Specific antitoxin may be helpful if given very early after onset of weakness.[7] Some snake venoms, e.g., cobra, produce similar weakness.

Organic phosphate anticholinesterase insecticides, such as parathion, mipafox, and malathion, are highly toxic to man. Their effects are attributable to accumulation of acetylcholine in smooth and cardiac muscle and secretory glands (muscarine-like effects), in motor nerves to striated muscle and preganglionic nerves to autonomic ganglia (nicotine-like effects), and in the central nervous system. Exposure of the eyes and respiratory tract to vapor or liquid results in marked pupillary constriction, headache, rhinorrhea, and tightness in the chest. Systemic absorption by any route, including the respiratory tract and skin, results in sweating, nausea, abdominal cramps, increased salivation and bronchial secretion, muscular fasciculations, severe generalized weakness, including weakness of the muscles of respiration, giddiness, headache, drowsiness, confusion, ataxia, coma, and generalized convulsions. Poisoning by an anticholinesterase compound should be suspected when unexplained weakness or coma is accompanied by miosis, muscular fasciculations, and excessive sweating, salivation, and bronchorrhea. Management relies on large doses of atropine, 2-PAM, and assisted ventilation.

Antibiotics. Muscular weakness attributed to neuromuscular block has been reported following the parenteral administration of therapeutic doses of polymyxin B or E (colistimethate, colistin), neomycin, kanamycin, and streptomycin to patients with renal insufficiency. Manifestations have included paresthesias of the face and hands, ptosis, diplopia due to external ophthalmoplegia, dysarthria, dysphagia, ataxia, areflexia, dyspnea and other signs of respiratory insufficiency, and even complete respiratory paralysis.

Hypokalemia may develop when there is deficient intake or absorption of potassium, excessive loss in vomitus, stool, or urine (diuretics, renal tubular dysfunction, hyperaldosteronism or hyperadrenocorticism), or excessive intracellular movement of the ion, into the liver following administration of glucose and insulin in the treatment of diabetic acidosis, or into the muscle in hypokalemic periodic paralysis.[6, 9] This rare disorder, which is usually familial, is characterized by periodic attacks of weakness. Onset of the disease usually occurs during puberty. Attacks almost always occur while the patient is asleep, 4 to 9 hours after supper, particularly after a meal high in carbohydrate.

Severe hypokalemia results in impairment of skeletal, cardiac, and, to a lesser extent, smooth muscle. This is more likely to occur after rapid reduction in plasma potassium concentration than after gradual reduction. Weakness caused by hypokalemic periodic paralysis occurs following less marked depression of serum potassium (usually to less than 3 mEq per liter) than in other causes of hypokalemia (usually to less than 2 mEq per liter), and is much more severe at comparable levels of hypokalemia. Weakness arising from hypokalemia characteristically involves the extremities, trunk and neck, and sometimes respiration. The muscles innervated by the cranial nerves are rarely affected. Both the tendon reflexes and the muscle contraction in response to direct percussion are diminished. If weakness is severe, there may be flaccid paralysis and, rarely, respiratory failure. The effect of hypokalemia on cardiac muscle may be recognized by electrocardiographic changes: first the appearance of a positive afterpotential on the falling limb of the T wave with broadening, later lowering, and still later inversion of the T wave, and depression of the ST segment. The interval between the Q or S wave and the termination of the T wave may be prolonged, but the interval between the Q or S wave and the origin of the T wave is not prolonged, in contrast to the prolongation produced by hypocalcemia. Extrasystoles and other arrhythmias may develop. There is increased sensitivity to the arrhythmic effects of digitalis, and, when these are present, the possibility of hypokalemia should be investigated. In very severe hypokalemia, cardiac dilatation and even arrest of the heart in systole may occur.

The relaxant effect of hypokalemia on smooth muscle may result in anorexia, nausea, abdominal distention, ileus, bladder atony, and vasodilation. Hypokalemia due to loss of potassium results in metabolic alkalosis, and alkalosis aggravates hypokalemia. When sodium ions are reabsorbed from the renal tubules they are normally exchanged for potassium and hydrogen ions, and if potassium is not available for this exchange an excess of hydrogen ions is lost. Furthermore, potassium ions lost from muscle are replaced by sodium and hydrogen ions from the extracellular fluid. The alkalosis that results from potassium loss is difficult to correct until potassium is replaced, since administered hydrogen ions will be lost in the urine until potassium ions are available for exchange with sodium.

Hypokalemia is treated by administration of potassium salts, preferably by mouth. The daily normal dietary intake of 80 mEq can be supplemented by 20 to 40 mEq after each meal, in solution, since tablets, unless enteric coated, may cause local vasoconstriction and mucosal ulceration. In patients with hypokalemic periodic paralysis, this amount can be given hourly until strength returns. Oral administration is safe as long as urinary output is adequate, since 80 per cent is normally excreted in the urine. Intravenous administration should be reserved for patients who cannot swallow, or have severe diarrhea or diabetic ketoacidosis, when large amounts may have to be replaced. Administration should not be more rapid than 25 mEq per hour and the electrocardiogram and serum level should be monitored. Oliguria mandates cautious replacement and anuria is a contraindication.

Hyperkalemia. Emergency treatment of hyperkalemia is reviewed elsewhere in this issue by Kunis and Lowenstein.

Normokalemic periodic paralysis resembles the hypokalemic type in onset during sleep, and the hyperkalemic type in onset following administration of potassium, and differs from both in the normal level of serum potassium present during attacks and in the amelioration of weakness following sodium chloride administration. The muscle contains vacuoles, and, during attacks, increased sodium concentration, and decreased potassium. Attacks of normokalemic periodic paralysis appear to be preceded by urinary loss of sodium and retention of potassium, and have been prevented by high salt intake and the administration of acetazolamide or 9-fluorohydrocortisone, which causes renal retention of sodium and loss of potassium.

Myasthenia gravis causes either transient or persistent weakness and abnormal fatigability. While weakness of the oculomotor muscles or levator palpebrae may develop within minutes or hours, weakness of the bulbar or peripheral muscles develops more slowly, over days, weeks, or months, usually with exacerbations and remissions. The initial symptom is ptosis in approximately 25 per cent, diplopia in 24 per cent, weakness of the legs in 13 per cent, and, in the remainder, blurring of vision, difficulty in swallowing or chewing, slurred or nasal speech, weakness of arms, hands, neck, face, or trunk, generalized fatigue, or rarely shortness of breath.[5] The extraocular muscles are affected at some time in the course of the disease in almost every patient. Impairment of these muscles occurs unilaterally or bilaterally and in almost all combinations of functional disturbance. Elevation of the lids and upward deviation of the eyes are usually most affected, and downward deviation is least affected. Occasionally there is complete limitation of extraocular movement. When ptosis is present, the orbicularis oculi is also usually affected, resulting in weakness of closure of the lid. This is a helpful sign in distinguishing between ocular palsy of neurogenic origin, which is usually not accompanied by orbicularis oculi weakness, and that due to myasthenia gravis or primary muscle disease. In about 20 per cent of patients with myasthenia gravis the disease remains localized to the extraocular muscles and orbicularis oculi. In 80 per cent the disease progresses to involve numerous muscles, and usually becomes generalized within 2 years after onset. The most common sequence is muscles of the eyes, face, swallowing, speech, jaw, tongue, neck, shoulders, arms, hands, hips, upper legs, lower legs, trunk and respiration.

The diagnosis is suggested from the history, distribution, and fluctuating nature of the weakness, which usually increases following exercise of involved muscles, and is confirmed by the improvement in

strength which occurs following the administration of an anticholinesterase compound, such as edrophonium (Tensilon), 10 mg intravenously, or neostigmine (Prostigmine) 1.5 mg intramuscularly with 0.6 mg of
atropine, when the patient is in a "basal" state at least 6 hours after the
last medication.[5-7] The improvement is often incomplete even after
maximum doses, but careful measurement reveals a significant change
in all except a few patients with localized ocular myasthenia and a rare
patient with generalized myasthenia. In these a response can sometimes
be elicited later in the course of the disease.

Symptomatic *management* relies on anticholinesterase medication:
if the patient is able to swallow, pyridostigmine (Mestinon) 60 to 120 mg
orally every 3 to 4 hours when awake, and the long acting preparation
180 mg at bedtime if necessary; or if unable to swallow, neostigmine 0.5
to 1 mg intramuscularly every 2 to 3 hours.[5-7] A higher dose should be
carefully evaluated and continued only if it results in an increase in
strength, since the optimal dose is the smallest amount that produces a
maximal level of strength. Determination of the effect of 2 mg edrophonium intravenously 1 hour after the last dose can serve as an aid in
adjusting the dose: upward if strength increases and downward if it
decreases. Small doses of atropine may be administered as needed to
reduce parasympathomimetic side-effects such as abdominal cramps,
diarrhea, and salivation. Exacerbation may follow from upper respiratory infection and may result in weakness of cough, pooling of secretions,
and airway obstruction. When this becomes severe, an endotracheal
catheter must be inserted, suctioning and assisted ventilation begun,
and tracheostomy performed over the tube. The patient often becomes
less responsive to anticholinesterase medication during exacerbation,
presumably because more end-plates have become insensitive to acetylcholine. This insensitive state often leads to confusion as to whether
the patient is overdosed (in "cholinergic crisis") or underdosed (in
"myasthenic crisis"). If the dose of anticholinesterase medication is
progressively increased without careful observation of the effect on
strength, overdose will result and this tends to render the patient more
insensitive. If respiration is being supported mechanically, the dose
should be reduced to the smallest amount necessary to sustain respiration in case of failure of mechanical support, and the patient should be
tested periodically with 1 to 2 mg of edrophonium intravenously to
ascertain when responsiveness returns. Atropine should be administered
only if absolutely necessary to diminish excessive secretions, and then
used in small doses to avoid inspissation.

For patients who are responding poorly to anticholinesterase medication, the next step is administration of corticosteroid. If the patient is
severely weak, an initial dose of 100 mg or more of prednisone is
administered daily. This usually causes exacerbation of weakness during the first week, followed by progressive improvement in subsequent
weeks. If the patient is not severely weak, an initial dose of 25 mg every
other day can be progressively increased until improvement occurs. This
may avoid the initial exacerbation, but may not result in improvement
for many weeks. Since prolonged administration of corticosteroid may

cause peptic ulcer, osteoporosis, aseptic necrosis of the femoral heads, cataracts, and other manifestations of hyperadrenocorticism the dose should be reduced when feasible, and discontinued if possible.

If the severely ill patient does not respond to corticosteroid, repeated plasmaphoresis can be employed. This provides temporary improvement, but must be combined with corticosteroids and possibly immunosuppressive drugs, such as azathioprine or cyclophosphamide, to achieve more lasting benefit.

Thymectomy is performed in patients who are not able to carry out normal activity on anticholinesterase medication. Tracheostomy should be performed over an endotracheal tube at operation. Most patients improve slowly over months or years. The 10 per cent of patients who have a thymoma should have thymectomy performed to prevent local invasion, even though the course of the myasthenia is not affected.

WEAKNESS WITH PAIN

Relatively few causes of weakness result in muscle pain or tenderness (Table 6), which must be distinguished from pain in the joints, tendons, bursae, or bones. Disorders of the upper motor neuron rarely cause pain, from thalamic injury or vasomotor changes. Pain is more common in some disorders of the lower motor neuron such as poliomyelitis and diseases affecting sensory roots (disc, tumor, spondylosis, or tabes) or peripheral nerves (neuropathy). Only a few disorders of muscle are accompanied by pain or tenderness.[6] When muscle pain or tenderness is not accompanied by objective evidence of weakness, it is usually due to trauma (especially stretch), viral disease, polymyalgia rheumatica, or tension-anxiety state.

Polymyalgia rheumatica is characterized by myalgia, arthralgia, increased sedimentation rate, and usually headaches, temporal artery tenderness, low grade fever, and/or ocular manifestations.[3] If temporal artery biopsy discloses arteritis, corticosteroid should be administered to prevent occlusion of ophthalmic or cerebral arteries. This also provides prompt symptomatic relief.

Table 6. *Disorders Characterized by Weakness with Muscle Pain or Tenderness*[6]

Rare disorder of upper motor neuron	Thalamic syndrome, vasomotor
Some disorders of lower motor neuron:	
Anterior horn cells	Poliomyelitis
Nerve roots	Disc, tumor, spondylosis, tabes
Nerves	Peripheral neuropathy (sensory plus motor)
Some disorders of muscle	Some viral diseases (epidemic myalgia, epidemic neuromyasthenia, influenza), brucellosis, leptospirosis, trichinosis, paroxysmal myoglobinuria, phosphorylase deficiency, polymyositis, alcoholic or clofibrate myopathy, trauma, polymyalgia rheumatica, tension-anxiety state

Table 7. *Disorders Characterized by Weakness with*
Increased Tone or Abnormal Movements[6]

Upper motor neuron	Spasticity, clonic movements, convulsions (cortex)
Extrapyramidal motor system	Rigidity
Basal ganglia	Resting tremor, chorea, athetosis, hemiballism
Cerebellum	Intention tremor
Olivary nucleus and tegmental and dentate connections	Myoclonus
Lower motor neuron	Reflex spasm (irritation of anterior horn cells in tetanus or poliomyelitis; of nerve roots in disc, tumor, or spondylosis; of nerves in tetany; or of muscles in myalgia or trauma)
	Fasciculations (slowly progressive injury of anterior horn cells in progressive muscular atrophy or syringomyelia; of nerve roots in disc, tumor, or spondylosis; or of peripheral nerves in chronic neuropathy)
Neuromuscular junction	Fasciculations (in anticholinesterase intoxication)
Muscle	Cramps in hyponatremia, vascular insufficiency, hypothyroidism, paroxysmal myoglobinuria, phosphorylase deficiency, black widow spider bite
	Stiffness in scleroderma, stiff man syndrome, myosclerosis, trauma, and occasionally in trichinosis, sarcoidosis, myalgia, and polymyositis
	Tremor or twitching in uremia, hypocalcemia, alkalosis, hyperthyroidism, alcoholism, drugs (barbiturate, bromide, penicillin), tension-anxiety state
	Myotonia in myotonic dystrophy and occasionally in hypothyroidism or hyperkalemic periodic paralysis

WEAKNESS WITH INCREASED TONE OR ABNORMAL MOVEMENTS

Weakness is accompanied by increased tone or abnormal movements in certain disorders of the motor system (Table 7), so that these signs often aid in diagnosis.[6]

Spasticity of affected muscles results from upper motor neuron lesions. It is greater in flexors of the arms and extensors of the legs, absent at rest or on slow movement, increased by rapid movement, and may be associated with spontaneous clonic movements. Myoclonic contractions may also occur after lesions of the olivary nucleus or of its tegmental and dentate connections. Convulsions may occur in cerebral disorders of almost any etiology.

Rigidity of affected muscles results from disease of the extrapyramidal motor system, especially the basal ganglia, or from certain drugs, including phenothiazines. It is greater in flexors of the arms and legs, is present at rest, and is not associated with increased tendon reflexes. It is often accompanied by *resting tremor.* Much less commonly lesions of the basal ganglia result in *chorea, athetosis,* or, rarely, *hemiballism. Intention tremor* results from lesions of the cerebellum or brain stem.

Ataxia may result not only from lesions of the cerebellum and its connections, but also from interruption of sensory proprioceptive pathways in the peripheral nerves (neuropathy), sensory roots (tabes dorsalis), or spinal cord (subacute combined degeneration, disseminated sclerosis, spondylosis, cervical disc protrusion, or syringomyelia), as well as from intoxication by alcohol, barbiturates, or other depressant drugs. Cerebellar ataxia, as well as that due to drug intoxication, is due to failure of central coordinating mechanisms, and is present with the eyes either open or closed. Sensory ataxia, on the other hand, is aggravated when the eyes are closed (positive Romberg sign), since the patient must rely on visual appreciation of the position of his extremities and body in space because of the absence of proprioceptive impulses.

Tetanic spasms occur in tetany (due to hypocalcemia, alkalosis, or rarely hypomagnesemia) and tetanus. In the former there is carpopedal spasm and positive Chvostek and Trousseau signs, and in the latter tonic and clonic spasms, trismus, and sometimes seizures. Local reflex spasm of muscle also occurs in poliomyelitis, pressure lesions of nerve roots due to disc, tumor, or spondylosis, and inflammatory or traumatic lesions of muscle.

Muscular cramps may result from hyponatremia, hypothyroidism, or black widow spider bite. Cramps occur following exercise in normal individuals, as well as in patients with vascular insufficiency or the rare muscle diseases phosphorylase deficiency and paroxysmal myoglobinuria.

Phosphorylase deficiency (McArdle's syndrome) is characterized by the appearance of muscle pain, stiffness, cramps and weakness within minutes after exercise is carried out, especially under ischemic conditions, such as after occlusion of the circulation of a limb. There is a fall in the concentration of lactate and pyruvate in the venous return from ischemic muscle performing work, in contrast to the rise which occurs in normal subjects under similar conditions. Exhausted muscle may continue in the contracted state, even at rest, owing to the persistence of localized contractures which are not accompanied by electrical activity. In half the patients, myoglobinuria occurs after exercise. The muscle contains excessive glycogen, and homogenates of muscle are unable to form lactate from endogenous or added glycogen unless muscle phosphorylase is added.

Paroxysmal myoglobinuria is characterized by intermittent attacks of muscle pain and cramping, usually precipitated by exercise, and followed by muscle firmness, tenderness, weakness, and darkening of the urine as a result of excretion of myoglobin from degenerating muscle fibers. The calf muscles are most often involved. Systemic manifestations, such as chills, fever, vomiting, abdominal pain, leukocytosis, and hypotension may occur. Occasionally the muscles of respiration may be involved, leading to respiratory paralysis. The myoglobinuria usually does not cause renal impairment, but, when very marked and accompanied by hypotension, it may result in tubular damage, anuria, and renal failure. The disease appears to be caused by intermittent degeneration of muscle fibers of unknown cause, with release into the blood of muscle constituents, including myoglobin, potassium, creatine, amino acids, glutamic oxalacetic transaminase, aldolase, and creatine phosphokinase. The serum levels of these compounds increase markedly following attacks.

SUBJECTIVE WEAKNESS

Subjective weakness, usually without objective evidence at the time of examination after subsidence of the episode, may occur acutely or recurrently when there is a decrease in the blood supply to the brain or skeletal muscles from any cause, such as decreased venous return (postural hypotension), decreased blood volume, tachyarrhythmia, myocardial ischemia or infarction, and/or cerebral vascular disease. Sufficient decrease in blood supply to the brain results in giddiness and syncope, varying degrees of loss of consciousness, and finally convulsions. Observation or history of these complaints facilitates identification of cerebral ischemia as the cause, but when the ischemia is mild or transient the patient may complain only of weakness, and the cerebral origin of the symptoms may not be readily recognized.

Acute, recurrent subjective weakness can also result from hyperventilation or hypoglycemia. Blowing off carbon dioxide and resulting alkalosis also causes giddiness, paresthesias, and sometimes tetany. Hypoglycemia may result in other central nervous symptoms: headache, giddiness, confusion, visual disturbances including diplopia, and if severe and prolonged, coma, convulsions, and paralysis. Both hyperventilation resulting from anxiety, and hypoglycemia, cause epinephrine release, which produces tachycardia, palpitations, sweating, and dilated pupils.

Subjective or objective weakness of the legs which recurs on walking, with or without pain, and is relieved by rest, is usually due to peripheral arterial insufficiency.

Impairment of volition may result in the complaint of local weakness or paralysis, as in hysteria; generalized weakness and fatigue, as in neurasthenia; weakness with catatonia, as in schizophrenia; or weakness with wasting resulting from inanition, as in anorexia nervosa. The diagnosis of weakness or fatigue of emotional origin can be made only after careful exclusion of other causes, but is often suggested by a history of anxiety and increased muscle tension, fatigue on awakening, early evening drowsiness, and improvement in symptoms following suggestion or placebo administration. However, it must be kept in mind that any disability may lead to emotional disorder. In such instances part of the disability may be relieved following hypnosis, placebo, or other forms of suggestion, but evidence of the underlying disease process remains.

REFERENCES

1. DeMyer, W.: Anatomy and clinical neurology of the spinal cord. *In* Baker, A. B. and Baker, L. H.: Clinical Neurology. Hagerstown, Maryland, Harper and Row, 1979, Vol. 3, No. 31, pp. 1–32.

2. Dimant, J., and Grob, D.: Electrocardiographic changes and myocardial damage in patients with acute cerebrovascular accidents. Stroke, 8:448–455, 1977.
3. Dimant, J., Grob, D., and Brunner, N. G.: Ophthalmoplegia, ptosis and miosis in temporal arteritis. Neurology, 1980, in press.
4. Goldstein, N. P., and Dyck, P. J.: Diseases of peripheral nerves. In Baker, A. B., and Baker, L. H.: Clinical Neurology. Hagerstown, Maryland, Harper and Row, 1978, Vol. 3, No. 38, pp. 1–72.
5. Grob, D.: Myasthenia gravis. A review of pathogenesis and treatment. Arch. Intern. Med., 108:615–638, 1961.
6. Grob, D.: Weakness. In Barondess, J. A., ed.: Diagnostic Approaches to Presenting Syndromes. Baltimore, Maryland, Williams and Wilkins, 1971, pp. 197–300.
7. Grob, D.: Use of drugs in myopathies. Ann. Rev. Pharmacol. Toxicol., 16:215–229, 1976.
8. Lichtenfeld, P.: Autonomic dysfunction in the Guillain-Barré syndrome. Amer. J. Med., 50:1971, 772–780.
9. Nardone, D. A., McDonald, W. J., and Girard, D. E.: Mechanisms in hypokalemia. Clinical correlation. Medicine, 57: 1978, 435–446.
10. Toole, J. F., and Cole, M.: Ischemic cerebrovascular disease. In Baker, A. B. and Baker, L. H.: Clinical Neurology. Hagerstown, Maryland, Harper and Row, 1977, Vol. 1, No. 10, pp. 1–45.

Maimonides Medical Center
4802 Tenth Avenue
Brooklyn, New York 11219

Hepatic Encephalopathy

Prem Misra, M.D.*

Hepatic encephalopathy ("hepatic coma")[9, 23, 26] is a commonly encountered problem in patients with liver disease. It is defined as a neuropsychiatric syndrome characterized by intellectual deterioration, altered state of consciousness, and neurologic abnormalities in a patient with advanced liver disease or portasystemic shunting. It is a complication of both acute and chronic liver diseases, such as viral hepatitis, drug-induced or toxin-induced liver disease, acute fatty liver of pregnancy, or cirrhosis of the liver. Rarely, it may be found in children with congenital abnormalities of ammonia metabolism, or patients with surgically induced portacaval shunts who have no parenchymal liver disease.

Patients with acute hepatic encephalopathy are usually younger and present with hyperactivity, delirium, and mania; many of these patients may scratch or bite while agitated and show physical and sexual aggressiveness. Patients with chronic hepatic encephalopathy, and older patients with fulminant hepatic failure, manifest only subtle signs in the early stages of hepatic coma: sleeping longer, day night reversal in sleep-rhythm, deterioration in personal care in previously well-groomed patient, intellectual deterioration, or worsening of handwriting. These changes may occur in the absence of overt signs of liver disease such as jaundice, ascites, or bleeding and therefore make the diagnosis more difficult — even though most patients manifest clinical signs of liver disease as well as abnormal bilirubin levels, prothrombin time, serum albumin, and other parameters of liver disease. A number of psychometric tests[21] have recently been devised to detect earliest changes of hepatic encephalopathy so that the mildest forms of intellectual deteriorations may be corrected early but from a clinical point of view subtraction of serial 7's, number connection test, and making a star with a set of matches all detect early changes.

For a diagnosis of hepatic encephalopathy, five elements must be present: abnormal mental and neuromuscular states, parenchymal liver

*Physician-in-Charge, Division of Gastroenterology, Department of Medicine, Queens Hospital Center Affiliation of Long Island Jewish-Hillside Medical Center; Assistant Professor of Medicine, School of Medicine, State University of New York at Stony Brook

Table 1. *Diagnosis of Hepatic Encephalopathy*

1. An abnormal mental state (altered judgment, personality, mood, behavior, sleep disturbances, precoma, coma)
2. An abnormal neuromuscular state (asterixis, spasticity, hyperreflexia clonus, hepato-cerebral degeneration, spastic paraparesis)
3. Parenchymal liver disease or portacaval shunting, most often both
4. Characteristic laboratory findings
   a. Increased ammonia levels in blood and cerebrospinal fluid
   b. Cerebrospinal fluid: Increased glutamine and alpha-ketoglutaramate levels
   c. Electroencephalographic changes: (normal 8 to 13 cycles per sec): generalized slowing (1½ to 3 cycles per sec; symmetrical, synchronous) high voltage and paroxysmal slow waves
5. Variable clinical features:
   a. Fetor hepaticus
   b. Hypothermia
   c. Hyperventilation

disease or portacaval shunting, characteristic laboratory findings, and characteristic clinical findings. These are outlined in Table 1.

Early in the course of hepatic encephalopathy the alterations in mood (euphoria, depression, agitation), behavior, personality or sleep disturbances are mild, but they worsen as the disease progresses. The patient becomes more confused, difficult to awaken, and finally lapses into coma. It is most interesting to note that usually during this earlier phase, when there is an inversion of sleep rhythm, these patients are commonly prescribed sedatives and hypnotics to ensure their nightly sleep.

Most patients with this syndrome have a musty, fishy, sweetish odor called fetor hepaticus, believed to be produced by mercaptans,[14] and specific for liver disease when present.

Hepatic encephalopathy progresses from a prodromal stage to pre-coma (impending coma), stupor, and finally into semi-coma and coma stages.

In most cases in precoma, asterixis or flapping tremor is elicited when the arms are outstretched, wrists hyperextended, and fingers are separated. The flap is bilateral, asynchronous, and occurs in bursts, once every 1 or 2 seconds. It can also be shown to occur in the closed eyelids, protruded tongue, pursed lips and in the toes. It reflects an inability to maintain sustained postures and is believed to result from impairment of afferent flow of joint, position and other sensations to the reticular formation in the brain stem, causing electrical lapses in the responsible muscles. Though characteristic, asterixis is by no means specific for hepatic encephalopathy: it may be seen in hypokalemia, uremia, poly-cythemia, congestive heart failure, pulmonary insufficiency, and seda-tive overdose.

During precoma, neurologic signs include hyperreflexia, spasticity and extensor plantar responses. Usually these are transient. With the onset of coma, they disappear and the extremities become flaccid, except in patients who develop chronic hepatocerebral degeneration and spastic paraparesis. In contrast, patients with coma due to acute fulminant hepatic failure may have convulsions, cerebral edema and decerebrate rigidity; the last is reversible. Also in coma due to fulminant hepatic failure, the various stages of progressive hepatic encephalopathy may get telescoped into a day or two and may not be easily identifiable. Table 2 outlines the various neurologic syndromes encountered in hepatic encephalopathy.[19]

While the features enumerated above are common to all types of hepatic encephalopathy, the clinical picture in individual patients may be considerably different and the diagnosis should be based on criteria in Table 1 as well as exclusion of other causes of coma and response to appropriate therapy. Patients with portasystemic encephalopathy usually have a well-defined precipitating factor. It may be excessive protein ingestion, gastrointestinal bleeding, diuretics, sedatives, anesthetics, infection, uremia, or constipation. It has been estimated that 36 per cent of all patients with cirrhosis of the liver die in hepatic coma.

It needs to be reemphasized that each of the components listed in Table 1 that are essential for diagnosis is nonspecific, and may be induced by varied metabolic abnormalities. Therefore exclusion of other causes is of paramount importance. Electroencephalographic changes suggestive of portasystemic encephalopathy may also be seen in hypoglycemia, vitamin B_{12} deficiency, carbon dioxide narcosis, and uremia, for example.

Table 2. *Neurological Manifestations of Hepatic Encephalopathy*

ENCEPHALOPATHY IN CHRONIC LIVER DISEASE

A. Portasystemic encephalopathy with prodrome, impending coma with pyramidal signs — hyperreflexia, ankle clonus, extensor plantar response, and coma
B. Chronic hepatocerebral degeneration
   1. Cerebellar signs: intention tremor, ataxia
   2. Extrapyramidal signs:
      a. Tremor: resting, flapping
      b. Choreoathetosis: facial grimacing, lip smacking, tongue protrusion, writhing sinuous or tortuous convulsions of the arms and legs, intention or action myoclonus
      c. Cogwheel rigidity and mask-like facies
   3. Pyramidal signs:
      a. Bilateral: as above
      b. Unilateral signs: hemiplegia or hemiparesis (transient or permanent) and focal epilepsy
C. Spastic paraplegia: with late retention of flexor plantar responses
D. Peripheral neuropathy
E. Acute psychosis
F. Dementia

ENCEPHALOPATHY IN ACUTE LIVER DISEASE (FULMINANT HEPATIC FAILURE)

A. Guillain-Barré syndrome
B. Asterixis
C. Convulsions, cerebral edema, coma
D. Decerebrate rigidity

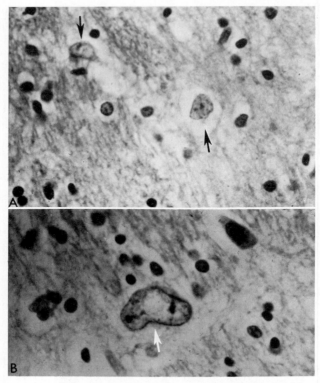

Figure 1. *A*, Section from the cerebral cortex of a teenaged girl with hepatic coma due to Wilson's disease showing swollen astrocytes (arrows) with markedly enlarged and prominent nuclei and well defined nucleoli (Alzheimer type II cell). In the background normal astrocytes and oligodendroglia are seen (×400). *B*, Another section from the cerebral cortex of the same patient shows a giant Alzheimer type II cell (arrow) with large nucleus and two prominent nucleoli (×400) and a background of normal glial cells.

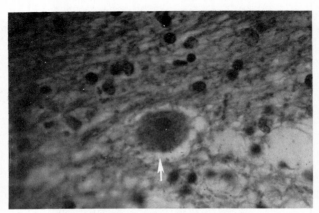

Figure 2.   Section from substantia nigra in the same patient with Wilson's disease showing a large oval cell with nucleus and foamy cytoplasm (opalski cell). Found in Wilson's disease, this rare cell is probably not derived from the astrocytes. The background shows astrocytes and oligodendroglia (×400). (Photomicrographs courtesy Dr. Z. Wessely, Department of Pathology, Queens Hospital Center.)

Table 3. *Neuropathologic Changes in Hepatic Coma*

ENCEPHALOPATHY IN CHRONIC LIVER DISEASE

1. Portasystemic encephalopathy
   a. Astrocytic changes: Alzheimer type II–astrocytes increase in size and number–
      in cerebral and cerebellar cortex, basal ganglia, dentate nucleus, etc.
   b. Neuronal degeneration: rare, in deeper layers of cerebral cortex
2. Acquired hepatocerebral degeneration
   a. Astrocytic changes (as above)
   b. Cortex and subcortical white matter: loss of neurons and myelin leading to spongy
      degeneration and microcavitation. (parieto-occipital, cortex basal ganglia, and
      cerebellum)
3. Spastic paraparesis
   a. Demyelination of corticospinal tracts both crossed and direct and of spinocerebellar
      pathways and dorsal columns
   b. Axonal degeneration
   c. Gliosis
4. Peripheral neuropathy: segmental demyelination of nerves

ENCEPHALOPATHY IN FULMINANT HEPATIC FAILURE

1. Cerebral edema (large swollen glial cells)
2. Herniation of cerebellar tonsils/temporal lobes

PATHOLOGY

An increase in the size and number of protoplasmic astrocytes, an otherwise nonspecific finding, is often encountered in the brain. This may represent metabolic activity necessary for detoxification of ammonia, since glutamic dehydrogenase activity in the same cells is also increased in hyperammonemic states. Later on degeneration to Alzheimer type II astrocyte may occur (Figs. 1 and 2), possibly because of a critical reduction in these cells of essential substances such as ATP, NADH and alpha-ketoglutarate as a consequence of excessive ammonia metabolism. Other histologic changes of the central nervous system encountered in hepatocerebral degeneration and fulminant hepatic failure are listed in Table 3.

PATHOGENESIS

The precise pathogenesis of hepatic encephalopathy is not well understood because of the functional heterogeneity and subcellular metabolic compartmentalization in different areas of the brain, and technical difficulties in the study of these areas in experimental models. The animal models studied, so far, have been akin to conditions existing in human fulminant hepatic failure rather than chronic portal systemic encephalopathy, and, despite greatly improved techniques of deep freezing, the deeper areas of the brain do not always reflect changes during life. The problems are compounded by our poor understanding of the complex mechanisms involved in the maintenance of consciousness.

However, the following facts are generally agreed upon in the causation of hepatic encephalopathy:

1. Metabolic and/or neurophysiologic abnormalities are involved since a complete reversal of the neuropsychiatric syndrome usually occurs with treatment (except in hepatocerebral degeneration and spastic paraparesis).

2. Several toxins, such as ammonia, mercaptans, fatty acids, amino acids, and so forth, are simultaneously involved because none of them alone can readily account for the clinical picture in all patients.

3. No critical protective substance produced in healthy liver and missing in hepatic coma has so far been identified.

4. The toxins mentioned above may alter (a) neuronal membrane function, (b) cerebral energy consumption, or (c) neurotransmitter balance resulting in interference with synaptic transmission.

5. Increased cerebral sensitivity to toxins or even to normal metabolites may exist.

6. In fulminant hepatic failure, changes in blood-brain barrier have been shown, and, at least in rats,[11] an increased transport of neutral amino acids across this barrier has been shown to exist after a portacaval shunt. The same has not been consistently shown in humans when plasma/cerebrospinal fluid ratios were determined in encephalopathic patients.

Ammonia is regarded as the most likely toxin and may cause encephalopathy either alone or acting together with short chain fatty acids or amino acids. Three facts suggest this: (1) NH_3 levels in blood and cerebrospinal fluid are elevated in most patients with PSE, (2) ammonia or substances that produce ammonia in the gut (e.g., proteins and blood) may induce coma in susceptible patients; and (3) the coma is frequently alleviated by measures aimed at reducing an influx of ammonia into the brain. Blood ammonia levels, usually elevated, though not always diagnostic — and often normal in encephalopathy caused by fulminant hepatic failure — are nevertheless a good way to follow the course of PSE in most comatose patients with this syndrome. Though arterial and cerebrospinal fluid ammonia levels correlate better, they may still lag behind the clinical changes because of the time needed for equilibration with plasma. Furthermore, in the presence of portacaval shunt, excess ammonia depresses cerebral blood flow and oxygen consumption. No parameter correlates better with the clinical severity of disease than the spinal fluid glutamine and alpha ketoglutaramate, both of which accumulate as a result of excess brain ammonia. It should also be kept in mind that the reasons blood ammonia levels, routinely determined in hospital chemistry laboratories, do not correspond to the clinical severity of encephalopathy are: these levels do not reflect the concentration in the brain; subtle changes in pH can affect the dissociation of $NH_4 \rightleftharpoons NH_3 + H$ and transfer of ammonia from blood to brain; and, finally, most routine hospital estimations of blood ammonia are inaccurate.

It may be recalled that the gastrointestinal tract, kidneys and skeletal muscle are major sources of ammonia. The ammonia from the gastrointestinal tract is both preformed ammonia present in the food and that produced by hydrolysis of urea by bacterial ureases. Kidneys are the second important source of NH_3, with renal venous ammonia concentration being higher than the arterial concentration. Both hypokalemia and renal tubular acidosis increase renal venous ammonia levels. In cirrhosis the muscle mass is also decreased and since brain, liver and muscle are normal organs for ammonia uptake, muscle wasting and hepatic injury lead to greater ammonia uptake in the brain.

Short-chain fatty acids, the plasma concentrations of which reflect the severity of liver disease rather than the presence of coma, are by themselves not causative in portasystemic encephalopathy but may inhibit the detoxification of ammonia via urea synthesis and glutamate formation and may have a synergistic role. Besides, the blood concentration of fatty acids in patients with portasystemic encephalopathy is usually not markedly elevated.

Plasma amino acids in portasystemic encephalopathy[5, 6, 17] show an increase of straight-chain alpha amino acids and aromatic amino acids (i.e., lysine, glycine, histidine, cysteine, ornithine, citrulline, aspartate, glutamine, methionine, phenylalanine, tyrosine, and tryptophan) and a decrease in the branched-chain amino acids (i.e., leucine, valine, isoleucine, arginine). The molar ratio of plasma branched chain amino acids to phenylalanine plus tyrosine decreases from a normal of 3 to 4 to approximately 1 or less. A synthetic mixture of amino acids low in methionine, phenylalanine and tryptophan and high in branched-chain amino acids has reversed encephalopathy both in dogs and man. It should be emphasized that phenylalanine and tyrosine are precursors of catecholamines, and tryptophan[17] is a precursor of serotonin. The changes in amino acid levels may therefore lead to depletion of some true neurotransmitters, or formation of false neurotransmitters, or to increased aromatic amino acid transport due to change in the blood-brain barrier and decreased competition from branched chain amino acids. It is possible that the balance of these neurotransmitters in a critical area of brain is upset by these changes. The reasons why the plasma amino acid profile is altered in portasystemic encephalopathy are far from clear but the catabolic state of these patients, poor protein intake, decreased rate of hepatic urea synthesis as well as alterations in insulin and glucagon levels may be contributory. It should be remembered that plasma amino acid levels are inversely related to the rate of hepatic urea synthesis for any one level of protein intake. It has been shown that there is approximately 50 per cent increase in insulin and 400 per cent increase in serum glucagon levels, causing a net decrease in insulin/glucagon ratio to one third the normal; this may indicate the catabolic state. In fulminant hepatic failure with extensive hepatic necrosis the amino acid abnormalities are different; all the amino acids in plasma are increased more than in portasystemic encephalopathy, especially methionine, phenylalanine, tyrosine, and tryptophan. The branched chain amino acids are normal or only slightly lower, but the ratio of (leucine + isoleu + val)/(Phe + ty) remains low. Brain aspartate and glutaramate are also increased in contradistinction to their low

values of experimental encephalopathy following hepatectomy or ischemic hepatic necrosis. Taurine is not increased. The reason for this is not
clear.

Some monoamines that act as neurotransmitters, such as norepinephrine,[28] are decreased; others, such as serotonin, are increased or
normal. However, most of the data are based on whole brain studies and
the amounts may vary in different areas of the brain. The greatest
amounts of serotonin and 5-hydroxyindolacetic acid are found in the
brain stem of rats. Moreover, there is an increase in amounts of false
neurotransmitters such as tyramine and octopamine, and it has been
suggested that the increased phenylalanine concentration in portasystemic encephalopathy impairs tyrosine hydroxylation to DOPA and
excess tyrosine is decarboxylated to tyramine and then converted to
octopamine. Because of a lack of DOPA, norepinephrine is not synthesized. These false neurotransmitters replace catecholamines at the
synapses and may explain the neurologic changes. However, infusion of
octopamine into the lateral ventricle of rats even in astronomical
amounts, does not result in coma, though it also results in fall of brain
dopamine and norepinephrine concentrations to 10 per cent of normal,
levels much lower than even recorded in portasystemic encephalopathy.
However, 0.5 mg of NH_4^+ similarly instilled causes convulsions and
coma in one minute.

Methyl mercaptan has been isolated from the urine of a patient in
hepatic coma and is increased several-fold in the breath, as are dimethyl-
sulfide and dimethyldisulfide. They cause reversible coma in animals
and enhance the toxicity of ammonia and fatty acids. However, the
encephalopathic effects of mercaptans[14] still await confirmation and
determination of their blood and tissue levels on a large scale.

Most of the toxins tested above may induce coma by one of the
following postulated mechanisms:

1. Direct effect on nerve cell membrane (e.g., ammonia, mercaptans, short-chain fatty acids)

2. Alteration in NADH/NAD ratio and malate aspartate shuttle in
cytoplasm/mitochondria, thus leading to lactate accumulation in the
cytoplasm and reduction in the excitatory neurotransmitter level.

3. Reduction of cerebral energy metabolism.

4. Synergistic impairment of ammonia detoxification, e.g., by mercaptans and short-chain fatty acid.

Finally it should be emphasized that under experimental conditions
the electrical activity of the brain is significantly affected by hepatectomy; however, when cytidine and uridine (nucleotides synthesized in
the liver) are administered, normal cerebral activity is restored. Therefore there still remains the possibility that the lack of a key substance (so
far unidentified) may be important in causing hepatic encephalopathy.

TREATMENT

The management of patients presenting with hepatic encephalopathy is somewhat different in those presenting with portasystemic en-

cephalopathy[5, 6, 12] and those whose coma is due to fulminant hepatic failure.[2, 22] A general outline for treatment of both is given in Table 4.

Portasystemic Encephalopathy

In a patient with preexisting liver disease who starts to show signs of hepatic encephalopathy, efforts must be made to identify and treat the precipitating cause for hepatic coma. When such a cause is not found, the patient is considered to have "spontaneous nitrogenous portal systemic encephalopathy" which implies that patient cannot handle "normal" amounts of protein in the diet because of at least a 50 per cent reduction in hepatic capacity to synthesize urea. This label also has a prognostic implication: that patient cannot be a candidate for shunt surgery for esophageal varices, since the likelihood of post-shunt encephalopathy in this group is 100 per cent. In case a precipitating factor cannot be readily recognized, the diagnosis should be re-evaluated and causes such as subdural hematoma and meningitis should be excluded.

Table 4. *Treatment of Hepatic Encephalopathy*

PORTASYSTEMIC ENCEPHALOPATHY

A. Recognition and treatment of precipitating factors
B. Reducing nitrogen load and ammonia production and absorption from the gut
  1. Dietary protein restriction
  2. Bowel cleansing
  3. Bowel sterilization
C. Supportive treatment
  1. Correction of fluid and electrolyte abnormalities
  2. Provision of caloric and nutritional needs (e.g. vitamins)
D. Treatment of the underlying liver disease where possible (e.g. steroids in chronic active hepatitis)
E. Experimental therapy
 1. Levodopa
 2. Bromocriptine
 3. Aminoacid infusions

FULMINANT HEPATIC FAILURE

A. Intensive nursing and medical care
  1. Adequate fluid and electrolyte balance
  2. Preventing overhydration/cerebral edema
B. Measures aimed at reducing ammonia production and absorption from the gut (protein restriction, bowel cleansing, lactulose/neomycin)
C. Prevention and treatment of complications
  1. Aspiration
  2. Infections
  3. Cardiac
  4. Pulmonary (adult respiratory distress syndrome)
  5. Renal failure
  6. Gastrointestinal bleeding, pancreatitis
  7. Clotting abnormalities and DIC
D. Nutritional support (maintenance of blood glucose levels especially)
E. Specific measures (in drug/toxin-induced fulminant hepatic failure: Use of acetylcysteine in acetaminophen hepatitis)
F. Special procedures: exchange transfusion, polyacryonitrile membrane hemodialysis, high dose steroids

CT scans can now be used to exclude the former, when bleeding contraindicates using other techniques.

In all other patients where diagnosis of portasystemic encephalopathy has been firmly established and a precipitating factor identified, the latter should be corrected. Each of the common precipitating factors is discussed in some detail in the following paragraphs.

GASTROINTESTINAL BLEEDING. The episode of bleeding reduces cerebral, hepatic, and renal perfusion and increases the nitrogen load in the gut — thereby increasing the plasma NH_3 and amino acid levels. The liver cannot detoxify enough ammonia because of poor perfusion and function while at the same time reduced renal perfusion further raises the blood urea nitrogen, thereby increasing the substrate for production of ammonia. Ammonia is also present in stored blood given to these patients, which contributes to the increased load. The rational therapy therefore involves: (1) expansion of blood volume by transfusing fresh blood where possible; (2) enemas and laxatives to remove the stored blood from the gut; (3) use of oral neomycin to reduce intestinal urease activity of bacterial origin; (4) rational treatment of the cause of bleeding — esophageal varices, gastritis, Mallory Weiss tears or peptic ulcer disease (intravenous pitressin 20 mg intravenously over a 20 minute period followed by a slower intravenous drip has been helpful in variceal bleeding and also produces vigorous peristalsis which may be purgative); (5) lactulose where neomycin will not or cannot be used because of contraindications.

INFECTION. When fever supervenes, increased protein and amino acid turnover due to increased metabolism results in increased nitrogen load and more ammonia production. This is potentiated by dehydration and resultant prerenal azotemia. Furthermore hyperthermia and associated hypoxia may enhance ammonia toxicity in cirrhotic patients. Patients with cirrhosis — especially those with alcoholic liver disease — are particularly prone to many bacterial infections. Appropriate cultures should be obtained and a sensitive antibiotic administered. Ascitic fluid should be examined and cultured even in the absence of signs or symptoms of peritoneal involvement, because infection of the fluid is frequently found.

RENAL FAILURE. Excessive diuresis and water restriction are common reasons for the development of renal failure in patients with ascites and liver disease. The prerenal azotemia resulting from excessive diuresis increases blood urea nitrogen and results in increased enterohepatic circulation of urea and consequently increased production of ammonia. Thiazides and other potassium-wasting diuretics produce hypokalemic alkalosis, which also increases renal ammonia production probably by increasing renal tubular glutaminase activity or carbonic anhydrase activity. Hypokalemic alkalosis further enhances transfer of ammonia across the blood brain barrier. In some cases an incomplete renal tubular acidosis may impair renal ammonia secretion, thereby increasing renal venous ammonia levels. The therapy consists of cessation of diuretics (no patient with hepatic coma should be on diuretics), repletion of potassium chloride, and plasma volume correction.

DIETARY EXCESSES.   Hepatic encephalopathy develops in some patients after periods of excessive protein intake. Sometimes the difference between the amount of protein well tolerated and the one resulting in portasystemic encephalopathy may be as little as one extra meatball ("one meatball syndrome"). This situation is more likely to be encountered in patients who had shunt surgery before. However control of dietary protein is one of the cornerstones of therapy for portasystemic encephalopathy. When oral feeding is not possible, as in severely ill and comatose patients, at least 1200 carbohydrate (sucrose or polycos) calories should be given daily. Three to 6 gm of essential amino acids may be added. Fats are avoided because they delay gastric emptying. If nasogastric feeding is not possible because of gastrointestinal bleeding or slow emptying or other reasons, intravenous hyperalimentation may be necessary. When the patient can tolerate oral feedings, dietary proteins are restarted, 10 to 20 gm per day, and increased every 2 to 5 days till either the optimum amount of protein is ingested daily or the patient becomes encephalopathic and dietary protein has to be reduced to a lower level. Recent studies have shown that vegetable proteins[7] and those from milk and cheese are tolerated better than meat proteins. Vegetable proteins are less ammoniagenic. This may be because they contain less methionine and aromatic amino acids, or because the vegetable diets change the gut bacterial flora, or simply because there is less absorbable protein in a vegetable diet. Since lactulose was not withheld during the study on vegetable protein, the final judgment on the usefulness of this diet should be reserved. It has also been shown that vegetable proteins contain lower amounts of ammonia, group A amino acids and mercaptans, the compounds usually cited in the causation of portasystemic encephalopathy.

SEDATIVES AND DRUGS.   Sedatives, narcotic analgesics, tranquilizers, and hypnotics are the second most important cause of precipitation of hepatic encephalopathy after gastrointestinal bleeding/diuretics. The mechanism appears to be either impaired hepatic metabolism leading to prolonged blood levels or increased cerebral sensitivity to the drug. Oxazepam (Serax), which is not metabolized by the liver but is excreted by the kidneys, is a safe sedative in cirrhotic patients — if a sedative must be used. Paraldehyde is wrongly considered a safe drug: even though the pungent aroma of the drug on a patient's breath is very impressive, most of the drug is metabolized by the liver. Sometimes, in a patient who is delirious and violent, physicians are called upon to prescribe sedatives. It should be emphasized at this point that the delirium in portasystemic encephalopathy usually lasts only a few hours to a maximum of 1½ days and does not in every instance, call for sedatives. Restraining the patient may be enough; if not, phenobarbitol and/or thorazine may be prescribed. Lorazepam (Ativan) and oxazepam (Serax) are also useful since they are not metabolized by the liver, particularly in patients with abnormal liver function tests. Chlordiazepoxide (Librium) should not be used in liver disease because unlike diazepam (Valium), chlordiazepoxide has a long half-life.

CONSTIPATION.   Constipation may lead to increased production and absorption of ammonia by increasing the contact time between the bacteria and the nitrogenous products in the gut. Rarely, excessive straining at stool may increase portal pressure and may even cause variceal bleeding. Therefore, these patients should receive enemas, purgatives, or laxatives as the situation demands. Tap water enemas are preferable to soap suds enemas because the latter may increase absorption of ammonia. Saline enemas may likewise increase sodium levels. Cool water enemas at 16° C have a sedative effect in manic patients. Magnesium sulfate may be a good cathartic in patients with history of alcoholism in helping to replete the magnesium stores.

METABOLIC FACTORS. Hypoxemia, hypoglycemia, and myxedema can all augment ammonia toxicity or may by themselves produce coma the treatment of which calls for specific measures.

NEUROLOGIC DISEASE. Subdural hematoma, meningitis, Wernicke-Korsakoff's disease, and other neurological disorders can occur in patients with or without liver disease and may precipitate coma. Their recognition and management is therefore important.

After the precipitating factors have been identified and treated, dietary protein restriction and bowel cleansing should be instituted in order to further reduce the intestinal nitrogen load. To prevent tissue protein degradation, adequate calories and vitamin supplements are given. Based on the recent recognition of amino acid abnormalities in the plasma of patients with portasystemic encephalopathy, solutions containing high concentrations of branched chain amino acids and low levels of aromatic amino acid have been infused in dog models and man. Early results are promising, but even though arousal has been achieved; the outcome of liver disease has not been affected. The poor nitrogen balance and the ill effects of ammonia in the patients with portasystemic encephalopathy also prompted the use of ketoanalogues of essential amino acids. Ketoanalogues have the structure of corresponding amino acids but have no amino group and therefore are non-nitrogenous compounds. When the ketoanalogues were administered to patients with portasystemic encephalopathy or to children with urea cycle abnormalities, thus providing nutrition via amination of these compounds without production of additional ammonia, there was often improvement in mental state, plasma ammonia, and glutamine levels. Oral feedings with appropriate amino acid composition (hepatic-aid) are now finding their way into the market for patients with liver disease.

NEOMYCIN. Neomycin, an unabsorbable antibiotic, has been in use for a long time. It is given orally in a 2 to 4 gm per day dose or as a 1 per cent solution in enema once or twice a day. The drug acts by reducing the population of urease-producing and other bacteria in the gut. One to 3 per cent of the administered amount of neomycin may be absorbed and is excreted by the kidney by glomerular filtration. Levels of 10 μg per ml in the urine, a therapeutic level for many bacterial pathogens of the urinary tract, are not uncommon. Where neomycin-resistant Klebsiella or proteus strains have developed, ampicillin, tetracycline, paramomycin, kanamycin, or sulfonamides may be tried. Ampicillin can be used orally or intravenously and unlike neomycin is not ototoxic or nephrotoxic.

LACTULOSE.   This drug is as effective as neomycin in both acute and chronic portasystemic encephalopathy.[4] The oral administration of lactulose is adjusted so that 50 to 150 ml per day in divided doses produces two to three soft stools daily. The drug is safe, and side-effects (nausea, vomiting, anorexia, bloating, abdominal cramps and diarrhea) are usually mild. When lactulose is not initially effective, the dose may be increased till a stool pH of about 5.0 is achieved. Lactulose is ideally suited for patients with renal disease or where ototoxicity is a concern.

Upon oral administration, lactulose passes unchanged to the ileum and colon where bacterial hydrolysis of the compound results in production of lactic and acetic acids, and other organic acids, thus reducing the intraluminal pH. In effect, an "acid dialysis" is produced by trapping ammonia, amines, various amides, and other basic nitrogenous substances, thus reducing their absorption into the blood. Lactulose may also favor the growth of lactobacillus acidophilus rather than E. coli, a more efficient ammonia-producing bacterium. The diarrheal action of lactulose is also synergistic. In lactase deficient patients lactose (milk sugar) ingestion may do the same. One mechanism common to lactulose and lactose in lactase-deficient patients is shortened intestinal transit time. However, it has recently been suggested that lactulose may stimulate incorporation of ammonia into bacterial proteins or decrease urea production and urea degradation, thus reducing the amount of ammonia generated.

In patients with hearing problems or renal disease — or when prolonged usage is anticipated — lactulose is preferable to neomycin. In some situations the two drugs administered together are more effective than either one alone. The reason for this effect is not clear; nor is the precise mechanism of action of lactulose,[3] even though it is possible that bacteria most active in lactulose fermentation are relatively resistant to neomycin.

Other Measures

LEVODOPA.[15]   Since decrease in cerebral catecholamines and accumulation of inert amines (false neurotransmitters) supposedly interfere with synaptic transmission in hepatic encephalopathy, it was suggested that use of levodopa will replenish normal neurotransmitters (dopamine and norepinephrine) and displace the false neurotransmitters octopamine and phenylethanolamine from synaptosomes. But in oral doses larger than 750 to 1000 mg daily, which produce gastrointestinal upset, consistent improvement has not followed levodopa therapy. In one controlled double-blind study involving 58 patients, those receiving levodopa did no better than those on placebo. It does have a short-lived arousal effect though.

BROMOCRIPTINE.[16]   Since hepatic encephalopathy may in part be due to a defect in dopaminergic neurotransmission, bromocriptine, which is a specific dopamine receptor agonist with prolonged action, has been tried in its treatment. Two out of 3 recent studies suggest that in doses of up to 15 mg daily orally, it may have some role. However, a full endocrine assessment of every patient and effective contraceptive measures in women of child-bearing age will be required prior to initiating therapy. Furthermore, the outcome of liver disease is not altered by this therapy and the standard therapy must be continued along with bromo-criptine.

Other therapeutic measures such as the use of steroids, hemodialysis, peritoneal dialysis, and hyperbaric oxygen have no proven role in treatment of chronic portasystemic encephalopathy.

FULMINANT HEPATIC FAILURE

It has been estimated that in the United States there are approximately 2000 cases of fulminant hepatic failure per year (versus 35,000 deaths per year from chronic liver disease), and the incidence is decreasing. The results of treatment of encephalopathy caused by fulminant hepatic failure are much less rewarding than those with portasystemic encephalopathy. Most cases (85 per cent) of fulminant hepatic failure are viral (hepatitis A, B, non A, non B); however, about 15 per cent of all cases may be due to drugs (isoniazid, rifampin, acetaminophen), mushroom poisoning (Amanita phalalloides), or toxins (phosphorus, hydrocarbons), ischemic necrosis, secondary to Budd Chiari syndrome and acute Wilson's disease. In general the therapy is directed at the following:

Protein restriction.
Bowel cleansing.
Lactulose/neomycin.
Frequent monitoring of vital signs/depth of coma.
Fluid, electrolyte, and acid base balance.
Nutritional support.
Prevention and treatment of complications: cardiac, pulmonary, renal, gastrointestinal, clotting abnormalities, infections.
Intensive nursing care.
Special procedures including charcoal hemoperfusion, polyacrylonitrile membrane hemodialysis, and exchange transfusions.

The aim of treatment of coma or encephalopathy caused by fulminant hepatic failure is to support a failing liver and allow time for it to regenerate. This will, of course, depend upon the severity of injury and cause, in addition to other variables, such as, in the case of a patient with viral hepatitis, the patient's age and the size of the liver. When the necrosis is drug-induced, every attempt should be made to eliminate the offending agent, reduce its absorption and if possible help in its metabolism (e.g., use of acetyl cysteine in case of acetaminophen induced hepatic necrosis). A younger patient with viral hepatitis causing fulminant hepatic failure has a much better prognosis than an older one, in the 40's for example. The first four of the measures listed above are self-explanatory. The others will be discussed in some detail.

In fulminant hepatic failure, serum sodium is often low but the total body sodium is usually normal; the hyponatremia, therefore, at least in early stages should be treated with fluid restriction. Hypokalemia usually is due to urinary losses and reduced intake, and potassium replacement may be needed. Only rarely is the patient hyperkalemic. From an acid-base point of view, either respiratory alkalosis resulting from hyperventilation or metabolic alkalosis is frequent. The former requires no treatment, the latter does require treatment since it enhances formation of ammonia and facilitates its entry into the brain. In some cases, severe metabolic alkalosis may require infusion of an isotonic solution of 150 ml of 1N HCL diluted in one liter of sterile water through a central vein catheter.

Hypoglycemia also requires treatment with intravenous hypertonic glucose as well as monitoring of urine and blood sugar levels. At times it may be severe and need close attention.

During the course of fulminant hepatic necrosis acute tubular necrosis or hepatorenal syndrome may supervene, necessitating hemodialysis and other standard measures, while liver regeneration proceeds.

Cerebral edema is a major complication usually seen in younger patients (under 30 years) with fulminant hepatic failure. It may present with coma, convulsions or even decerebrate rigidity or changes in pulse and blood pressure suggestive of shock without overt hemorrhage. Even though steroids, glycerol and mannitol have been tried, none has been helpful. It is important to remember that decerebrate rigidity in this setting is often reversible and does not imply the same hopeless prognosis as it does in other neurologic diseases. Some patients with fulminant hepatic failure develop hypothermia secondary to the brain stem affliction or may suddenly become apneic, resulting in respiratory failure; management of hypothermia and tracheostomy for respiratory failure may be needed.

Coagulation abnormalities are not uncommon in fulminant hepatic failure and are usually manifested as bleeding from the puncture sites. When disseminated intravascular coagulation (DIC) occurs, fresh frozen plasma is helpful; clotting factors should not be given because they enhance the process. Heparin has not been helpful. Some patients have developed fulminant hepatic failure when given factor IX complex (Konyne). These are probably patients with chronic liver disease — possibly non-A, non-B hepatitis, because Konyne comes from donors in Germany, who were screened for hepatitis B. No screening test is presently possible for non-A, non-B hepatitis. If bleeding is due to thrombocytopenia, platelet concentrates should be given. In the management of most coagulation problems vitamin K is of little help in increasing the levels of factor II, VII, IX, and X. When disseminated intravascular coagulation (DIC) is suspected it should be easy to diagnose because a prolonged prothrombin time along with a *slight* reduction in factor VIII levels implies DIC, while prolonged prothrombin time with normal factor VIII levels means only the presence of liver disease.

When gastrointestinal bleeding ensues, it should be managed according to the standard principles. Prophylactic use of cimetidine in fulminant hepatic failure may reduce bleeding from hemorrhagic gastritis. In patients with high blood urea nitrogen or creatinine, cimetidine may contribute to encephalopathy.

Hard to recognize sepsis, arrhythmias, acute pancreatitis, adult respiratory distress syndrome, hypotension, and brain edema all require continuous vigilance for prevention and early treatment. Fulminant hepatic failure is one entity in which .25 N saline should not be given, and in which it is better to stay somewhat behind in fluid replacement, if cerebral edema is to be avoided. Aspiration of oral secretions, and so forth, is also a continuous threat and necessitates intensive nursing care, reverse Trendelenberg positioning, continuous nasogastric suction, and 2 hourly turning on the sides.

STEROIDS. A double blind trial with high dose steroid therapy did not show any clear-cut effect on prognosis when steroids were given in large dosage. However, on the basis of animal experiments, it has been claimed that prophylactic use of steroids may "tighten" the blood-brain barrier and thus prevent the development of encephalopathy.

Before further discussion of other heroic measures sometimes used to save the life of a patient with fulminant hepatic failure, it should be emphasized that simple supportive measures outlined above can result in a 40 per cent survival. Other than the fact that (at least in viral hepatitis) survival is age-related (at age 15 mortality is 65.8 per cent; at age 45 it is 95 per cent), no indices have been identified that clearly are predictive of poor prognosis except falling plasma concentrations of prothrombin and complement. Hepatocyte volume fraction of less than 35 per cent (normal is 85 per cent) determined in a liver biopsy specimen, galactose elimination capacity, bile acid conjugation, ligandinemia, factor VII levels, as well as serum alpha-fetoprotein levels have all been suggested as indicators of prognosis but are not reliable. It has also been pointed out that patients who lose their oculovestibular reflex[8] die while those who have a positive reflex survive.

Special procedures such as exchange transfusion,[10, 20] plasmaphoresis, cross circulation (either with a primate or human volunteer) extracorporeal liver perfusion, charcoal hemoperfusion and polyacrylonitrile membrane hemodialysis have not resulted in higher rates of recovery even though the comatose state has often been reversed. Of the procedures mentioned only exchange transfusion has been subjected to a controlled trial and failed to show significantly better results. Only 21 per cent of patients survived, not unlike those treated without exchange transfusion.

Total body washout (which consists of asanguinous hypothermic total body perfusion while the patient is on extracorporeal bypass) similarly has failed to show consistently improved results. In one study of 12 patients a response was noted in 5, but only 3 survived.

Activated charcoal hemoperfusion, originally reported from Kings College Hospital in London showed that 10 out of 22 patients in grade IV coma survived. However, the subsequent experience has not been so good, in fact in a series total of 100 cases subjected to this modality of treatment the last 18 patients died and the series had to be terminated. The deaths may have been related to removal of epinephrine, norepinephrine, T$_3$, aldosterone, insulin, and other normally present compounds from the blood.

The ordinary hemodialysis, similarly, has no salutary effect on hepatic coma. However, using polyacrylonitrile membrane hemodialysis,[18] which permits the removal of compounds with a molecular weight of up to 15,000 (middle molecules) three uncontrolled studies[9] have been performed and only Silk[24] et al. felt that survival was improved, the other two studies only showed a transient improvement in consciousness. In 81 per cent of failures cerebral edema was present at autopsy. In one series of 25 patients reported from Paris, France, prothrombin time worsened, more than in patients who underwent charcoal hemoperfusion, but 9 patients survived. Hypotension, another complication of this procedure, occurred in only one patient and responded to volume expansion. The procedure removes ammonia, free fatty acids, amino acids, and bile acids to a significant degree. Patients' consciousness seems to correlate to plasma phenylalanine and tyrosine levels. This parameter may in future help determine the frequency and duration of such dialysis.

Faced with a dismal outcome in patients with fulminant hepatic failure, it is heartening to note that special liver units focusing on the intensive care of these patients have achieved survival rates of 30 to 40 per cent by meticulous attention to symptomatic management and nursing care. This fact needs to be emphasized in the care of these patients.

Newer modalities of treatment such as hepatitis B immune globulin for hepatitis B antigen–positive cases have not been helpful either. In experimental animal models, e.g., fulminant murine hepatitis, combined insulin/glucagon administration appears to be promising. No human studies are available. The small number of country-wide cases of fulminant hepatic failure makes it imperative to conduct multicenter trials in order to have meaningful data and success in devising temporary biologic support systems needed to tide the patient over the acute phase of the disease and to allow the necessary time for the liver to regenerate. What is needed most is work along three lines: (1) development of systems for removal of toxic substances from the blood, including development of more selective and better adsorbents; (2) better understanding of the factors promoting liver regeneration. At present, it appears that identification of conditions or substances that promote liver regeneration is the most hopeful avenue to follow; and (3) overcoming immunologic and other barriers to successful liver transplantation, should that turn out to be the only choice.

REFERENCES

1. Abouna, G.. M., Veasey, P. R., and Terry, D. B.: Intravenous infusion of hydrochloric acid for treatment of severe metabolic alkalosis. Surgery, 75:194–202, 1974.
2. Auslander, M. O., and Gitnick, G. L.: Vigorous medical management of acute fulminant hepatitis. Arch. Intern. Med., 137:599–601, 1977.
3. Conn, H. O.: Lactulose: A drug in search of a modus operandi. Gastroenterology, 74:624–626, 1978.
4. Conn, H. O., Leevy, C. M., Vlahcevic, Z. R., et al.: Comparison of lactulose and neomycin in the treatment of chronic portal systemic encephalopathy: A double blind controlled trial. Gastroenterology, 72:573–583, 1977.

 5. Fischer, J. F., and Baldessarini, R. J.: Pathogenesis and therapy of hepatic coma. *In*
    Popper, H., and Schaffner, H., eds.: Progress in Liver Disease. New York, Grune &
    Stratton, Vol. 5, 1976 pp 363–397.
 6. Galambos, J. T.: Evaluation and therapy of encephalopathy. *In* Cirrhosis. Philadelphia,
    W. B. Saunders Co., 1979.
 7. Greenberger, N. J., Carley, J., Schenker, S., et al.: Effect of vegetable and animal protein
    diets in chronic hepatic encephalopathy. Dig. Dis., *22*:845–855, 1977.
 8. Hanid, M. A., Silk, D. B. A., and Williams, R.: Prognostic value of the oculovestibular
    reflex in fulminant hepatic failure. Brit. Med. J., *1*:1029, 1978.
 9. Hoyumpa, A. M., Jr., Desmond, P. V., Avant, G. R., et al.: Hepatic encephalopathy.
    Gastroenterology, *76*:184–195, 1979.
10. Lewis, J. D., Hussey, C. V., Varma, R. R., et al.: Exchange transfusion in hepatic coma.
    Factors affecting results with long term follow up data. Amer. J. Surg., *129*:125–129,
    1975.
11. Livingstone, A. S., Potvin, M., Goresky, C. A., et al.: Changes in the blood brain barrier in
    hepatic coma after hepatectomy in the rat. Gastroenterology, *73*:697–704, 1977.
12. Maddrey, W. C., Weber, F. L., Jr.: Chronic hepatic encephalopathy. Med. Clin. N. Amer.,
    59:937–944, 1975.
13. Maddrey, W. C., Weber, F. L., Jr., Coulter, A. W., et al.: Effects of keto analogues and
    essential amino acids in portal systemic encephalopathy. Gastroenterology, *71*:190–
    195, 1976.
14. Mc Clain, C. J., Zieve, L., Doizaki, W., et al.: Mercaptans in portal systemic encephalopa-
    thy due to alcoholic liver disease. Gastroenterology, *74*:1064, 1978.
15. Michel, H., Cauvet, G., Granier, P. M., et al.: Treatment of cirrhotic hepatic encephalopa-
    thy by L-dopa. A double blind study of 58 patients. Digestion, *15*:232–233, 1977.
16. Morgan, M. Y., Jakobovits, I. M. J., and Sherlock, S.: Successful use of bromocriptine in
    the treatment of chronic hepatic encephalopathy. Gastroenterology, *78*:663–670,
    1980.
17. Ono, J., Hutson, D. G., Dombro, R. S., et al.: Tryptophan and hepatic coma. Gastroen-
    terology, *74*:196–200, 1978.
18. Opolan, P., Ropin, J. R., Hugult, C., et al.: Hepatic failure coma (HFC) treated by
    polyacrylonitrile membrane (PAN) hemodialysis (HD). Trans. Amer. Soc. Artif. Intern.
    Organs, *22*:701–710, 1976.
19. Read, A. E., Sherlock, S., Laidlaw, J., et al.: The neuropsychiatric syndromes associated
    with chronic liver disease and extensive portal systemic collateral circulation. Quart. J.
    Med., *36*:135–150, 1967.
20. Redeker, A. G., and Yamahiro, H. S.: Controlled trial of exchange transfusion therapy in
    fulminant hepatitis. Lancet, *1*:136, 1973.
21. Rikkers, L., Jenko, P., Rudman, D., et al.: Subclinical hepatic encephalopathy: Detec-
    tion, prevalence and relationship to nitrogen metabolism. Gastroenterology, *72*:1119,
    1977.
22. Scharschmidt, B. F.: Approaches to the management of fulminant hepatic failure. Med.
    Clin. N. Amer., *59*:927–935, 1975.
23. Schenker, S., Breen, K. J., and Hoyumpa, A. M., Jr.: Hepatic encephalopathy: The
    current status. Gastroenterology, *66*:121–151, 1974.
24. Silk, D. B. A., Trewby, P. N., Chase, R. A., et al.: Treatment of fulminant hepatic failure
    by polyacrylonitrile membrane haemodialysis. Lancet, *2*:1–3, 1977.
25. Ward, M. E., Trewby, P. N., Williams, R., et al.: Acute liver failure: Experience in a
    special unit. Anesthesia, *32*:228–239, 1977.
26. Zieve, L.: Hepatic encephalopathy: Summary of present knowledge with an elaboration
    on recent developments. *In* Popper, H., and Schaffner, H., eds.: Progress in Liver
    Disease. New York, Grune & Stratton, 1979.
27. Zieve, L., and Nicoloff, D. M.: Pathogenesis of hepatic coma. Ann. Rev. Med., *26*:143–
    157, 1975.
28. Zieve, L., Olsen, R. L.: Can hepatic coma be caused by a reduction of brain noradrenaline
    or dopamine. Gut, *18*:688–691, 1977.

Queens Hospital Center
82-68 164th Street
Jamaica, New York 11432

Acute Life-Threatening Dermatologic Disorders

*Howard M. Simons, M.D.**

As the environment becomes more complex, as people are exposed more to greater numbers of drugs and chemicals, the frequency of life-threatening skin conditions appears to be increasing. Indeed, anaphylaxis, toxic epidermal necrolysis, and erythema multiforme — three of the conditions discussed below — are frequently the result of exposures to adverse or hostile environmental factors.

Accurate diagnosis and subsequent treatment of these life-threatening conditions require thorough understanding of occasionally subtle cutaneous changes. For this reason, the discussion which follows puts heavy stress on diagnostic clues that can be gleaned from history, from signs, and from symptoms. Background information is largely omitted; it can be found easily in standard dermatologic texts.

ANAPHYLAXIS

Anaphylaxis is a symptom complex, potentially life-threatening, that involves the integumentary, respiratory, cardiovascular, and digestive systems, singly or (more commonly) in combination. As with serum sickness, anaphylaxis frequently displays the two cutaneous changes of urticaria and angioedema, thus meriting its inclusion in a discussion of dermatologic conditions. Urticaria is an eruption of "hives" or welts, transient swellings of the skin which are well circumscribed, erythematous, and usually pruritic. As they enlarge, their raised irregularly rounded borders surround paler centers. The term "angioedema" suggests a more severe form of urticaria with larger lesions and involvement of subcutaneous or deeper structures.

In anaphylaxis, angioedema usually predominates, and typically is manifested in swollen eyelids, tongue, and lips. Edema of the larynx or

---

*Instructor in Dermatology, Hospital of the University of Pennsylvania, Physician-in-Chief, Dermatology, Abington Memorial Hospital, Abington, Pennsylvania

lower bronchial tree can produce shortness of breath and a feeling of tightness in the chest. Wheezing may be severe. Cyanosis and more severe respiratory distress may be followed by asphyxiation. Hypotension occurs frequently in more severe cases, whereas gastrointestinal symptoms are seen less often. Anaphylaxis usually occurs immediately or within hours of antigenic exposure.

The most common type of anaphylaxis is the so-called immunologic (or allergic) type, resulting from an antigen-antibody reaction in which histamine and other substances are released from mast cells and basophils. The production of this type of anaphylaxis requires the individual to form specific antibodies of the IgE class following exposure to an antigen. These specific antibodies become fixed to the surfaces of mast cells and, upon subsequent exposure to the antigen, act in some poorly understood manner to cause release of histamine from mast cell granules. Histamine, along with other chemical mediators, then acts pharmacologically and/or activates other mediators or reflex actions that result in clinical anaphylaxis.

Serum sickness, on the other hand, usually begins 7 to 14 days after antigenic exposure, and its usual symptoms of urticaria, arthralgia, fever, and lymphadenopathy begin insidiously. Serum sickness, which derived its name from its onset following injection of non-human serum, is now seen most frequently as a complication of drug therapy. When the antigenic substance has been injected, an intense reaction of urticaria or edema will often occur at the site of injection.

Etiology

DRUGS.   Although many drugs can cause anaphylaxis, penicillin is notorious in this regard because of the frequency and explosiveness of its reactions (Fig. 1). Even more sinister is the danger of occult sensitization

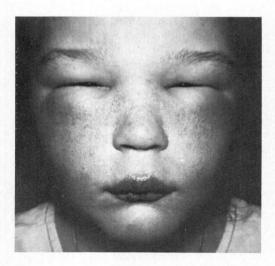

Figure 1. Angioedema occurring two hours after an injection of penicillin. The chest tightness and severe apprehension responded rapidly to an injection of epinephrine.

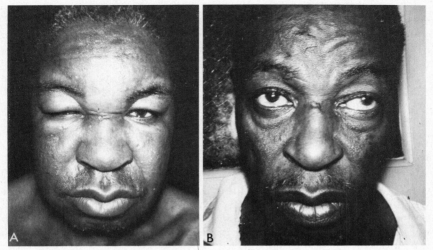

Figure 2. *A*, Angioedema from aspirin, developing over several days. *B*, Same patient following treatment with systemic corticosteroids and antihistamines.

to penicillin in hospital and pharmaceutical personnel, and from dairy products.[1] Cephalosporin antibiotics display cross hypersensitivity with penicillin, and should be used cautiously in persons with a history of allergy to penicillin. On the other hand, anaphylactic reactions from ampicillin are rare, suggesting that the frequently seen maculopapular eruptions caused by ampicillin are nonallergic and not indicative of "penicillin" allergy. Aspirin holds a unique position in the production of urticaria and anaphylaxis. As an antigen, it produces angioedema and anaphylaxis (Fig. 2); and it causes exacerbations in 20 to 40 per cent of patients with urticaria,[7] almost certainly on a non-immunologic basis.

ACTH, insulin, other hormones, diagnostic agents, serums, vaccines, and blood can produce anaphylaxis, although recent advances in the manufacture and preparation of some of these materials appear to have reduced the incidence. Much less common are anaphylactic reactions following topical applications of such drugs as mechlorethamine hydrochloride[5] — used to treat mycosis fungoides — and topical antibiotics.

INSECTS. Urticaria and anaphylaxis from insect stings result primarily from hymenoptera (bees, wasps, hornets, and yellow jackets), and should not be confused with either the *normal reaction* to stings or the *delayed reaction*. Most persons will experience swelling, redness, and burning pain at the site of the sting, occurring almost immediately and usually subsiding within several hours. The delayed or localized reaction is much less common, occurs from a few hours to a few days after the sting, and may be manifested by extension of the local swelling, increasing discomfort, varying distortions of the stung part, or vesicles. It does not result from an immunologic reaction but appears to depend instead on pharmacologic reactions of chemicals or toxins in the venom.

Anaphylaxis may occur independently of the preceding normal or delayed reaction, in that a severe delayed reaction is not necessarily a forerunner of anaphylaxis.

FOODS. Although many foods may cause anaphylaxis, those most commonly cited are seafood, fish in general, seeds and berries, and nuts. A secondary group of less frequent offenders includes eggs, chocolate, pork, and milk. Anaphylactic reactions to foods are more likely to be associated with gastrointestinal symptoms, fatigue, or headache.

Recognition

Early recognition of anaphylaxis can be life-saving, and this early recognition depends to a great extent on the proper evaluation of patients with urticaria or angioedema. These patients should be questioned about the presence of gastrointestinal symptoms, of lightheadedness or dizziness, of feelings of generalized warmth, and of soreness or tightness in the throat or chest. As nonspecific as these symptoms may be, other vague symptoms may be described by the patient: mild apprehension or weakness, a "queasy stomach," or an itchiness of the nose or mouth.

More severe angioedema of the bronchial tree leads to varying degrees of airway obstruction. Chest tightness may progress to shortness of breath, expiratory wheezing, and pulmonary hyperinflation. Untreated, dyspnea, cyanosis, and hypotension may be followed by respiratory failure and unconsciousness.

Signs and symptoms of circulatory collapse may overshadow those of pulmonary obstruction, as seen by fainting or lightheadedness, followed by hypotension, pallor, and loss of consciousness. In the absence of urticaria or angioedema, these changes might suggest cerebral ischemia, seizure, or cardiovascular emergency. History of recent injection might enable recognition of anaphylaxis, as the latter is much more likely to occur following parenteral administration than following oral medication. Also the patient or his family should be questioned about recent skin tests and the possibility of an occult insect sting in which the normal reaction was inapparent.

The following conditions may be confused with immunologic (allergic) urticaria and must be considered in the differential diagnosis of the patient with urticaria:

COLD URTICARIA. At least two clinical forms exist. In the more common acquired cold urticaria, lesions usually appear within minutes of exposure to cold. Histamine appears to be the mediator of the reaction, but other agents almost certainly are involved. The production of a pruritic wheal following the application of an ice cube to normal skin for at least 5 minutes will confirm the diagnosis. Familial cold urticaria, a rare condition, appears to be a systemic reaction in which urticarial lesions are delayed in onset (with negative ice cube test), nonpruritic, and associated with arthralgias and a leukocytosis.

CHOLINERGIC URTICARIA. In this condition, sweating or exertion, emotional stress, and eating spicy foods produce characteristic 1 to 3 mm wheals surrounded by a large red flare. The diagnosis is based on the observation of the small wheals, along with supporting history. Surprisingly, it is difficult to confirm this diagnosis by injecting cholinergic drugs intradermally, although vigorous exercise or a hot bath are almost always able to reproduce the characteristic skin changes.[4] A recent study has shown significant airway obstruction in cholinergic urticaria, a condition generally thought to be limited to the skin.[10]

DERMATOGRAPHISM. About one third of the normal population shows the triple response of Lewis following firm stroking of the skin. The term dermatographism is applied when the triple response is persistent or exaggerated or produces a pruritic syndrome. Although dermatographism may be seen following emotional stress or drug reactions, the cause in most patients is not apparent. When a pruritic syndrome is present, scratching induces further dermatographism, and the appearance may mimic urticaria.

HEREDITARY ANGIOEDEMA. This dominantly inherited condition is characterized by recurrent episodes of nonpruritic swellings of the skin and angioedema of the mucosa of the respiratory and gastrointestinal tracts. Severe abdominal pain and vomiting can simulate a surgical emergency, and laryngeal obstruction may be life-threatening. Patients with this disorder have deficient amounts of an inhibitor of C1 esterase.

Although relatively rare, hereditary angioedema should be considered in the evaluation of every patient with these symptoms. Recognition is aided by the presence of (1) a familial history, (2) severe abdominal pain, which is unusual in anaphylaxis, and (3) angioedema *without* urticaria. Until recently, treatment of the acute attacks had been symptomatic: analgesics for abdominal pain and tracheostomy for severe laryngeal edema. However, a recent report has described effective specific treatment of the acute episodes with intravenous administration of C1-inhibitor concentrate.[6]

Treatment

Although the initial treatment of anaphylaxis (and urticaria) is epinephrine, its use depends upon the severity of the reaction. In the absence of hypotension, 0.3 ml of 1:1000 dilution should be injected subcutaneously and repeated at 5 to 10 minute intervals if needed. An antihistamine like diphenhydramine hydrochloride should be administered intramuscularly. If the anaphylaxis is caused by medication injected into an extremity, proximal tourniquets, along with ice applications and injection of epinephrine into the injection site should reduce absorption of the antigenic substance. Caution must be used if the patient has cardiac disease or is hypertensive, in which cases smaller initial doses of epinephrine are indicated.

If respiratory symptoms persist or progress, intubation, administration of oxygen, and intravenous aminophylline may be indicated. Emergency tracheostomy should be considered if conservative measures are unavailable or unsuccessful in relieving severe laryngeal edema.

Since hypotension will delay the absorption of epinephrine from a subcutaneous site, epinephrine should be given intramuscularly to these patients. An intravenous infusion should also be started to facilitate administration of such drugs as levarterenol, antihistamines, and even corticosteroids. The latter may neutralize the delayed effects of the causative antigen but are of little or no value in the early management of anaphylaxis.

Since intravenously administered epinephrine increases greatly the risk of cardiac arrhythmia, this route is reserved for life-threatening situations, and only 1:100,000 dilution of epinephrine should be used. Diphenhydramine hydrochloride should be given cautiously if broncho- spasm is suspected, and in patients with asthma it should be replaced by another antihistamine such as promethazine hydrochloride.

When possible, a tourniquet should also be applied proximal to the site of a sting; and if the stinger remains, it should be scooped out carefully with a dull blade to avoid injection of more venom into the skin. All patients with anaphylaxis should be observed and treated until the symptoms have abated, preferably in a hospital setting.

TOXIC EPIDERMAL NECROLYSIS

Toxic epidermal necrolysis is a cutaneous syndrome heralded by erythema, fever, bullae, and widespread exfoliation of the skin. This desquamation is probably its most characteristic feature and is similar in appearance to wet paper peeling off a wall (Fig. 3). The Nikolsky sign, where gentle pressure on normal skin causes bullae or further des- quamation, is invariably present (Fig. 4). As the exfoliation progresses, the denuded surface appears moist, erythematous, and glistening, simi- lar in appearance to a severe thermal burn — hence the alternative term for this condition, *scalded skin syndrome*. The process begins suddenly, and initial lesions usually appear around the eyes, oronasal areas, and genitalia before becoming generalized.

The most common symptom, skin tenderness, is often severe. Even before clinical changes are seen in the skin, infants and younger children will remain very still because of the discomfort produced by movement. Other symptoms include anorexia, lethargy, diarrhea, and vomiting.

Etiology

The causes of toxic epidermal necrolysis fall into two main groups. In infants and children up to 7 years of age, most cases are caused by epidermolytic toxin elaborated by staphylococci. In almost all cases of this milder form of the disease, the toxin is produced by group 2 staphylococci, usually phage type 71 or 55/71, but more recent reports have implicated group 1 as well. The mortality rate for infants is high, but drops to around 5 per cent in the 1 to 6 year age group.

In adults, various drugs and chemicals cause a more severe form of toxic epidermal necrolysis characterized by more extensive mucous membrane involvement and a mortality rate of 30 to 40 per cent. The

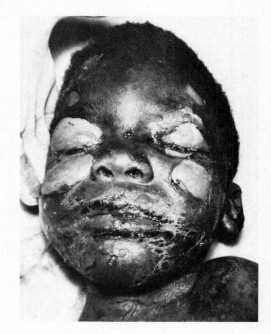

Figure 3. The "peeling wall paper" appearance of toxic epidermal necrolysis. Note the severe periorifacial involvement and loss of fluid through the skin.

drugs most often cited are sulfonamides, phenylbutazone, salicylates, penicillins, and barbiturates, although a complete list of all drugs mentioned in the literature would exceed 100 preparations. One patient in whom the syndrome developed following the ingestion of gin and tonic was exquisitely sensitive to small quantities of quinine.[3] Carbon monoxide and a fumigant containing acrylonitrile have been reported to produce toxic epidermal necrolysis following inhalation.[8]

Although this syndrome is reported in adults with a variety of diseases, it is not clear whether the skin changes are related to these

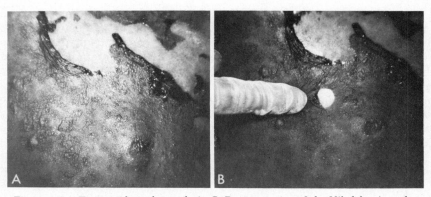

Figure 4.   A, Toxic epidermal necrolysis. B, Demonstration of the Nikolsky sign where gentle pressure produces further desquamation. The Nikolsky sign is also "positive" in pemphigus, but not in erythema multiforme.

diseases or caused by one of the many medications that these patients received.

Recognition

In more severe forms of toxic epidermal necrolysis, the combination of widespread painful erythema and sheetlike exfoliation with flaccid bullae usually permits a rapid clinical diagnosis. Erythema multiforme also has peri-orificial involvement (Fig. 5), but often shows typical iris or target lesions (Fig. 6), a negative Nikolsky sign, and discrete lesions rather than widespread exfoliation. Erythema multiforme and toxic epidermal necrolysis are both reaction patterns, and in cases which cannot be separated clinically, both entities may be present at the same time.

Milder cases of toxic epidermal necrolysis that occur in children may be less easy to recognize clinically, and a high index of suspicion is essential. About 90 per cent of children are febrile and 50 per cent show leukocytosis, circumstances suggesting an infectious process but otherwise nonspecific. Although erythema may be absent, skin tenderness is an almost constant finding, resulting in an irritable, febrile child who appears afraid to move. There is usually a history of sore throat, ear ache, or rhinorrhea.

Division of toxic epidermal necrolysis into two major types should aid recognition. The milder staphylococcal type is seen mainly in children, whereas the more severe "drug" type shows more mucous membrane involvement and may be confused clinically with erythema multiforme. It should be remembered, however, that the "drug" type may be seen in children as well as adults and that a few staphylococcal cases have been reported in adults.

It is noteworthy that the histology of the two types differs in the level of epidermal separation. The staphylococcal type shows epidermal cleavage high in the malpighian layer, whereas the drug type shows epidermal necrosis with subepidermal cleavage.

Treatment

As soon as the presumptive diagnosis of toxic epidermal necrolysis is made, cultures should be obtained from the nasopharynx, blood, urine, unruptured bullae, skin, eyes, and ears. An intravenous drip should be started immediately to facilitate therapy and maintenance of fluid balance and nutrition. Patients under 10 years of age (and most older patients as well) should be treated for penicillinase-producing *Staphylococcus aureus* infection. Hospitalization is almost always advisable when the condition is diagnosed in an early phase, although it is surprising how many milder patients escape hospitalization because they are diagnosed retrospectively as they are improving.

In drug-induced cases, systemic steroids are clearly indicated, and moderate to high doses should be given, depending on the presence of relative contraindications to their use. The intravenous route should be used initially. One of the most challenging problems is the severely ill child whose history and clinical appearance do not permit differentiation between toxic epidermal necrolysis and erythema multiforme, even though one or the other seems more likely. The child may be toxic, febrile, and dehydrated and have already received small doses of numerous medications. In such a patient, high-dose steroids should be combined with appropriate antibiotics, keeping in mind the possibility of a drug-induced syndrome. Systemic steroids do not appear to affect *Staphylococcus aureus*–induced toxic epidermal necrolysis adversely, provided that an effective antibiotic is given simultaneously.

Local care of the skin may be life-saving in the seriously ill patient with the drug-induced type. Warmed silver nitrate, 0.5 per cent aqueous, should be applied as compresses to denuded areas in order to reduce the numbers of gram-negative organisms. Use of a rotating frame will aid compressing and also reduce trauma to the intact skin. Loss of heat can be reduced by placing the patient in a warm humidified room, and strict isolation procedures will reduce the chances of a life-threatening secondary infection. Fluids, electrolytes, and nutrition must be monitored and maintained, especially in infants.

ERYTHEMA MULTIFORME

Erythema multiforme is an acute disorder affecting the skin and mucous membranes and displaying distinctive clinical lesions. It occurs most commonly in a mild form, but for unknown reasons it also may appear as a more severe toxic process often referred to as the Stevens-Johnson syndrome. Episodes of both forms resolve spontaneously in 2 to 4 weeks. However, rarely a fulminating course with secondary infection may have a fatal outcome.

Etiology

The causes of erythema multiforme are many, and each year several new "causes" are added to the list. Although little is known about the mechanisms of production of the disease, recent investigations suggest that small blood vessels in the skin become sensitized by bacterial, viral, or chemical products. A large number of recurrent cases are caused by, or at least are associated with, *Mycoplasma pneumoniae* and the virus of herpes simplex, and this may include the common "idiopathic" erythema multiforme that occurs in children and young adults during the winter and early spring. Other infections that may be related include histoplasmosis, trichomonas, influenza, ECHO and coxsackie viremias, orf, and fungal infections. Vaccinations with the viruses of vaccinia, mumps, and poliomyelitis have also been incriminated.

Although many drugs have been reported to produce erythema multiforme, those most often cited are the penicillins, sulfonamides, and barbiturates. Phenolphthalein, used as a laxative or as a dye in inexpensive red wines, produces a localized erythema multiforme reaction of the genitalia or lips. X-ray therapy, internal malignant disease, and collagen diseases are other causes.

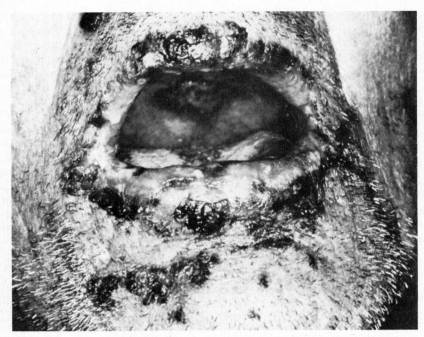

Figure 5.   Erythema multiforme occurring in a patient receiving sulfamethoxazole. Note the involvement of the tongue and palate as well as the hemorrhagic crusting of the lips and perioral skin.

Recognition

Early lesions are bright red macules that typically appear suddenly on the hands and feet in a symmetric distribution. Other common sites are the forearms, elbows, and lower legs, and all these sites may be involved together. The lesions may coalesce and become generalized, but rarely is the trunk involved before the extremities. Mucosal lesions, present in about 30 per cent of cases, begin as vesicles or bullae that become eroded or crusted (Fig. 5).

The red macules evolve to violaceous papular swellings or more frequently to the characteristic iris (or target) lesions. The latter are pathognomonic of erythema multiforme and show a thin peripheral red border, a middle pale zone, and a dusky center which may be vesicular (Fig. 6). Iris lesions are edematous at first but later persist as macules until they fade, 8 to 12 days after their initial appearance. Resolution occurs without scarring, but hyperpigmentation may persist for weeks to months. Pruritus is variable.

The Stevens-Johnson syndrome is characterized by severe mucosal involvement, especially of the mouth and eyes, although the vagina and urethra often show changes as well. The palate and oral mucosa show raw, tender surfaces covered by a sticky gray exudate; the lips may be swollen, bloody, crusted, and exquisitely tender. The patient cannot eat

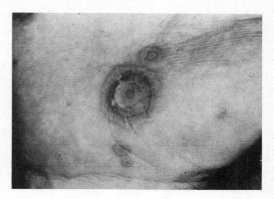

Figure 6. Characteristic target or iris lesions of erythema multiforme.

or drink or open his mouth to permit examination. The eyes are bilaterally involved with a purulent conjunctivitis; the lids are edematous, and crusting causes them to stick together. Corneal involvement with ulceration may occur, probably due to secondary bacterial infection. Genital lesions show a similar exudative clinical pattern, but the anal and nasal mucosae are rarely involved.

The skin may show the iris and maculoedematous lesions of the milder form or may display severe vesiculobullous lesions, frequently with hemorrhage. In other cases, severe mucosal involvement will occur without skin changes. Stevens-Johnson syndrome may be ushered in with fever, malaise, prostration, and a prodrome of flu-like symptoms; but these changes, along with pneumonitis, may be due to an underlying respiratory virus.

Recognition of erythema multiforme depends on the characteristic appearance of the eruption, and diagnosis is almost impossible during the prodromal period. If the patient is seen during the prodrome, an upper or lower respiratory infection may be suspected. On the other hand, erythema multiforme is often recurrent in children and young adults, and taking a thorough history may enable the astute physician to predict the appearance of the eruption.

In sum, erythema multiforme is recognized by its characteristic symmetry, acral and mucosal distribution, and cutaneous iris or vesiculobullous lesions. With the use of rigorous clinical standards, false-positive diagnosis may be avoided. There are no specific laboratory tests for erythema multiforme, and any abnormal findings usually reflect an underlying process or secondary infection. Recognition of erythema multiforme occasionally will require consideration of the following mucocutaneous disorders.

PEMPHIGUS.   In this more chronic and indolent process, the bullae are larger, break easily, and leave eroded lesions which tend to enlarge by detachment of the epidermis at the periphery. Involvement of the trunk is common, and erythema is rarely prominent. Mouth lesions are the first site of activity in more than one-half of cases; however, they are typically erosive and show little tendency toward crust formation. The

Nikolsky sign is present and may account for the localization of skin lesions to areas of the trunk that are exposed to friction or pressure. If pemphigus is suspected, a Tzanck test performed on material scraped from the floor of a bulla will show acantholytic cells, swollen epidermal cells whose cytoplasm has condensed peripherally at the cell walls.

BEHÇET'S DISEASE. This rare clinical entity reported most often from eastern Mediterranean countries is characterized by recurrent oral and external genital ulcerations in association with iritis and other destructive inflammatory changes of the eyes. The mouth lesions are quite similar to the erosions of recurrent aphthous stomatitis, and Behçet's disease is more easily confused with the latter than with erythema multiforme. Ocular involvement is usually progressive and severe, although it is initially unilateral in half the cases in contrast to erythema multiforme, where eye lesions are symmetric. Behçet's disease may show varying multisystem involvement. Its other skin lesions are described as acneiform or pyodermatous when present.

BULLOUS PEMPHIGOID. In this skin disease of the elderly, large tense bullae appear in association with erythema in a wide distribution, although the axillae, groin regions, and flexor arm areas are more commonly involved. Oral mucosal lesions occur in one third of patients, but are few in number, are rarely very painful, and never progress to severe stomatitis. Bullous pemphigoid may be further differentiated from erythema multiforme by: (a) its gradual onset and more chronic course; (b) the absence of iris lesions, although gyriform erythematous lesions are seen; (c) the sparing of acral areas; and (d) its rarity in patients under age 50, even though occasional childhood cases have been seen.

TOXIC EPIDERMAL NECROLYSIS. In most cases, the sheetlike exfoliation of this entity contrasts well with the more discrete vesiculobullous eruptions of erythema multiforme, and yet confusion between the two entities does occur. Favoring toxic epidermal necrolysis are a positive Nikolsky sign, exfoliation around the mouth rather than crusting of the lips, unilateral eye involvement, and the symptom of tender skin.

Treatment

In severe forms of erythema multiforme, systemic steroids are indicated and should be started immediately: hydrocortisone 80 to 120 mg every 8 hours intravenously; or prednisone orally 60 to 90 mg daily if oral ingestion is tolerated. Thorough history and physical examination must aim at uncovering latent infections and must record all medications (including "over-the-counter" preparations) that the patient has taken. It seems unnecessary to suggest that any medication which might be the cause of this severe reaction must be discontinued. Antibiotics should be reserved for treatment of specific infections.

Mild forms of erythema multiforme usually require little more than symptomatic treatment, reassurance about the benign course, and an explanation to the patient about likely causes of this mucocutaneous disorder. The discomfort of oral lesions may be reduced by warm saline gargles, aspirin, and viscous lidocaine. The tablespoon of lidocaine

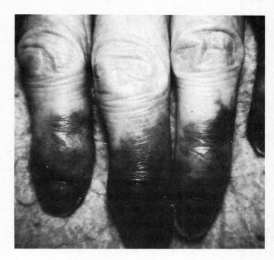

Figure 7. Acral ecchymotic changes of purpura fulminans.

should be swished around in the mouth, held there for one minute, and then swallowed, just before meals. Applications of Vaseline will soften superficial crusting around the eyes and lips.

PURPURA FULMINANS

This rare entity is characterized by the sudden appearance of large ecchymotic areas which often become necrotic or gangrenous (Fig. 7). These fulminating ecchymoses usually are on the extremities, although acral parts of the face may be involved. The skin changes are accompanied or soon followed by fever, chills, and vascular collapse, which may lead to death within one or two days. In patients who survive, gangrenous digits often will either self-amputate or require surgical amputation.

The etiology of purpura fulminans is better understood by its relationship to the syndrome of disseminated intravascular coagulation. Although purpura fulminans is most often described as occurring in children recovering from mild viral or bacterial infections, it is also seen in certain obstetric disorders, following pulmonary surgery, in prostatic carcinoma, and following certain snake bites. All of these conditions have been reported to show altered intravascular coagulation and increased fibrinolytic activity.

Apparently, clots form continuously in blood vessels as a normal occurrence, and this process may increase in various conditions, even without clinical thrombotic disease. In purpura fulminans and the diseases mentioned above, intravascular clotting is more extreme, more generalized, and results in the consumption of circulating fibrinogen. Thus, coagulation in distal vessels and generalized defibrination explain the acral gangrene and large ecchymotic areas, respectively, that occur in purpura fulminans.

Recognition

The combination of rapidly progressing hemorrhagic skin lesions with signs of prostration, hypovolemic shock, and fever is very suggestive of purpura fulminans. The ecchymoses are palpable and usually limited to the extremities initially, although they often spread centripetally, show some blistering necrosis, and may be followed by gangrene of the digits.

Less severe forms of purpura fulminans merge with the syndrome of disseminated intravascular coagulation, and it seems appropriate to use the latter term in such cases, reserving purpura fulminans for the more explosive, life-threatening condition described above. The diagnosis of disseminated intravascular coagulation is most often made on hospitalized patients with conditions such as septicemia, leukemia, carcinoma, burns, extensive trauma, and premature separation of the placenta. As more sophisticated hematologic testing becomes available, it seems likely that patients with these ailments will be shown to have increased clotting tendencies even in the absence of clinical bleeding.

On the other hand, patients with this intravascular coagulation syndrome may seek medical attention either because of hemorrhage (purpura, hemoptysis, hematuria, etc.) or because of their underlying disease (septicemia, carcinoma, etc.); but without both present together, the correct diagnosis is easily missed. Indeed, in almost 50 per cent of cases of disseminated intravascular coagulation, cutaneous lesions are the presenting sign.[9] Any patient with palpable purpura should be questioned thoroughly in regard to underlying cardiopulmonary conditions which could produce hypoxia, the presence of cancers, especially of the prostate, recent treatment with chemotherapeutic agents, and infections of any kind. Acral or facial cyanosis is seen occasionally and is sharply outlined and usually gun-metal or purplish in color. It does not blanch with pressure.

The diagnosis of purpura fulminans or disseminated intravascular coagulation can almost always be confirmed by laboratory tests which show a prolonged prothrombin time and decreased fibrinogen and platelets. In patients with liver disease or in milder cases where tests are equivocal, a skin biopsy is helpful.

Treatment

Although the intravascular coagulation syndrome usually is managed by treating the underlying disease, purpura fulminans produces such severe hemorrhage that it should be treated immediately with anticoagulation. Although the dose of intravenous haparin has not been clearly established for this condition, somewhere in the range of 60 to 100 units per kg every 4 hours seems reasonable. The hemorrhage will continue for at least 18 to 24 hours before responding to heparin; treatment is usually continued for 3 or 4 days longer. Monitoring of the hemostatic factors usually shows a more rapid return to normal of fibrinogen than of platelets.

Supportive measures are essential, and acidosis and hypotension in particular should be treated vigorously in order to increase the already decompensated tissue perfusion. Blood transfusion may be indicated. Local skin care is aimed at preventing and treating infections which are expected to occur as the large ecchymotic areas become necrotic or gangrenous. Gentle compression with an antibacterial soap and applications of gentamicin ointment will be helpful.

Milder forms of disseminated intravascular coagulation rarely require heparin, since therapy for the primary process usually is available. An exception is in acute leukemias where heparin may halt a hemorrhagic episode until the malignant disease can be brought under effective long-term control by chemotherapy.

LOXOSCELISM

The bite of the brown house spider, *Loxosceles reclusa,* may produce a necrotic slough at the site of envenomation in association with systemic toxicity of variable severity. The spider is found in the southern and central parts of the United States, where its natural habitat appears to be rocky or wooded areas. However, in colder regions it has moved indoors, where it lives unnoticed in closets, attics, and basements. Its tendency to live in old clothes and trunks no doubt accounts for sporadic cases in such nonendemic areas as Pennsylvania and California.

The brown spider is 8 or 9 mm long and is fairly easily identified by the violin-shaped band on its cephalothorax.

Recognition

The spider bite either is not felt or produces only a slight stinging discomfort initially. However, pain may appear within 2 to 10 hours, followed by erythema, tenderness, and occasionally blister formation. Subsequently an ischemic zone appears around the site, and the latter becomes indurated and hemorrhagic. An irregular, often stellate eschar slowly becomes demarcated over the next 5 to 10 days, and with separation of the eschar an ulcer is seen (Fig. 8).

Systemic toxic reactions occur in a small number of patients and are more severe in children. Chills, fever, weakness, nausea, vomiting, and restlessness have been described in association with a faint maculopapular erythematous eruption that is occasionally petechial. Hemolytic reactions are a rare complication that can be fatal in children.

Mild cutaneous changes with little or no systemic reactions may follow recluse spider bites and probably are much more common than the severe cases. If the spider is not observed, an itchy or mildly painful erythematous reaction that is not followed by necrosis might be ascribed to a hymenoptera sting. These milder forms are difficult to recognize, except in endemic areas.

The differential diagnosis of an early spider bite may include cellulitis, pyoderma, or hymenoptera sting. Severe pain that requires narcotics for control, a central vesicle or bleb, and a 2-hour or longer delay in the onset of the local reaction favor recluse spider bites over stings. The generalized eruption after spider bites is usually morbilliform rather

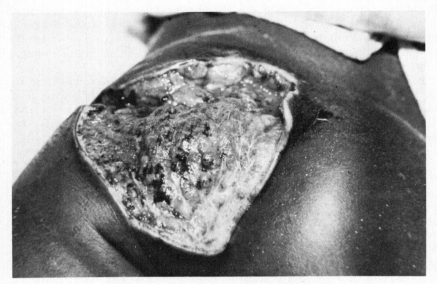

Figure 8.   Large ulceration of the buttock eight days after a *Loxosceles reclusa* bite.

than urticarial. Although no laboratory tests are helpful early in the course, evidence for hemolysis may be found later: hemoglobinemia, thrombocytopenia, and bilirubin elevation. Subsequent necrotic ulceration is often *late* confirmatory evidence of the diagnosis.

A somewhat similar painful necrotic ulceration may occur 3 to 10 days after initiation of coumarin anticoagulants. This "coumarin necrosis" occurs almost exclusively in women and produces multiple asymmetric lesions. It begins as painful red areas which evolve rapidly into purpuric swellings, followed by ulceration and formation of hemorrhagic eschars. The history of recent coumarin anticoagulation helps separate this rare entity from loxoscelism.

Treatment

Pain, a delayed but common feature, is usually the reason for seeking medical treatment. The pain typically intensifies over several days before diminishing. Although non-narcotic analgesics should be tried initially, narcotic preparations frequently are needed. The pain appears to be unrelated to the amount of tissue damage, in that extremely painful spider bites may show no necrosis.

Immediate or early excision with primary closure is a suggested therapy, but seems rather heroic when many recluse spider bites will resolve without necrosis. However, if elliptical excision of a small site is technically feasible, it is probably a valuable form of therapy since it guarantees that a much larger, perhaps massive, necrotic slough will not occur.

The value of systemic corticosteroids in preventing necrosis is disputed, and animal investigations have shown no benefit from this medication even when administered prior to envenomation.[2] On the other hand, systemic corticosteroids appear to reduce the systemic reaction and hemolytic syndrome, and high doses seem indicated in cases where surgical excision is impractical. Lymphangitis and cellulitis are occasional complications that should be treated with a suitable antibiotic.

REFERENCES

1. Almeyda, J., and Levantine, A.: Adverse cutaneous reactions to the penicillins. Brit. J. Dermatol., 87:293, 1972.
2. Berger, R. S.: A critical look at therapy for the brown recluse spider bite. Arch. Dermatol., 107:298, 1973.
3. Callaway, J. L., and Tate, W. E.: Toxic epidermal necrolysis caused by "gin and tonic." Arch. Dermatol., 109:909, 1974.
4. Commens, C. A., and Greaves, M. W.: Tests to establish the diagnosis in cholinergic urticaria. Brit. J. Dermatol., 98:47, 1978.
5. Daughters, D., Zackheim, H., and Maibach, H.: Urticaria and anaphylactoid reactions: After topical application of mechlorethamine. Arch. Dermatol., 107:429, 1973.
6. Gadek, J. E., Hosea, S. W., Gelfand, J. A., et al.: Replacement therapy in hereditary angioedema. New Eng. J. Med., 302:542, 1980.
7. James, J., and Warin, R. P.: Chronic urticaria: The effect of aspirin. Brit. J. Dermatol., 82:204, 1970.
8. Radimer, G. F., Davis, J. H., and Ackerman, A. B.: Fumigant-induced toxic epidermal necrolysis. Arch. Dermatol., 110:103, 1974.
9. Robboy, S. J., Mihm, M. C., Colman, R. W., et al.: The skin in disseminated intravascular coagulation. Brit. J. Dermatol., 88:221, 1973.
10. Soter, N. A., Wasserman, S. I., Austen, K. F., et al.: Release of mast-cell mediators and alterations in lung function in patients with cholinergic urticaria. New Eng. J. Med., 302:604, 1980.

1245 Highland Avenue
Abington, Pennsylvania 19001

Index

Note: Page numbers of article titles are in **boldface** type.